ALSO BY BOB GREENE

The Best Life Diet

The Best Life Diet Daily Journal

Bob Greene's Total Body Makeover

The Get With the Program! Guide to Good Eating

Get With the Program!

The Get With the Program! Daily Journal

Keep the Connection: Choices for a Better Body and a Better Life

Make the Connection: Ten Steps to a Better Body—and a Better Life

A Journal of Daily Renewal: The Companion to Make the Connection

BOB GREENE

THE BEST

LIFE DIET
COOKBOOK

More than 175 Delicious,
Convenient, Family–Friendly Recipes

With black-and-white photography by Erik Johnson
and color photography by Alan Richardson

SIMON & SCHUSTER

NEW YORK   LONDON   TORONTO   SYDNEY

Simon & Schuster
1230 Avenue of the Americas
New York, NY 10020

First Simon & Schuster hardcover edition January 2009

SIMON & SCHUSTER and colophon are registered trademarks of Simon & Schuster, Inc.

For information about special discounts for bulk purchases, please contact Simon & Schuster
Special Sales at 1-800-456-6798 or business@simonandschuster.com.

Designed by Joel Avirom and Jason Snyder

Manufactured in the United States of America

10   9   8   7   6   5   4   3   2   1

Library of Congress Cataloging-in-Publication Data
Greene, Bob (Bob W.)
   The best life diet cookbook / Bob Greene; with black and white photography by Erik Johnson
and color photography by Alan Richardson.
      p. cm.
   1. Reducing diets—Recipes. 2. Weight loss. 3. Nutrition. 4. Physical fitness. I. Title.
RM222.2.G7226 2008
641.5'635—dc22   2008029461

ISBN-13: 978-1-4165-8833-7
ISBN-10:   1-4165-8833-7

ACKNOWLEDGMENTS

I WANTED THIS COOKBOOK TO be something special. Often, recipe books that are health- and calorie-conscious use the same techniques and a narrow range of ingredients. But the collection of recipes that you're about to experience employs innovative techniques and unique combinations of ingredients to create meals that are respectful of calories, nutritionally rich, and delicious. Accomplishing this required the hard work of several talented, dedicated individuals who are part of the Best Life Team. First and foremost, Sidra Forman, www.thebestlife.com chef, whose hours spent in the kitchen creating, tasting, and tweaking led to the exciting array of recipes found, not only in this book but online at www.thebestlife.com. Sidra is the heart and soul of our recipe development program. I'd also like to thank Janis Jibrin, RD, the Best Life lead dietitian, who's meticulous oversight and passion for perfection ensures that all our recipes and meal plans not only conform to the Best Life Guidelines with respect to calories and nutrients but that they are delicious as well. Whether she is testing a recipe, educating our members online, shopping for innovative new products, or working with companies on their formulations, Janis has one goal in mind: to improve the way people eat. Special thanks also goes to Donna Fennessy, the exceptionally precise and hard-working editor of www.thebestlife.com, for the hours logged in on this project. I'd also like to thank Heather K. Jones, RD, Tracy Gensler, RD, Tamara Goldis, RD, Derrick Bullock, Erik Johnson, and Reggie Casagrande for their contribution to this book.

CONTENTS

THE BEST LIFE DIET

COOKBOOK

Introduction

EATING IS MEANT TO BE one of life's great pleasures. The simple act of sitting down to a meal can bring us joy, satisfaction, and, of course, nourishment; in a word, fulfillment—both physical *and* emotional. Just think of the many memorable events in your life: sharing an intimate, romantic dinner with your partner, toasting a job promotion with friends, celebrating your child's first birthday, or one of the many special holidays you've spent with family. You may or may not remember the delicious food you enjoyed on these occasions, but I'm willing to bet that you remember the moment, the ritual of eating with friends and family, the joy of sharing these events with your loved ones. Simply put, the pleasure of eating and the bonding experience of a meal shared with others is a truly gratifying experience, one that enriches and improves our lives.

Unfortunately, so many of us have lost that special connection with the experience of eating. The reality is that our busy schedules have prevented us from savoring the act of sitting down to a meal, whether it's just yourself or with those you care about. As a result, many of us have fallen into the trap of trying to satisfy the need for emotional fulfillment that once may have come from dining with friends and family by focusing on the quantity of food and eating more than we probably need or is healthy. That's where this cookbook can help: you can reclaim the experience of eating as a celebration by sitting down to enjoy these high-quality, delicious dishes without overdoing it. This book contains more than just recipes, though. You'll also find a few different two-week meal plans, all of which incorporate these delicious recipes into a day's worth of eating to ensure that you get all the nutrients you need and the right amount of calories.

I hope that you'll come to think of eating healthy, home-cooked meals made from the freshest, most natural ingredients as a gift that you give to yourself and your loved ones. This may require you to reconsider cooking a bit; I encourage you to try to think of whipping up a nutritious meal not as just another task you have to do at the end of a busy day, but as a ritual that provides important vitamins and minerals, promotes good health, and gives you a wonderful opportunity to spend quality time with your family. Nourishing yourself and your loved ones, especially with great, healthy foods, is simply one of the most effective ways to satisfy the body and soul.

To me, that's what eating is all about, and I'm challenging *you* to make an effort to embrace that experience, to stock your refrigerator with healthy foods, to make your kitchen a special place where friends and family gather, and to sit down and enjoy meals once again! This cookbook can help you make all of these things a reality and, in turn, improve the quality of your health and perhaps even your relationships.

I know that many people just don't have a lot of extra time to cook a meal, and I took that into consideration when choosing the dishes to include in this book. Sure, there are some recipes that will challenge your skills in the kitchen; in fact, there's a whole section devoted to recipes from some of the greatest chefs from across the world. But the majority of the recipes here take just 30 minutes or less, and they include ingredients that you likely already have in your kitchen or can easily find at your local grocery store. The perfect example is Rotisserie Chicken Salad with Oranges and Pistachios (page 77). It's so easy to pull together and takes just 20 minutes to make because you're starting with an already cooked chicken from your local supermarket. Plus, it offers a new way to serve a familiar dish: instead of pairing the chicken with the same old side dishes, you're creating a beautiful salad with juicy oranges and crunchy pistachios. And there are many more recipes just like this one!

This cookbook will help you get back on track in the kitchen, and still leave you with plenty of time to get through everything on your to-do list. But I know that time isn't your only concern when it comes to eating; many of us have also become very calorie-conscious. For those of you who are trying to maintain your weight or slim down, these recipes will also help you focus on the quality of your food instead of the quantity. When you use fresh, high-quality foods, you won't have to eat as much to get that taste payoff. You'll be satisfied with less food, which means you'll consume fewer calories each time you sit down to eat. If you're looking for another way to keep your calories in check, you might be interested in our meal plans, which start on page 269. We've created three different plans, each of which offers six calorie levels (1,500, 1,600, 1,700, 1,800, 2,000, and 2,500 calories per day; as you know, calorie needs vary per person, and should be determined by how active you are and a variety of other factors). Putting together a perfectly balanced diet that provides all the vitamins and minerals you need each day without going over a certain calorie limit is like solving a complex puzzle. Don't worry: we've taken all the guesswork out of it with these meal plans.

Here's a quick preview of the meal plan options you can choose from. If you're really time-pressed, the "Quick and Easy" Meal Plan (page 293) will be a dream come true. This plan doesn't require a lot of cooking, and all the recipes in this section take no more than 20 minutes to prepare. On a typical day you'll have yogurt, fruit, and nuts for breakfast, a chicken wrap for lunch, and Cornmeal-Crusted Catfish with Spicy Slaw (page 145) for dinner (another 20-minute recipe).

If you have more time to spend in the kitchen, check out the "Kitchen Connoisseur" Plan (page 272). While still relying on quickly prepared recipes, this plan has you spending just a little more time in the kitchen, and includes more adventurous recipes. Wednesday of Week 2 is typical: homemade muesli for breakfast, lunch (made in 10 minutes) is Shrimp, Avocado, and Sesame Seed Salad (page 74) and dinner is Vegetarian Baked Beans on Grits (page 158).

Cooking for a family? You'll love the "Family-Friendly" Plan (page 315), which uses recipes from this book that kids (and picky partners) can all enjoy. No one will turn up their nose at Ginger Waffles, Chicken Noodle Soup, Taco Salad, Cottage Pie (based on beef and potatoes), and other healthy versions of family favorites. In fact, don't be surprised if foods that weren't all that well liked by your family soon become welcome dishes. Take the Broccoli, White Bean, and Leek Tart (page 152) as an example. You may be thinking that your family doesn't eat white beans or broccoli, but when you put them into a creamy tart, they will not only eat these healthy foods but they'll actually *like* them! In terms of time, this plan falls somewhere between the "Quick and Easy" and the "Kitchen Connoisseur" plans. You don't have to follow the meal plans to the letter, of course. You can simply browse the section for recipes that will go over big at your dinner table.

No matter which plan you choose, you can be confident that you'll be getting all the nutrients you need. Each meal has been composed to ensure that you get the perfect balance of fat, carbs, and protein, and the plans are rich in vitamins, minerals, and phytonutrients. Why is this so important? Often, when someone fills up on empty calories (like a mound of French fries) or even has a relatively healthy dish that's missing a satisfying element, such as a whole grain roll, brown rice, or other complex carbohydrate, they tend to be more prone to grazing or snacking throughout the day. The end result: they take in more calories. These meals, on the other hand, will keep you satisfied and full, and will therefore help you cut your calorie intake. (Not to mention that these recipes also fit perfectly into the Best Life plan, a three-phased program to help you lose weight and live healthier. To learn more about the program, check out the revised and updated edition of *The Best Life Diet* [Simon & Schuster, 2009] or the companion Web site, www .thebestlife.com.)

This cookbook also includes an interesting mix of recipes. You'll notice a number of familiar classics (think chili and roasted potatoes), as well as comfort food with a healthy twist so you can enjoy these dishes every day, if you wish. I think you'll be pleasantly surprised with the results. For example, if you didn't know better, you'd think the Steel-Cut Oats "Polenta" (page 167) was a real splurge. But the recipe, which combines sage and oats to create a savory side dish with a crispy exterior and soft, indulgent interior, is high in fiber and uses no cream or butter. Basically, these dishes offer incredible flavor, but they're better for you! And we've also created fresh, new dishes by pairing basic ingredients that you may never have thought to combine. The Broiled Mahimahi with Grapes and Leeks (page 143) is the perfect example. You've probably never considered combining grapes and leeks, but the result is amazing; there's no need to add extra salt, butter, or cream. That means you can keep your intake of sodium and saturated fat down while enjoying fabulous, flavorful food.

I like to think of these dishes, most of which are a snap to prepare, as easy but elegant. That may seem like a bit of a contradiction, but it's not at all. The Broiled Mahimahi calls for just six ingredients, including salt and pepper! Don't mistake simple for boring, though. Many of these dishes may challenge your tastes and I hope that you'll try them with an open mind and enjoy them as much as I do. The recipes in this book—including those in Best Life Recipes from World-Class Chefs, which come from a number of chefs who just happen to be some of my personal favorites—may be a little different from what you're used to cooking and eating. For instance, chef Anita Lo's Barbecued Breast of Chicken, Suzanne Goin's Succotash Salad, and Nobu Matsuhisa's Parmesan Baked Small Scallops are unique yet accessible. I'm hoping that these foods will expand your eating horizons. (You'll also find dishes from Mollie Ahlstrand, Dan Barber, Thomas Keller, Sarma Melngailis, Vitaly Paley, Tal Ronnen, Charlie Trotter, Roy Yamaguchi, and Eric Ziebold in this section.)

With each recipe, you'll be reminded that eating is about so much more than simply satisfying your hunger. Cooking and enjoying healthy meals is a great way to take care of yourself and your family. I know that we are all doing our best to live the healthiest life we can. Eating a nutritious diet can and should be a part of this process because it's a key component of living a happy and fulfilled life. With the help of this book, I'm hoping you'll find a little more joy in cooking, a little more satisfaction in eating, a little more nutrition in your meals, and a little more time to sit down and experience the smells, flavors, and textures of your food. I want you to discover the pleasure of eating again and to allow healthy foods to enrich your life. The recipes in this book can play a part in helping you achieve this wonderful and fulfilling experience.

Recipes

IN MANY OF THE FOLLOWING recipes, you'll notice I've given brand-name suggestions for a variety of ingredients, including soymilk, whole grain crackers, and healthy spreads. Many of these recommended brands carry my Best Life Seal of Approval, meaning they're rich in good-for-you elements, such as whole grains, healthy fats, fiber, vitamins, calcium and other minerals, and phytonutrients. In addition to the commonly used ingredients on the next page, the following products are Best Life approved: Benefiber, Edy's and Dreyer's Fruit Bars; Hershey's cocoa and Extra Dark chocolates; Lean Cuisine; Libby's 100% Pure Pumpkin; Nestlé Pure Life Purified Waters; Nonni's Biscotti; Skinny Cow bars, sandwiches, and cones; Slim-Fast bars and shakes; and Wish-Bone Salad Spritzers and Bountifuls. The California Table Grape Commission, Florida Grapefruit, and the Mushroom Council, are also food partners. Products carrying the Best Life seal or Best Life Treat seal are available in most supermarkets nationwide.

In order to keep sodium within a healthy range, these recipes use moderate amounts of salt, deriving their flavor from herbs and other ingredients. If you need to add a little extra salt, follow the guidelines on page 271.

COMMONLY USED INGREDIENTS

BEANS: All of these recipes work with both boiled-from-scratch and canned beans. No particular brand was used consistently; we like the low-sodium Goya beans and the no-salt-added Eden Organic beans. If you have the choice, opt for either of these brands or any other no-salt-added or low-sodium (no more than 130 milligrams per ½ cup) variety. Otherwise, you can use regular canned beans, but drain and rinse them well in a colander before adding to a recipe to rid the beans of excess salt. Note that cooking times for recipes that contain beans assume you're using canned beans; you'll have to factor in more time if you soak and boil them. See page 345 for instructions.

CRISPBREAD: Recipes using this ingredient were developed with Wasa Multi Grain, Light Rye, or other whole grain Wasa crispbreads carrying the Best Life seal.

HEALTHY SPREAD: This refers to margarines or spreads made with no partially hydrogenated oil. We developed recipes using Smart Balance Buttery Spread.

LIQUID EGGS: These are pasteurized egg whites. The recipes were developed using All-Whites, which are 100 percent liquid egg whites, and Better'n Eggs (98 percent liquid egg whites with vitamins added), a fat-free, cholesterol-free replacement for whole eggs.

MAYONNAISE: These recipes use mayonnaise that has no more than 50 calories per tablespoon. We relied on two Hellmann's varieties: Canola Cholesterol Free and Light.

PEANUT BUTTER: Smart Balance Peanut Butter with omega-3 fats was used in recipes calling for peanut butter.

SOYMILK: If a recipe calls for soymilk, it's the plain variety; otherwise, you'll notice that we've specified the flavor, such as unsweetened, vanilla, or chocolate. We used Silk soymilk in these recipes.

WHOLE WHEAT OR FIBER-ENRICHED PASTA: Not everyone likes the grittiness of 100 percent whole wheat pasta, so we developed these recipes using two highly nutritious, fiber-rich Barilla pastas: Barilla Whole Grain, which is 51 percent whole grain, and Barilla PLUS.

WHOLE WHEAT TORTILLAS, WRAPS, OR FLATBREADS: We used Multi-Grain Flatout Flatbread throughout.

Breakfast

Blueberry Smoothie

SERVES 1

THIS INTENSE BLUEBERRY SMOOTHIE is full of disease-fighting antioxidants. The flax-seeds (or almonds) provide a nutty flavor and a source of healthy fat to keep you satisfied until lunch.

1 cup frozen blueberries, such as
    Cascadian Farm Organic Frozen
    Blueberries

1 cup light vanilla soymilk, such as Silk

2 tablespoons ground flaxseeds (or
    ground almonds; see page 348)

Combine all the ingredients in a blender until smooth, about 2 minutes.

PREP TIME: 5 minutes   **TOTAL TIME:** 5 minutes

PER SERVING, ABOUT: Calories: 238 Protein: 10 g Carbohydrate: 34 g Dietary Fiber: 9 g
Sugars: 19 g Total Fat: 9 g Saturated Fat: 1 g Cholesterol: 0 mg Calcium: 352 mg Sodium: 100 mg

Peanut Butter Banana Smoothie

SERVES 1

WHIPPING UP THIS QUICK recipe is a deliciously satisfying way to start your day. In fact, it's an entire meal in a shake!

1 frozen banana

2 tablespoons ground flaxseeds (see page
    348)

1 tablespoon chunky peanut butter, such
    as Smart Balance

1 cup light vanilla soymilk, such as Silk

¼ cup liquid egg whites, such as
    AllWhites

Combine all the ingredients in a blender until smooth, about 2 minutes. Serve.

PREP TIME: 5 minutes   **TOTAL TIME:** 5 minutes

PER SERVING, ABOUT: Calories: 416 Protein: 21 g Carbohydrate: 46 g Dietary Fiber: 9 g
Sugars: 22 g Total Fat: 18 g Saturated Fat: 2 g Cholesterol: 1 mg Calcium: 371 mg Sodium: 268 mg

Crunchy Yogurt with Fruit and Nuts

SERVES 1

THIS RECIPE MAKES A well-balanced, one-dish breakfast. It covers nearly 50 percent of your calcium needs (for those age 50 and under), and the walnuts give you a nice dose of omega-3 fats.

6 ounces light yogurt (blueberry, Key lime, or apple)

½ cup plain nonfat yogurt

1⅓ cups fresh fruit sliced (berries and banana for blueberry yogurt; mango, orange, and banana for Key lime yogurt; apple, pear, and banana for apple yogurt)

1 crispbread, such as Wasa Light Rye, Multi Grain, or other variety with the Best Life seal, crushed

2 tablespoons roughly chopped walnuts

Combine all the ingredients in a medium bowl and serve. (For a softer consistency, let sit for 15 minutes to 1 hour.)

PREP TIME: 5 minutes   **TOTAL TIME:** 5 minutes

PER SERVING, ABOUT: Calories: 409 Protein: 18 g Carbohydrate: 68 g Dietary Fiber: 11 g Sugars: 38 g Total Fat: 9 g Saturated Fat: 1 g Cholesterol: 2 mg Calcium: 491 mg Sodium: 261 mg

MORE THAN MILK: NEW CHOICES IN THE DAIRY SECTION

It seems that everyone is wearing milk moustaches these days, and with good reason. Milks—dairy and other varieties—provide a hefty dose of calcium, which not only strengthens your bones but also helps protect your heart and reduces your risk for certain types of cancer. Some research even suggests that calcium may make it a little easier to lose weight, although this benefit is still being studied. With all these perks, it won't come as a surprise that many of our breakfasts and even snacks call for milk or soymilk.

With so many milk options, you may be wondering which one is best. When it comes to nutrition, the two most popular choices—cow's milk and soymilk—are pretty close. As long as you choose a calcium- and vitamin D-enriched soymilk, it offers the same amount of these nutrients for just about the same amount of calories as cow's milk. You may choose one over the other simply because you like the taste better, or you have certain health issues that make one a smarter choice for you. Take a look at what each drink delivers:

COW'S MILK

Benefits: Aside from calcium, cow's milk provides B vitamins—critical for converting food to energy, protecting brain health, and preventing anemia—as well as a good amount of protein (1 cup offers about as much protein as 1 ounce of chicken).

Healthy Tip: Go for fat-free (skim) or 1% milk; you'll save up to 63 calories and 4 g of saturated fat per cup over 2% and whole. The carbohydrate in milk (lactose or milk sugar) can be a problem if you're lactose intolerant, a condition that affects 1 in 10 people. If you're just slightly lactose intolerant, you can usually handle ½ cup of milk at a time, but if you're severely intolerant, even a few tablespoons can cause gas and other digestive problems.

SOYMILK

Benefits: Soymilk doesn't contain lactose, so it's a great option for people who can't tolerate cow's milk. It's also high in protein; and the type of protein in soy has been shown to lower cholesterol. It has a vaguely nutty taste. The "original" flavor is closest to milk, and "unsweetened" is decidedly less sweet than milk.

Healthy Tip: Buy soymilk that's around 100 calories per cup; save the higher-calorie varieties, such as chocolate, for a treat. And make sure to shake well, as the calcium settles to the bottom. Most research shows that eating a moderate amount, 2 to 3 servings per day of soy food (as opposed to soy supplements), is safe and may even be protective against cancer and osteoporosis. One cup of soymilk equals 1 serving.

If you can't tolerate cow's milk or soymilk, you can try some of these varieties. Limit yourself to no more than 110 calories and opt for a brand that provides at least 30 percent of the Daily Value for calcium and 25 percent for vitamin D per cup. Almond milk is lower in calories so you can have a little more.

ALMOND MILK

This mildly rich tasting drink is low in fat and calories (40 to 60 calories per cup; vanilla has 90 calories and chocolate has 120 calories). The most widely available brand, Almond Breeze, is slightly lower in calcium (20 percent) and vitamin D (25 percent) than other milks. Try 1½ cups of the plain "original" or any of the unsweetened flavors with your cereal. You can also use it in shakes and soups or as a substitute for milk in most baked goods.

RICE MILK

It has a thinner consistency than other milks, and a slightly sweet taste, which makes it best for cereal and desserts. It's also higher in calories—120 to 130 per cup—so use only on occasion unless it's the only milk you can tolerate.

HEMP MILK

Made from hemp seeds (not the leaves, which is where the psychoactive ingredient in marijuana is found), this has a strong herbal and nutty taste that doesn't go well with everything. It is naturally rich in heart-healthy omega-3 fatty acids, which is why it's a little more caloric than other milks (110 to 130 calories per cup; chocolate has more). If you go with hemp milk, try to shave off a few calories elsewhere to make up for it.

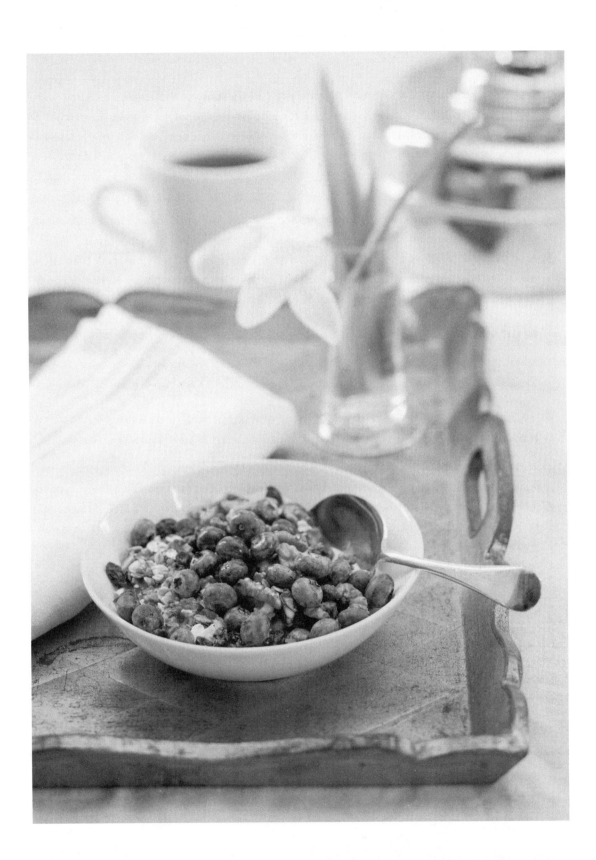

Quinoa Granola

SERVES 4

FORGET ABOUT SUGARY, LOW-FIBER cereals, they won't satisfy or give you much energy; instead, try whipping up your own healthful cereal. You can make this recipe ahead and store it in an airtight container or resealable baggy. Serve with fat-free milk, almond milk, or soymilk.

½ cup raw quinoa

½ cup rolled oats

2 tablespoons walnuts

⅛ teaspoon salt

2 tablespoons honey

2 tablespoons raisins

1. Preheat the oven to 225°F.

2. In a medium pot, add the quinoa and cover with water. Bring to a boil and cook for 7 minutes. Drain and rinse the quinoa with cold water.

3. Combine all the ingredients (including the quinoa) except for the raisins on a sheet pan and place in the oven. Mix often with a spatula to prevent sticking and to toast evenly. Cook until dry and lightly toasted, about 45 minutes. Mix in the raisins and serve.

PREP TIME: 10 minutes **TOTAL TIME:** 1 hour

PER SERVING, ABOUT: Calories: 188 Protein: 5 g Carbohydrate: 34 g Dietary Fiber: 3 g Sugars: 12 g Total Fat: 4 g Saturated Fat: 0 g Cholesterol: 0 mg Calcium: 25 mg Sodium: 79 mg

Muesli

SERVES 4

THIS HEARTY MUESLI CAN be made ahead and stored in a resealable baggy or an airtight container. It's an excellent way to include oatmeal, one of the healthiest, most satisfying foods available, into your diet.

1 cup rolled oats

½ cup raisins or other dried fruit

¼ cup chopped walnuts

¼ cup toasted wheat germ (available at most grocery stores)

¼ cup wheat bran

⅛ cup raw unsalted shelled sunflower seeds

⅛ cup ground flaxseeds (see page 348)

1 teaspoon cinnamon

½ teaspoon orange rind, very finely chopped

Mix all the ingredients thoroughly in a large bowl. Serve.

PREP TIME: 5 minutes   **TOTAL TIME:** 5 minutes

PER SERVING, ABOUT: Calories: 278 Protein: 9 g Carbohydrate: 40 g Dietary Fiber: 8 g Sugars: 13 g Total Fat: 13 g Saturated Fat: 1 g Cholesterol: 0 mg Calcium: 60 mg Sodium: 6 mg

Irish Oatmeal with Pears and Vanilla

SERVES 4

WARM CEREALS CAN BE especially comforting on a cool morning. The pears and vanilla add the ideal amount of flavor and sweetness to a hearty oatmeal.

3 cups water

⅛ teaspoon salt

1 cup raw steel-cut oats (regular or quick)

2 pears, cored and shredded

3 vanilla beans (add only the seeds scraped out of the middle; discard the bean) or 1½ teaspoons vanilla extract

1 teaspoon maple syrup

2 teaspoons healthy spread, such as Smart Balance Buttery Spread

4 tablespoons chopped toasted almonds (see page 346)

1. Bring the water to a boil in a medium pot. Add the salt and stir in the oats, pears, vanilla, and maple syrup.

2. Cook the oatmeal according to the package directions.

3. Divide into serving bowls, top with the spread and almonds, and serve.

PREP TIME: 5 minutes

TOTAL TIME: 12 to 30 minutes, depending on whether you use quick or regular oats

PER SERVING, ABOUT: Calories: 314 Protein: 9 g Carbohydrate: 43 g Dietary Fiber: 12 g Sugars: 9 g Total Fat: 12 g Saturated Fat: 1 g Cholesterol: 0 mg Calcium: 68 mg Sodium: 91 mg

Carrot Muffins

MAKES 12 MUFFINS

THESE DAIRY-FREE, MOIST, AND filling muffins are incentive to get out of bed in the morning. The batter can be made the night before; simply pour it into muffin cups and store the pan in the refrigerator covered with plastic wrap for morning baking. If you put them directly into the oven from the refrigerator, add 5 minutes to the cooking time. Now *that's* a good morning!

½ cup silken tofu

½ cup soymilk

¼ cup honey

¼ cup sugar

3 tablespoons canola oil

¼ cup fresh pineapple or canned in its own juice, mashed

1 cup whole wheat flour

1 cup wheat bran

2 teaspoons baking soda

1 teaspoon baking powder

1 teaspoon cinnamon

3 cups grated carrots

½ cup coarsely chopped walnuts

1. Preheat the oven to 350°F.

2. Puree the tofu in a food processor for 1 minute.

3. With a standing or hand mixer, combine the tofu, soymilk, honey, sugar, oil, and pineapple, until completely incorporated, about 1 minute. (You can also do this in a large bowl with a wooden spoon.) Once completely mixed, add the flour, bran, baking soda, baking powder, cinnamon, carrots, and walnuts and mix until just combined, about 30 seconds in a mixer or 1 to 2 minutes by hand.

4. Divide evenly into muffin tins and bake until a toothpick inserted into the middle of a muffin comes out clean, about 25 minutes. Serve.

PREP TIME: 15 minutes   TOTAL TIME: 40 minutes

PER MUFFIN, ABOUT: Calories: 179 Protein: 5 g Carbohydrate: 25 g Dietary Fiber: 5 g Sugars: 12 g Total Fat: 8 g Saturated Fat: 1 g Cholesterol: 0 mg Calcium: 131 mg Sodium: 277 mg

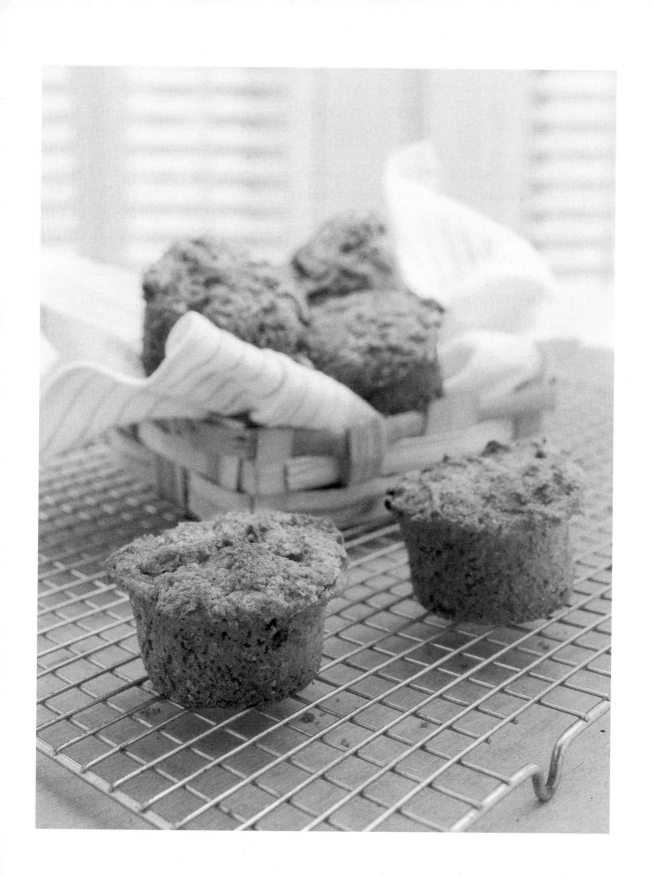

Brown Rice Pudding

SERVES 4

INSTEAD OF THROWING OUT leftover brown rice, why not use it to make a tasty and nutritious breakfast? You can enjoy this dish warm or cold.

2 cups soy or fat-free milk

2 tablespoons sugar

1 teaspoon vanilla extract

1/2 teaspoon cinnamon

1/2 cup liquid eggs, such as Better'n Eggs,
    or 2 eggs

2 cups cooked brown rice

1/4 cup raisins

1/4 cup ground flaxseeds (see page 348)

1. Combine the milk, sugar, vanilla, and cinnamon in a medium pot. Bring to a boil, stirring constantly.

2. Beat the eggs in a small bowl, then slowly add to the milk mixture while whisking continuously.

3. Immediately stir in the rice and return the mixture to a boil, stirring constantly. Reduce the heat to a simmer, add the raisins and flaxseeds and cook for 15 minutes, stirring every 5 minutes. Serve.

PREP TIME: 5 minutes   TOTAL TIME: 20 minutes

PER SERVING, ABOUT (analyzed with Better'n Eggs): Calories: 260 Protein: 10 g
Carbohydrate: 42 g Dietary Fiber: 4 g Sugars: 16 g Total Fat: 5 g Saturated Fat: 1 g
Cholesterol: 0 mg Calcium: 185 mg Sodium: 125 mg

BENEFICIAL BREWS

You probably already know that tea is good for you, but so is your daily java fix, according to new research. Both beverages are rich sources of antioxidants, which have been linked with a decreased risk for a number of different diseases. Your cup may help:

Cut Your Cancer Risk. Numerous studies link tea, especially green tea, to a reduced risk for colon cancer, and possibly breast cancer. Coffee drinkers may have a reduced risk for colon cancer and liver cancer.

Protect Your Pumper. Tea seems to offer the most benefit; studies suggest that drinking about 3 cups daily is associated with a lower risk for heart disease and heart attacks. The coffee connection is a little more tenuous. Some studies show that coffee drinkers may be more likely to get heart disease possibly because coffee temporarily spikes blood pressure (it goes back down after the caffeine wears off) and may trigger arrhythmias. However, other studies indicate that drinking coffee is linked to a lower risk for heart disease, likely the result of coffee's many antioxidants. The American Heart Association says that drinking 1 to 2 cups per day doesn't seem to be harmful.

Boost Brain Health. Studies generally show that coffee drinkers are less likely to get Parkinson's disease than those who drink little to no joe. Possible reasons: Coffee contains caffeine, which has been shown to protect brain cells, and antioxidants, which are also protective. A few studies are also starting to suggest that tea may be beneficial as well, especially black tea, because like coffee, it contains caffeine and antioxidants. Coffee and tea drinkers also stay sharper with age, suffering less cognitive decline than non-drinkers. Sipping coffee also offers short-term perks, such as increased clarity and focus. Tea does the same thing, but because it has less caffeine and contains an amino acid called theanine, it can be more calming.

Decrease Diabetes Risk. Both coffee and tea drinkers have a decreased risk for developing diabetes compared to abstainers. Even decaf coffee drinkers have a lower risk, so researchers speculate that antioxidants are at work. A compound in coffee delays the rise in blood sugar and increases levels of hormones that help with blood sugar control. Tea's antioxidants appear to improve insulin sensitivity.

Zucchini Muffins

MAKES 12 MUFFINS

HERE'S A GREAT WAY to use this often overabundant summer veggie. You can make the batter the night before, put it in muffin cups, cover with plastic wrap, and store the pan in the refrigerator overnight. If you're putting the muffins directly in the oven from the refrigerator, add 5 minutes to the baking time.

½ cup liquid eggs, such as Better'n Eggs,
   or 2 eggs

½ cup fat-free milk

¼ cup honey

¼ cup sugar

3 tablespoons olive oil

1 cup whole wheat flour

1 cup wheat bran

2 teaspoons baking soda

1 teaspoon baking powder

1 teaspoon cinnamon

Pinch of salt

3 cups shredded zucchini (using a grater)

½ cup walnuts

1. Preheat the oven to 350°F.

2. With a standing or hand mixer, combine the eggs, milk, honey, sugar, and oil until completely incorporated, about 1 minute. (You can also do this in a large bowl with a wooden spoon.) Once completely mixed, add the remaining ingredients and mix until just combined, about 30 seconds in a mixer or 1 to 2 minutes by hand.

3. Divide the batter into muffin tins, and bake until a toothpick inserted into the middle of a muffin comes out clean, about 25 minutes. Serve.

PREP TIME: 15 minutes   **TOTAL TIME:** 40 minutes

PER MUFFIN, ABOUT (analyzed using Better'n Eggs): Calories: 158 Protein: 4 g Carbohydrate: 23 g Dietary Fiber: 4 g Sugars: 11 g Total Fat: 7 g Saturated Fat: 1 g Cholesterol: 0 mg Calcium: 71 mg Sodium: 302 mg

Ginger Waffles

SERVES 4

THIS SPICED-UP VERSION OF the standard waffle is simply mouthwatering. Add a little sweetness by topping it with some fresh fruit.

2 tablespoons molasses

1½ cups nonfat plain yogurt

½ cup liquid eggs, such as Better'n Eggs, or 2 eggs

2 tablespoons melted healthy spread, such as Smart Balance Buttery Spread

½ cup all-purpose unbleached flour

½ cup whole wheat flour

½ cup bran

⅛ teaspoon salt

1¼ teaspoons baking powder

2 tablespoons sugar

¾ teaspoon ground ginger

TOPPING

4 teaspoons healthy spread, such as Smart Balance Buttery Spread

6 teaspoons maple syrup

3 cups berries or sliced pears

4 tablespoons nonfat plain yogurt

1. Heat a waffle iron. If your waffle iron has settings, put it at medium-high.

2. Whisk together the molasses, yogurt, eggs, and spread in a large bowl. Add the flours, bran, salt, baking powder, sugar, and ginger and whisk until just combined, about 30 seconds.

3. Depending on the size of your waffle maker, pour ¼ to ½ of the waffle batter in the iron and cook according to the waffle iron instructions, usually about 5 minutes per waffle.

4. Spread each waffle with 1 teaspoon healthy spread, top with 1½ teaspoons maple syrup, ¾ cup fruit, and 1 tablespoon yogurt. Serve.

PREP TIME: 5 minutes   TOTAL TIME: 10 minutes

PER SERVING, ABOUT (analyzed using Better'n Eggs): Calories: 402 Protein: 15 g Carbohydrate: 71 g Dietary Fiber: 10 g Sugars: 27 g Total Fat: 9 g Saturated Fat: 2 g Cholesterol: 2 mg Calcium: 357 mg Sodium: 439 mg

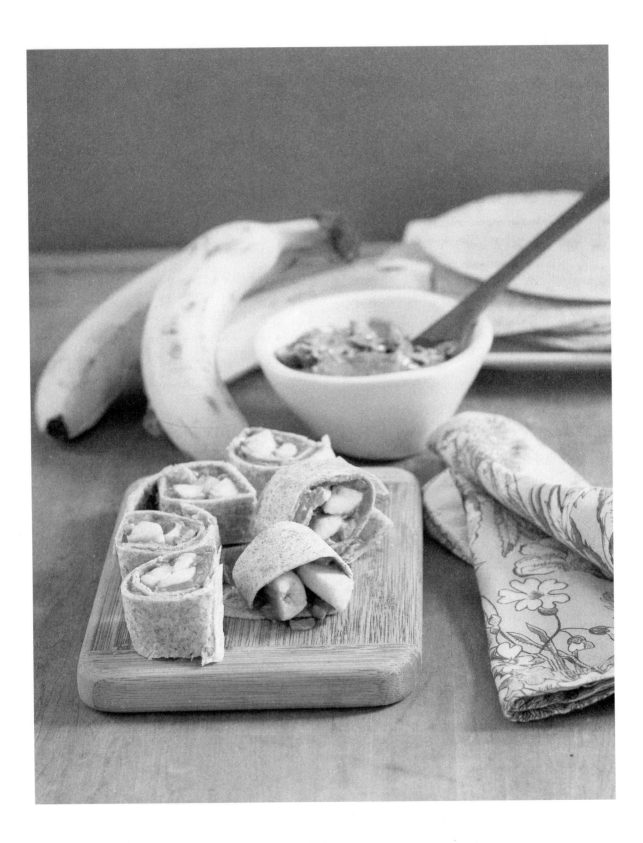

Peanut Butter and Banana "Sushi"

SERVES 1

YOU CAN EAT THIS in-a-snap wrap at home or on-the-go. It will keep you energized until lunch.

1 whole wheat tortilla

1½ tablespoons chunky peanut butter,
    such as Smart Balance

½ banana, sliced

1. Spread the tortilla with peanut butter. Top with the sliced banana.

2. Roll the tortilla into a log and cut into 1-inch pieces with a sharp knife. Serve.

PREP TIME: 5 minutes   **TOTAL TIME:** 5 minutes

PER SERVING, ABOUT: Calories: 303 Protein: 15 g Carbohydrate: 35 g Dietary Fiber: 11 g Sugars: 9 g Total Fat: 15 g Saturated Fat: 2 g Cholesterol: 0 mg Calcium: 23 mg Sodium: 463 mg

---

LABEL LOOKOUT! FAIR TRADE CERTIFIED

To protect workers, especially those in developing countries, the international Fair Trade Labelling Organizations (the U.S. arm is TransFairUSA) developed stringent worker welfare guidelines. These ensure that farmers and farm workers get a fair price, safe working conditions, and a living wage. Not to mention, food producers partnering with TransFair invest a portion of the profits back into community and professional development projects, such as scholarship programs. Not necessarily certifiably organic, Fair Trade products adhere to a number of organic principles, such as promoting sustainable agriculture and limiting the use of harmful pesticides.

Turkey Bacon and Egg White Wrap

SERVES 1

LOVE BREAKFAST SANDWICHES? TRY this healthful version to save yourself extra fat and calories. It's easy to make, and the combo of protein and fiber will nourish you.

Vegetable oil cooking spray

1 tablespoon diced onion

1 slice turkey bacon, chopped into small pieces

½ red pepper, diced

¼ cup liquid egg whites, such as AllWhites, or 2 egg whites

Black pepper to taste

One ¼-inch-thick tomato slice, chopped

1 whole wheat 100-calorie wrap, tortilla, or flatbread, such as Multi-Grain Flatout Flatbread

1. Heat a heavy-bottomed skillet over medium heat.

2. Coat the skillet with cooking spray. Add the onion and bacon to the pan and cook for 2 minutes. Add the red pepper and cook for 2 more minutes. Add the egg whites and cook for 2 more minutes, stirring constantly. Season with pepper.

3. Place the egg mixture and tomato on a tortilla and roll up. Serve.

PREP TIME: 5 minutes   TOTAL TIME: 12 minutes

PER SERVING, ABOUT (analyzed using AllWhites): Calories: 159 Protein: 12 g Carbohydrate: 27 g Dietary Fiber: 4 g Sugars: 5 g Total Fat: 3 g Saturated Fat: 1 g Cholesterol: 8 mg Calcium: 21 mg Sodium: 458 mg

Tofu Mushroom Scramble on Whole Wheat Tortilla

SERVES 1

THIS IS A HEALTHFUL, satisfying breakfast that you can take with you. When choosing tofu at your supermarket, look for one prepared with calcium sulfate so you'll enjoy the added benefit of up to 400 milligrams of calcium with each ½ cup of tofu.

Vegetable oil cooking spray

2 tablespoons minced onion

1 cup sliced mushrooms

½ cup firm tofu

⅛ teaspoon salt

Black pepper to taste

1 whole wheat tortilla

1. Heat a heavy-bottomed skillet over medium-high heat.

2. Coat the skillet with cooking spray. Add the onion and mushrooms and cook for 3 minutes. Add the tofu and stir, breaking the tofu up and incorporating it with the onion and mushrooms. Cook until the tofu is slightly browned, about 5 minutes, stirring often. Add the salt and pepper.

3. Place the tofu mixture on the tortilla. Roll the tortilla, tucking in the ends as you roll. Serve.

PREP TIME: 5 minutes   **TOTAL TIME:** 13 minutes

PER SERVING, ABOUT: Calories: 332 Protein: 23 g Carbohydrate: 33 g Dietary Fiber: 8 g Sugars: 2 g Total Fat: 12 g Saturated Fat: 1 g Cholesterol: 0 mg Calcium: 147 mg Sodium: 524 mg

Spinach and Roasted Garlic Tart

SERVES 4

THIS EGGLESS, FRITTATA-LIKE DISH makes a filling, savory breakfast. It is delicious just out of the oven, reheated, or served at room temperature.

1 cup raw quinoa, rinsed

1 pound silken tofu

3 cloves roasted garlic (see page 344)

2 tablespoons olive oil

2 cups raw spinach, coarsely chopped

2 tablespoons finely chopped fresh herbs, such as sage, rosemary, thyme, and oregano

½ teaspoon salt

Black pepper to taste

Vegetable oil cooking spray

1. Preheat the oven to 375°F.

2. Place the quinoa in a medium pot and cover with water. Bring to a boil and cook for 5 minutes. Drain the quinoa and place in a large bowl.

3. Process the tofu, roasted garlic, and oil in a food processor until completely smooth, about 2 minutes.

4. Add the tofu mixture to the quinoa and stir in the spinach, herbs, salt and pepper.

5. Coat a 9-inch pie pan with cooking spray. Pour the quinoa mixture into the pan and cook for 30 minutes. Serve.

PREP TIME: 10 minutes   **TOTAL TIME:** 30 minutes

PER SERVING, ABOUT: Calories: 290 Protein: 12 g Carbohydrate: 34 g Dietary Fiber: 3 g Sugars: 2 g Total Fat: 12 g Saturated Fat: 2 g Cholesterol: 0 mg Calcium: 84 mg Sodium: 318 mg

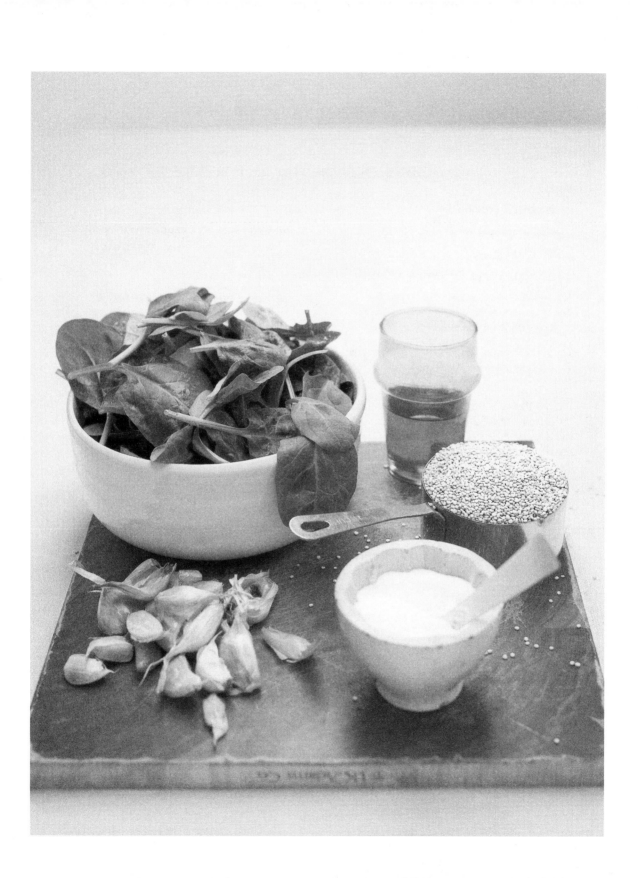

Leek and Mushroom Breakfast Pie

SERVES 4

THIS CLASSIC QUICHE-LIKE PIE works for breakfast, lunch, or dinner.

Vegetable oil cooking spray

2 leeks, white part only, thinly sliced,
   well washed

3 cups (about 8 ounces) mushrooms,
   sliced

4 Wasa crispbreads (any variety with the
   Best Life seal), crushed

1 cup liquid eggs, such as Better'n Eggs, or
   4 whole eggs

1 cup fat-free milk

1/8 teaspoon nutmeg

1/8 teaspoon salt

Black pepper to taste

1/2 cup cubed reduced-fat Swiss cheese

1. Heat a heavy-bottomed skillet over medium heat. Preheat the oven to 375°F.

2. Coat a skillet with cooking spray. Cook the leeks in the skillet for 5 minutes, stirring often. Add the mushrooms and cook for 3 more minutes.

3. Coat a 9-inch pie plate with cooking spray. Cover the bottom of the pie plate with the crispbread crumbs. Cover the crackers with the leek and mushroom mixture.

4. Beat together the eggs, milk, and nutmeg in a large bowl. Season with salt and pepper. Pour the egg mixture over the mushrooms. Distribute the cheese over the top.

5. Bake for 40 minutes. Serve.

PREP TIME: 10 minutes   TOTAL TIME: 60 minutes

PER SERVING, ABOUT (analyzed using Better'n Eggs): Calories: 153 Protein: 16 g
Carbohydrate: 21 g Dietary Fiber: 3 g Sugars: 7 g Total Fat: 1 g Saturated Fat: 1 g
Cholesterol: 6 mg Calcium: 240 mg Sodium: 256 mg

Savory Cracker Pudding

SERVES 4

HAVE PUDDING FOR BREAKFAST with this savory dish!

1 onion, sliced

Vegetable oil cooking spray

1 cup Better'n Eggs, or 4 eggs

2 teaspoons thyme

½ cup fat-free milk

3 crispbreads, such as Wasa (any variety with the Best Life seal), each broken into about 6 large pieces

1 tomato, sliced

4 tablespoons grated Parmesan

1. Preheat the oven to 375°F.

2. Coat the onion with cooking spray. Place on a sheet pan and bake for 5 minutes.

3. Mix together the eggs, thyme, and milk.

4. Coat a 9-inch pie plate with cooking spray. Place the crispbreads in the pie plate and pour the egg mixture on top. Cover with the cooked onion and tomato slices. Top with the Parmesan.

5. Bake for 20 minutes and serve.

PREP TIME: 10 minutes   TOTAL TIME: 35 minutes

PER SERVING, ABOUT (analyzed using Better'n Eggs) Calories: 122 Protein: 10 g Carbohydrate: 17 g Dietary Fiber: 2 g Sugars: 7 g Total Fat: 2 g Saturated Fat: 1 g Cholesterol: 5 mg Calcium: 122 mg Sodium: 190 mg

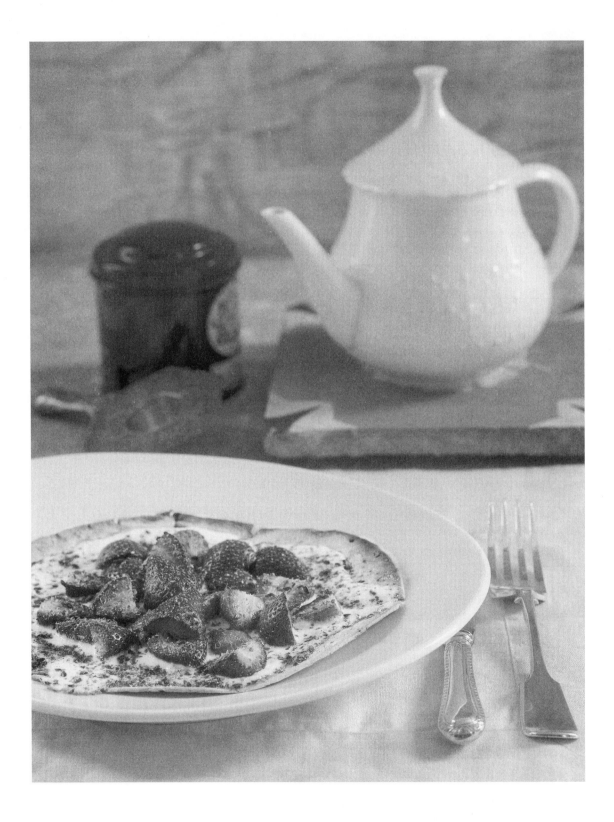

Breakfast Pizza

SERVES 1

YES, YOU CAN HAVE pizza for breakfast! This nutritious and satisfying version is low in fat and high in calcium and fiber, and, if you use Flatout Flatbread, omega-3 fats.

⅓ cup part-skim ricotta cheese

1½ teaspoons honey

1 whole wheat 100-calorie wrap, tortilla, or flatbread, such as Multi-Grain Flatout Flatbread

¾ cup fresh berries

2 tablespoons slivered (or roughly chopped) almonds

1. Preheat the oven to 375°F.

2. Mix the ricotta and honey in a small bowl. Spread the flatbread or tortilla with the ricotta and top with the berries and almonds.

3. Place on a sheet pan and bake for 4 minutes. Turn the oven to broil and cook for 2 more minutes. Serve.

PREP TIME: 4 minutes   **TOTAL TIME:** 10 minutes

PER SERVING, ABOUT (analyzed using Multi-Grain Flatout Flatbread): Calories: 385 Protein: 22 g Carbohydrate: 49 g Dietary Fiber: 11 g Sugars: 22 g Total Fat: 17 g Saturated Fat: 5 g Cholesterol: 25 mg Calcium: 412 mg Sodium: 293 mg

Soups

STARTER SOUPS

Sunchoke Soup

SERVES 4

SUNCHOKES OR JERUSALEM ARTICHOKES are not from Jerusalem nor are they a relative of the artichoke. These potato-like veggies, which taste similar to an artichoke, come from a specific type of sunflower, thus, the name sunchoke. (You might find them under either name at the grocery store.) Although they are cooked in this recipe, they can also be eaten raw and are a welcome addition to most salads. This recipe makes an incredibly rich and flavorful soup.

Vegetable oil cooking spray

1 large onion, chopped

4 cups sunchokes, washed thoroughly (if dirty, scrub with a brush)

3 cups water

1 tablespoon plus ½ teaspoon thyme, chopped

¼ teaspoon salt

Black pepper to taste

1. Heat a large, heavy-bottomed pot over medium heat.

2. Lightly coat the hot pot with cooking spray. Add the onion and cook until browned, about 10 minutes.

3. Add the sunchokes, water, and 1 tablespoon thyme. Bring the soup to a simmer and cook until the sunchokes are very tender, about 10 minutes.

4. Puree the soup in a blender until smooth, about 2 minutes.

5. Add the salt and pepper. Garnish with the remaining ½ teaspoon thyme and serve.

PREP TIME: 10 minutes   TOTAL TIME: 35 minutes

PER SERVING, ABOUT: Calories: 130 Protein: 3 g Carbohydrate: 30 g Dietary Fiber: 3 g Sugars: 16 g Total Fat: 0 g Saturated Fat: 0 g Cholesterol: 0 mg Calcium: 36 mg Sodium: 157 mg

Onion Broth

SERVES 4

THIS LIGHT BUT DELICIOUS soup is a great way to start a meal on a cold winter or fall day. Roasting the different types of onions creates a slightly sweet caramelized taste and the additional cooking harmonizes the different flavors.

1 yellow onion, sliced	1 bay leaf
1 white onion, sliced	½ teaspoon rosemary
4 shallots, peeled and sliced	4 cups water
2 leeks, white parts only, well washed and thinly sliced	¼ teaspoon salt
	Black pepper to taste
Vegetable oil cooking spray	¼ cup sliced green onions (scallions)

1. Preheat the oven to 375°F. Put a sheet pan in the oven to warm up. Coat the yellow and white onions, shallots, and leeks with cooking spray.

2. Put the onions, shallots, and leeks on the hot sheet pan and roast for 10 minutes.

3. Place the yellow and white onions, shallots, and leeks in a stockpot with the bay leaf, rosemary, and water. Bring the mixture to a boil. Reduce the heat to a simmer and cook for 10 minutes.

4. Using a spoon, remove the bay leaf and discard. Add the salt and pepper. Sprinkle the green onions on top and serve.

PREP TIME: 10 minutes   **TOTAL TIME:** 30 minutes

PER SERVING, ABOUT: Calories: 61 Protein: 2 g Carbohydrate: 14 g Dietary Fiber: 2 g
Sugars: 4 g Total Fat: 0 g Saturated Fat: 0 g Cholesterol: 0 mg Calcium: 48 mg Sodium: 158 mg

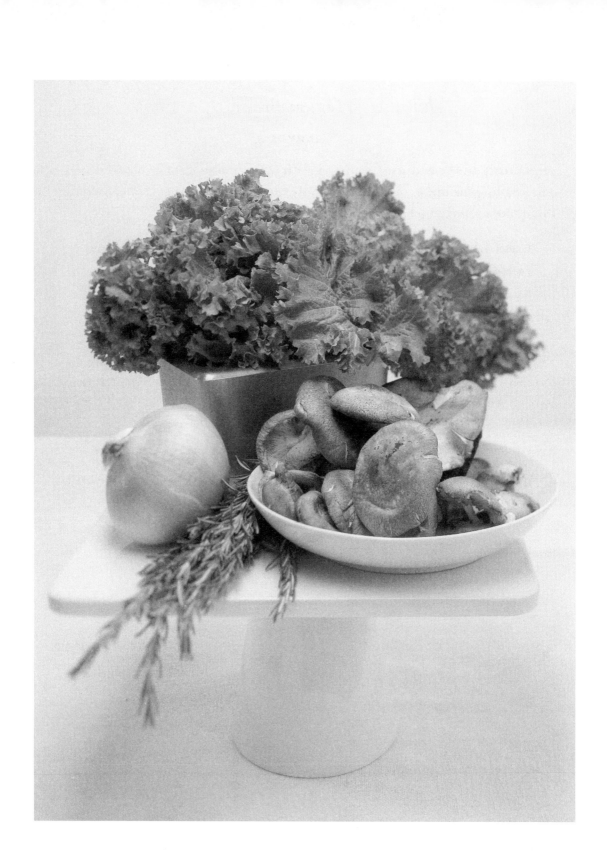

Shiitake Mushroom and Greens Soup

SERVES 4

ENJOY THE TASTE AND reap the nutritional benefits of mushrooms and leafy greens. The mushrooms make a delicious, slightly earthy tasting broth, which enhances whatever greens you choose to use in this soup.

6 cups water

1 onion, sliced

6 ounces shiitake mushrooms, stems removed and reserved, caps sliced

1 carrot, peeled and chopped

1 tablespoon herbs, such as sage, rosemary, or thyme

3 cups chopped hearty greens, such as mustard greens, kale, collard greens, or turnip greens, well washed

¼ teaspoon salt

1. In a medium pot, combine the water, onion, shiitake stems, and carrot. Bring to a boil and reduce to a simmer.

2. Simmer for 20 minutes, strain, and return the broth to the pot.

3. Add the sliced shiitake caps, herbs, and greens to the broth and bring to a boil. Reduce the heat to simmer for 5 minutes. Add the salt and serve.

PREP TIME: 10 minutes   **TOTAL TIME:** 40 minutes

PER SERVING, ABOUT: Calories: 75 Protein: 3 g Carbohydrate: 18 g Dietary Fiber: 3 g Sugars: 4 g Total Fat: 1 g Saturated Fat: 0 g Cholesterol: 0 mg Calcium: 83 mg Sodium: 181 mg

Warm Pea Soup

SERVES 4

THE SIMPLICITY OF THIS recipe highlights the sweet, unique taste of peas. The soup has an almost velvety texture on your tongue. If you are making it in the spring and have fresh sweet peas available, it will be well worth the extra trouble of removing them from their shells.

1 potato, peeled and diced	¼ teaspoon salt
8 cups water, divided	Black pepper to taste
2 cups chopped green onions (scallions), white and green parts	4 tablespoons low-fat sour cream
3 cups fresh peas removed from shell or frozen, defrosted at room temperature	

1. Place the potato in a saucepan, cover with water, and bring to a boil. Reduce the heat to a simmer and cook until the potato is tender, about 10 minutes. Remove the potato.

2. Fill a medium pot with 6 cups water, add the green onions, and bring to a boil. Add the peas and turn off the heat immediately. Let the pea mixture sit for 5 minutes. Drain the peas and green onions and puree in a blender with the potato, salt, pepper, and 2 cups water until very smooth, about 3 minutes.

3. Heat the soup over a low flame in a medium pot, stirring often, until warm, about 5 minutes. Garnish with the sour cream and serve.

PREP TIME: 5 minutes   TOTAL TIME: 25 minutes

PER SERVING, ABOUT: Calories: 169 Protein: 9 g Carbohydrate: 30 g Dietary Fiber: 8 g Sugars: 9 g Total Fat: 2 g Saturated Fat: 1 g Cholesterol: 8 mg Calcium: 95 mg Sodium: 171 mg

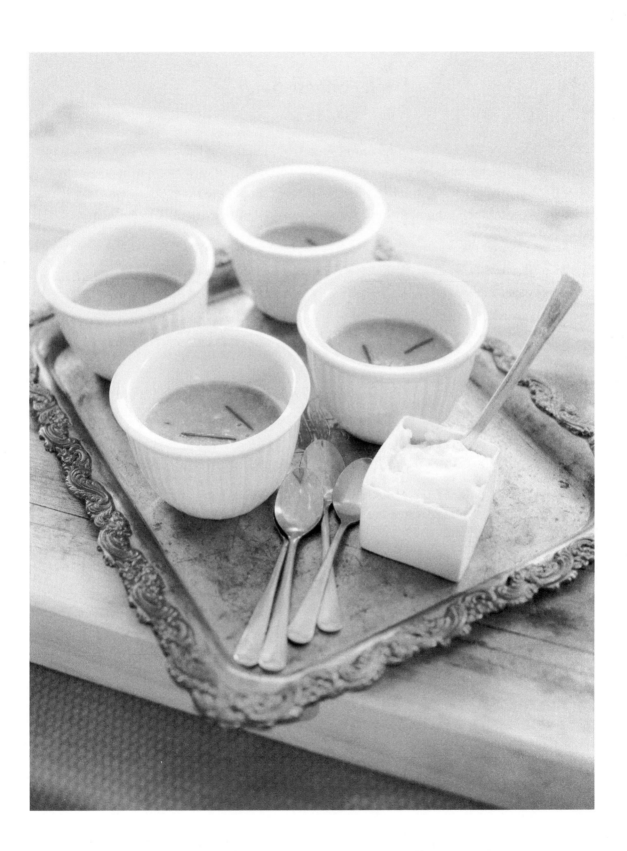

Winter Squash Soup

SERVES 4

YOU CAN ENJOY THIS rich and warming soup from fall through early spring, the peak season for winter squash. Feel free to experiment with different varieties of winter squash; all will work and each will result in a slightly different soup. One note: Some squash contains more water than others, so you may need to add a little extra milk to get to a thick soup consistency.

Vegetable oil cooking spray	½ teaspoon ground ginger
1 onion, sliced	1½ cups almond milk or fat-free milk
2 cups mashed, cooked winter squash, (see page 348)	¼ teaspoon salt
2 tablespoons fresh chopped sage	Black pepper to taste

1. Heat a stockpot over medium heat. Coat the stockpot with cooking spray. Add the onion and cook for 5 minutes.

2. In a blender combine all the ingredients (including onion) and puree until smooth, about 2 minutes. Return the mixture to the pot and heat thoroughly before serving.

   PREP TIME: 7 minutes using cooked squash (40 minutes if using raw squash)
   TOTAL TIME: 15 minutes (50 minutes)

PER SERVING, ABOUT: Calories: 72 Protein: 4 g Carbohydrate: 14 g Dietary Fiber: 2 g Sugars: 7 g Total Fat: 0 g Saturated Fat: 0 g Cholesterol: 2 mg Calcium: 232 mg Sodium: 125 mg

Cucumber Soup with Lime and Yogurt

SERVES 4

CREAMY, REFRESHING, QUENCHING, AND tart, this soup is perfect on a hot summer day.

3 cucumbers, peeled and seeded	⅛ teaspoon salt
Juice of 1 lime	¼ cup fresh dill
1 cup nonfat yogurt	

Combine all the ingredients in a blender and puree until smooth, about 2 minutes. Serve immediately or chill until you are ready to serve.

PREP TIME: 13 minutes   **TOTAL TIME:** 15 minutes

PER SERVING, ABOUT: Calories: 55 Protein: 4 g Carbohydrate: 9 g Dietary Fiber: 1 g Sugars: 2 g Total Fat: 0 g Saturated Fat: 0 g Cholesterol: 1 mg Calcium: 146 mg Sodium: 123 mg

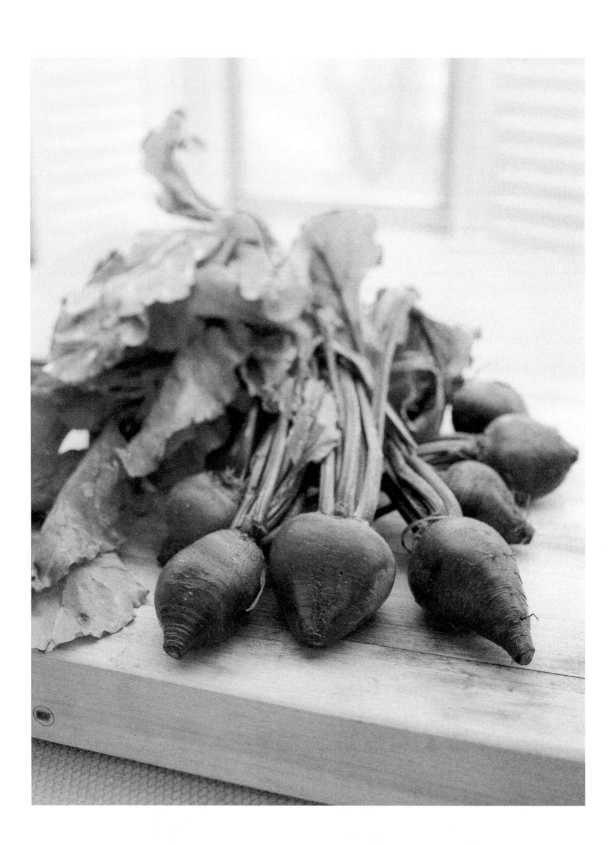

Beet Soup

SERVES 4

THIS BUTTERY, RICH, SWEET-TASTING soup is delicious cold or hot, depending on your mood or the weather. You can use large red beets, yellow, white, candy stripe, or baby beets if they are available.

3 cups shredded beets

1 onion, chopped

Vegetable oil cooking spray

2½ cups water

¼ cup white vinegar

⅛ teaspoon salt

4 teaspoons reduced-fat sour cream (with no more than 45 calories and 2 g saturated fat per 2 tablespoons)

Black pepper to taste

1. Preheat the oven to 375°F.

2. Place the beets and onion on a sheet pan and coat with cooking spray. Cook for 10 minutes, stirring once after 5 minutes.

3. Transfer the beets and onion to a large stockpot and add the water. Bring to a boil and reduce to a simmer for 5 minutes. Add the vinegar and salt. Puree the soup in a blender until very smooth, about 3 minutes.

4. Serve hot or cold, garnished with sour cream and generously seasoned with pepper.

PREP TIME: 12 minutes   **TOTAL TIME:** 35 minutes

PER SERVING, ABOUT: Calories: 68 Protein: 2 g Carbohydrate: 14 g Dietary Fiber: 3 g Sugars: 8 g Total Fat: 1 g Saturated Fat: 0 g Cholesterol: 2 mg Calcium: 31 mg Sodium: 157 mg

Carrot and Avocado Soup

SERVES 4

THE FLAVORS OF AVOCADO and carrot blend to create a creamy, sweet, and savory soup.

3 cups carrot juice (juice yourself or buy fresh carrot juice)

1 ripe avocado, skin and pit removed

1 tablespoon lime juice

¼ teaspoon salt

Black pepper to taste

Place all the ingredients in a blender. Season with pepper. Process until smooth, about 3 minutes. Serve.

PREP TIME: 5 minutes　　**TOTAL TIME:** 5 minutes

PER SERVING, ABOUT: Calories: 129 Protein: 2 g Carbohydrate: 20 g Dietary Fiber: 4 g
Sugars: 7 g Total Fat: 6 g Saturated Fat: 1 g Cholesterol: 0 mg Calcium: 48 mg Sodium: 200 mg

Chilled Mango Soup

SERVES 4

THIS CHILLED SOUP CAN be a refreshing change. It's best if the mangoes you use are ripe; check to see that it indents easily when you apply light pressure with your finger and that it's fragrant when held near your nose.

½ cup water

2 medium mangoes, peeled, seeds removed, and chopped

¼ cup rice wine vinegar

1 tablespoon extra virgin olive oil

¼ cup diced red onion

1 cucumber, seeded, peeled, and chopped

¼ cup fresh cilantro

⅛ teaspoon salt

2 tablespoons chopped fresh chives

1. Place all the ingredients except the chives in a blender and blend until smooth, about 2 minutes. Taste the soup; if it's stringy, pass it through a fine strainer to remove any mango strings.

2. Chill, garnish with chives, and serve.

PREP TIME: 10 minutes　**TOTAL TIME:** 10 minutes

PER SERVING, ABOUT: Calories: 111 Protein: 1 g Carbohydrate: 20 g Dietary Fiber: 2 g Sugars: 17 g Total Fat: 4 g Saturated Fat: 1 g Cholesterol: 0 mg Calcium: 23 mg Sodium: 78 mg

MAIN SOUPS AND STEWS

Corn and Lima Bean Chowder

SERVES 4

THANKS TO FROZEN VEGGIES you can make this recipe all year round, but for the most flavorful soup, whip this up in midsummer when you can get fresh corn and lima beans from your local farmers' market.

1 medium onion, chopped

Vegetable oil cooking spray

2 cups fresh or frozen lima beans

3 cups almond milk, soymilk, or fat-free milk

1 teaspoon chopped fresh thyme, or ½ teaspoon dried

2 cups corn, cut off the cob or frozen

Heaping ¼ teaspoon salt

Black pepper to taste

1. Heat a heavy-bottomed stockpot over medium heat.

2. Coat the onion with cooking spray and cook in the stockpot, stirring often, for 5 minutes.

3. Add the lima beans, milk, and thyme. Heat until the soup just begins to simmer, about 5 minutes, stirring frequently.

4. Add the corn, salt, and pepper. Serve.

PREP TIME: 15 minutes   TOTAL TIME: 25 minutes

PER SERVING, ABOUT: Calories: 245 Protein: 10 g Carbohydrate: 49 g Dietary Fiber: 8 g Sugars: 10 g Total Fat: 3 g Saturated Fat: 0 g Cholesterol: 0 mg Calcium: 189 mg Sodium: 352 mg

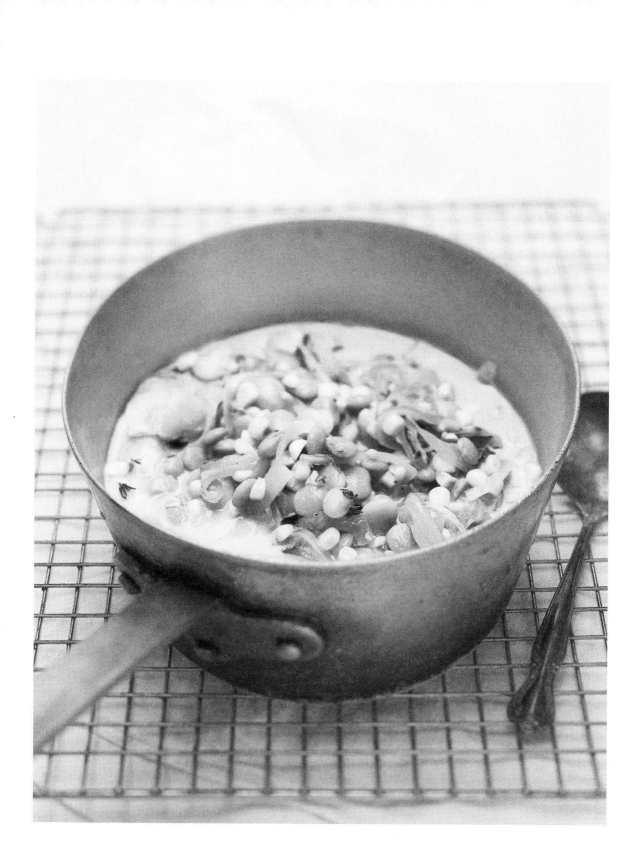

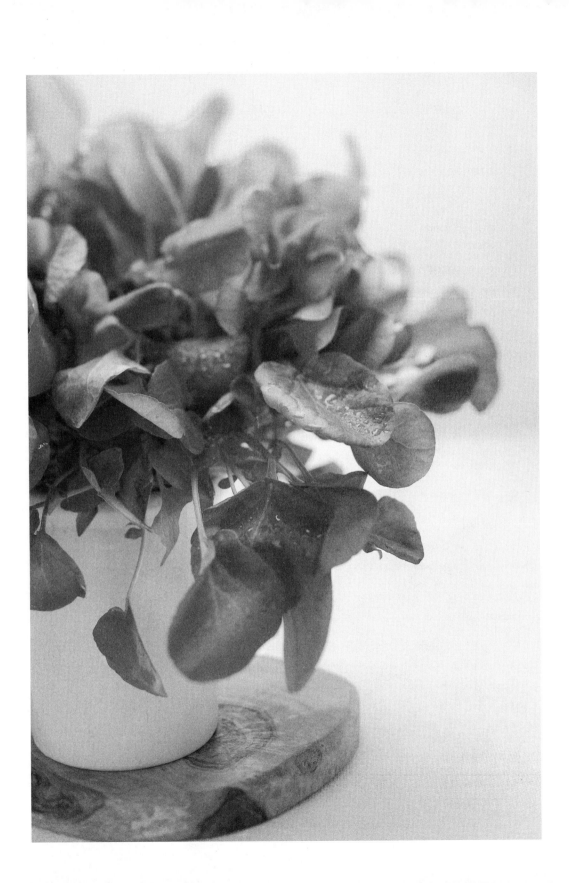

Beef Stew with Spring/Summer Vegetables

SERVES 4

THIS LIGHT BEEF STEW features vegetables that are at their best right when the weather is warm.

1 pound top round beef, cut into 1½-inch cubes

1 onion, chopped

4 leeks, well washed, top third and bulb end discarded; remaining part sliced

1 cup dry white wine

2 large carrots, sliced

2 large tomatoes, chopped

6 cups water

¼ cup fresh basil leaves

1 cup coarsely chopped fresh Italian parsley

1 cup fresh shelled peas, or frozen

1 cup fresh or frozen sugar snap peas

Heaping ¼ teaspoon salt

1 cup watercress or arugula

1. Heat a large heavy-bottomed pot over medium-high heat.

2. Place the beef in the pot and brown on all sides, about 3 minutes per side.

3. Remove the beef and cook the onion and leeks in the same pot until they are browned, about 5 minutes.

4. Add the wine to the pot and scrape the bottom of the pot using a wooden spoon or metal spatula to incorporate the browned onion and beef residue into liquid.

5. Add the beef back into the pot, along with the carrots, tomatoes, water, basil, and parsley. Bring to a boil, then reduce the heat to low, and simmer for 1 hour.

6. If serving immediately, add the peas, sugar snap peas, and salt. Cook for 2 more minutes. Garnish with the greens and serve. If serving later, refrigerate until ready to serve. Heat the stew over medium heat until heated through, about 5 minutes. Add the peas, sugar snap peas, and salt. Heat for 2 more minutes. Garnish with greens and serve.

PREP TIME: 20 minutes   TOTAL TIME: 1 hour 40 minutes

PER SERVING, ABOUT: Calories: 348 Protein: 32 g Carbohydrate: 31 g Dietary Fiber: 7 g Sugars: 12 g Total Fat: 7 g Saturated Fat: 2 g Cholesterol: 62 mg Calcium: 166 mg Sodium: 334 mg

Turkey Chili

SERVES 4

THIS WILL NOT ONLY be your most healthful chili recipe but also your all-time *favorite* chili recipe. It's so flavorful that you won't even realize it's low-fat. This freezes well. Or, you can keep it in the refrigerator for a few days.

Vegetable oil cooking spray

1 large onion, chopped

3 cloves garlic, minced

1 pound ground turkey breast

3 cups water

2 cups chopped fresh tomatoes, or canned no-salt-added tomatoes

1 sweet red pepper, seeded and finely chopped

1 stalk celery, chopped

1/8 teaspoon cayenne

1 1/2 teaspoons cumin

1 bay leaf

2 tablespoons chili powder

Heaping 1/4 teaspoon salt

1 1/2 cups canned no-salt-added kidney beans, such as Eden Organic, drained and rinsed, or cooked (page 345)

2 tablespoons chopped red onion

2 tablespoons shredded low-fat Cheddar, such as Cabot 50% Reduced Fat Cheddar

1. Lightly spritz a large heavy-bottomed stockpot with cooking spray. Heat over medium heat.

2. Add the onion and garlic and cook until golden brown, about 8 minutes, stirring regularly.

3. Add the turkey and cook until brown, about 10 minutes, stirring regularly.

4. Add the water, tomatoes, pepper, celery, cayenne, cumin, bay leaf, chili powder, and salt; stir and bring to a boil.

5. Reduce the heat to a simmer and cook for 30 minutes.

6. Add the beans and continue to cook until the beans are hot, about 5 minutes. Remove the bay leaf before serving.

7. Divide the chili evenly into 4 bowls. Top each with ½ tablespoon red onion and ½ tablespoon Cheddar. Serve.

PREP TIME: 20 minutes   **TOTAL TIME:** 1 hour 20 minutes

PER SERVING, ABOUT: Calories: 367 Protein: 29 g Carbohydrate: 28 g Dietary Fiber: 9 g Sugars: 7 g Total Fat: 17 g Saturated Fat: 4 g Cholesterol: 90 mg Calcium: 102 mg Sodium: 467 mg

---

LABEL LOOKOUT! BEST LIFE APPROVED

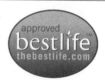

You'll find this seal on products that can help you eat healthfully and lose weight. Products carrying this seal must meet specific nutrition criteria for fiber, sodium, saturated fat, or other nutrients. For instance, pasta must contain at least 4 g fiber per 2 ounce dry serving. The ingredients list must also make the grade; for instance, cereal must be based on whole grains and soymilk must be enriched with calcium and vitamin D. The companies offering these products have made a commitment to removing, or substantially reducing, ingredients that are not in your best interest, such as trans fat and sodium. To check out the guidelines, and for a list of Best Life approved products, go to www.thebestlife.com.

Chicken Noodle Soup

SERVES 4

THIS QUICK AND HEARTY chicken noodle soup is great whether you're feeling under the weather or simply craving comfort food.

4 cups low-sodium chicken broth or 8 cups Chicken Stock (see page 338)

1 quart water (if using store-bought broth)

4 skinless boneless ½ chicken breasts (about 1 pound total), cut into bite-sized pieces

2 medium carrots, chopped

1 onion, finely chopped

1 stalk celery, chopped

½ cup fresh Italian parsley

1 teaspoon chopped fresh rosemary, or ½ teaspoon dried

1 teaspoon chopped fresh thyme, or ½ teaspoon dried

7 ounces (about ½ package) whole grain or fiber-enriched thin spaghetti, such as Barilla Whole Grain, cooked according to package instructions

Heaping ¼ teaspoon salt

1. In a large pot, bring the broth, water (if you're using store-bought broth), and chicken to a boil. Add the carrots, onion, celery, parsley, rosemary, and thyme.

2. Reduce the heat to low and simmer for 10 minutes.

3. Add the cooked pasta and salt. Serve as soon as it simmers.

PREP TIME: 20 minutes   **TOTAL TIME:** 30 minutes

PER SERVING, ABOUT: Calories: 337 Protein: 34 g Carbohydrate: 43 g Dietary Fiber: 7 g Sugars: 5 g Total Fat: 3 g Saturated Fat: 0 g Cholesterol: 66 mg Calcium: 45 mg Sodium: 214 mg

Beef Stew with Winter Root Vegetables

SERVES 4

WARM UP WITH A healthy, satisfying bowl of stew. This recipe incorporates the delicious flavors of root vegetables, which are at their peak when the weather is cool.

1 pound top round beef, cut into 1½-inch cubes

1 onion, chopped

8 shallots, skin removed and cut into 4 pieces

1 cup dry red wine

2 parsnips, peeled and sliced

2 turnips, peeled and sliced

1 rutabaga, peeled and sliced

8 cups water

1½ teaspoons chopped fresh rosemary, or ½ teaspoon dried

1½ teaspoons chopped fresh sage, or ½ teaspoon dried

1 slice whole wheat bread

Heaping ¼ teaspoon salt

2 cloves garlic, minced

1 cup fresh Italian parsley

1. Heat a large heavy-bottomed pot over medium-high heat.

2. Place the beef in the pot and brown on all sides, about 3 minutes per side.

3. Remove the beef. Cook the onion and shallots in the pot until browned, about 10 minutes.

4. Add the wine to the pot and scrape the bottom of the pot using a wooden spoon or metal spatula to incorporate the browned onion and beef bits into the liquid.

5. Add the beef back into the pot along with the vegetables, water, rosemary, and sage.

6. Bring to a boil. Reduce the heat to low, cover, and simmer for 1 hour.

7. Puree the bread, salt, garlic, and parsley in a food processor for 1 minute. Add the bread mixture to the stew and stir until combined. Serve.

PREP TIME: 20 minutes   **TOTAL TIME:** 1 hour 50 minutes

PER SERVING, ABOUT: Calories: 310 Protein: 30 g Carbohydrate: 33 g Dietary Fiber: 8 g Sugars: 12 g Total Fat: 6 g Saturated Fat: 2 g Cholesterol: 62 mg Calcium: 166 mg Sodium: 383 mg

Bean and Pasta Soup

SERVES 4

THE BARILLA PLUS PASTA in this soup adds protein, fiber, and omega-3 fatty acids to an already healthy and hearty soup.

1½ cups canned no-salt-added white beans, or cooked (see page 345)

1 bay leaf

1 large carrot, chopped

1 onion, chopped

2 cloves garlic, roughly chopped

1 red jalapeño or any other hot pepper variety, chopped

1 teaspoon chopped fresh rosemary, or ½ teaspoon dried

1 teaspoon chopped fresh sage, or ½ teaspoon dried

2 cups chopped tomatoes, or canned no-salt-added tomatoes

2 cups cooking greens, such as chard, collard greens, or escarole, well washed and broken into bite-sized pieces

6 cups water

7 ounces (about ½ package) Barilla PLUS Pasta elbows, cooked according to package instructions

¼ teaspoon salt

4 tablespoons grated Parmesan

1. In a large pot, combine the beans, bay leaf, carrot, onion, garlic, jalapeño, rosemary, sage, tomatoes, greens, and water and bring to a boil.

2. Reduce the heat until the soup is at a simmer and cook for 20 minutes.

3. Add the cooked pasta and salt; heat thoroughly.

4. Evenly divide the soup among 4 bowls, top each with 1 tablespoon Parmesan, and serve.

PREP TIME: 10 minutes　TOTAL TIME: 30 minutes

PER SERVING, ABOUT: Calories: 344 Protein: 19 g Carbohydrate: 60 g Dietary Fiber: 10 g Sugars: 7 g Total Fat: 4 g Saturated Fat: 1 g Cholesterol: 4 mg Calcium: 178 mg Sodium: 464 mg

Vegetable Chili

SERVES 4

THIS CHILI IS SO flavorful, you won't even miss the meat. It keeps in the refrigerator for a few days and freezes well.

Vegetable oil cooking spray

1 large onion, chopped

3 cloves garlic, minced

4 cups water

3 cups chopped fresh tomatoes, or canned no-salt-added tomatoes

2 sweet red peppers, seeded and finely chopped

2 stalks celery, chopped

2 carrots, chopped

1/8 teaspoon cayenne

1/2 teaspoon cumin

1 bay leaf

2 tablespoons chili powder

Heaping 1/4 teaspoon salt

2 cups canned low-sodium red kidney beans, such as Goya, drained and rinsed, or cooked (page 345)

1/2 cup cracked wheat or bulgur

2 tablespoons chopped red onion

1/4 cup shredded low-fat Cheddar

1. Lightly spritz a large heavy-bottomed stockpot with cooking spray. Heat over medium heat. Add the onion and garlic and cook until golden brown, about 8 minutes, stirring regularly.

2. Add the water, tomatoes, peppers, celery, carrots, cayenne, cumin, bay leaf, chili powder, salt, beans, and cracked wheat. Stir and bring to a boil.

3. Reduce the heat to low and simmer for 30 minutes.

4. Remove the bay leaf and divide the chili evenly among 4 bowls. Top each bowl with 1/2 tablespoon red onion and 1 tablespoon Cheddar. Serve.

PREP TIME: 20 minutes   TOTAL TIME: 50 minutes

PER SERVING, ABOUT (analyzed with Goya low-sodium red kidney beans):
Calories: 287 Protein: 15 g Carbohydrate: 54 g Dietary Fiber: 17 g Sugars: 12 g
Total Fat: 3 g Saturated Fat: 1 g Cholesterol: 4 mg Calcium: 184 mg Sodium: 409 mg

Sweet Potato Peanut Soup

SERVES 4

THIS UNUSUAL BUT COMPLEMENTARY combination of flavors hits the spot on a cold day. Sweet potatoes are an excellent source of vitamin A—you get nearly five times the daily requirement of this vitamin in a single serving of this soup! Sweet potatoes are also rich in vitamin C, fiber, and vitamin B6, while the peanut butter provides protein, and if you use Smart Balance, omega-3s.

Vegetable oil cooking spray

1 large onion, chopped

2 cloves garlic, minced

2 teaspoons minced fresh gingerroot

1½ teaspoons ground cumin

½ teaspoon ground cinnamon

Pinch of ground cloves

3 cups chopped fresh tomatoes, or canned no-salt-added tomatoes

1½ pounds sweet potatoes, peeled and chopped

4½ cups water

1 carrot, peeled and chopped

⅛ teaspoon salt

⅛ teaspoon cayenne

6 tablespoons (¼ cup plus ⅛ cup) peanut butter, such as Smart Balance

1 small bunch chopped fresh cilantro, leaves only

Red pepper flakes to taste

1. Heat a heavy-bottomed stockpot over medium heat.

2. Coat the pot with cooking spray and add the onion, garlic, and ginger. Stir constantly and cook for 5 minutes.

3. Add the cumin, cinnamon, and cloves and continue cooking for 2 more minutes, stirring constantly.

4. Add the tomatoes, sweet potatoes, and water. Bring to a boil. Reduce the heat to low and simmer for 20 minutes.

5. Add the carrot, salt, cayenne, and peanut butter and cook for 5 minutes.

6. Puree in a blender until smooth, about 3 minutes.

7. Garnish with the cilantro and red pepper flakes and serve.

PREP TIME: 10 minutes   **TOTAL TIME:** 50 minutes

PER SERVING, ABOUT: Calories: 338 Protein: 10 g Carbohydrate: 47 g Dietary Fiber: 9 g Sugars: 12 g Total Fat: 14 g Saturated Fat: 2 g Cholesterol: 0 mg Calcium: 106 mg Sodium: 276 mg

Lentil and Lamb Soup

SERVES 4

HEARTY AND SATISFYING, THIS soup is almost a complete meal; just add a whole grain roll and you're all set.

12 ounces lean lamb boneless sirloin, cut into 1-inch pieces

Vegetable oil cooking spray

1 onion, chopped

3 carrots, sliced

1 cup green or brown lentils

4 cups water

4 cloves minced garlic

1 tablespoon chopped fresh rosemary, or ½ teaspoon dried

1 tablespoon minced fresh ginger

1 tablespoon curry powder

3 cups chopped fresh tomatoes, or canned no-salt-added tomatoes

¼ teaspoon salt

1. Heat a heavy-bottomed stockpot over medium heat.

2. Coat the lamb with cooking spray and cook in the pot, turning often, until browned on all sides, about 5 minutes.

3. Add the onion, carrots, lentils, water, garlic, rosemary, ginger, curry powder, and tomatoes. Cook until the lamb and lentils are tender, about 1 hour.

4. Stir in the salt before serving.

PREP TIME: 20 minutes   TOTAL TIME: 1 hour 25 minutes

PER SERVING, ABOUT: Calories: 388 Protein: 34 g Carbohydrate: 47 g Dietary Fiber: 20 g Sugars: 9 g Total Fat: 8 g Saturated Fat: 2 g Cholesterol: 54 mg Calcium: 98 mg Sodium: 257 mg

Seafood Stew

SERVES 4

THIS STEW, WHICH IS loaded with sustainable healthful seafood, is easy enough for an everyday meal and impressive enough for a special occasion.

Vegetable oil cooking spray

1 onion, chopped

2 potatoes, peeled and cut into 1-inch chunks

2 stalks celery, chopped

2 cups chopped fresh tomatoes, or canned no-salt-added tomatoes

2 carrots, peeled and sliced

2 cups dry white wine

2 cups water

1 tablespoon chopped fresh thyme, or 1/2 teaspoon dried

1/3 pound bay scallops

1/3 pound shrimp, peeled and deveined

1/3 pound black or regular cod, cut into 1-inch chunks

1/8 teaspoon salt

Black pepper to taste

1. Heat a large heavy-bottomed stockpot over medium heat. Coat the bottom of the hot pot with cooking spray and add the onion, potatoes, and celery. Cook for 5 minutes, stirring frequently.

2. Add the tomatoes, carrots, wine, water, and thyme and bring to a boil. Reduce the heat to low and simmer for 10 minutes.

3. Add the scallops, shrimp, and cod and return to a simmer. Turn off the heat and add the salt and pepper. Serve immediately.

PREP TIME: 10 minutes   **TOTAL TIME:** 30 minutes

PER SERVING, ABOUT: Calories: 301 Protein:24 g Carbohydrate: 29 g Dietary Fiber: 4 g Sugars: 6 g Total Fat: 3 g Saturated Fat: 0 g Cholesterol: 85 mg Calcium: 83 mg Sodium: 265 mg

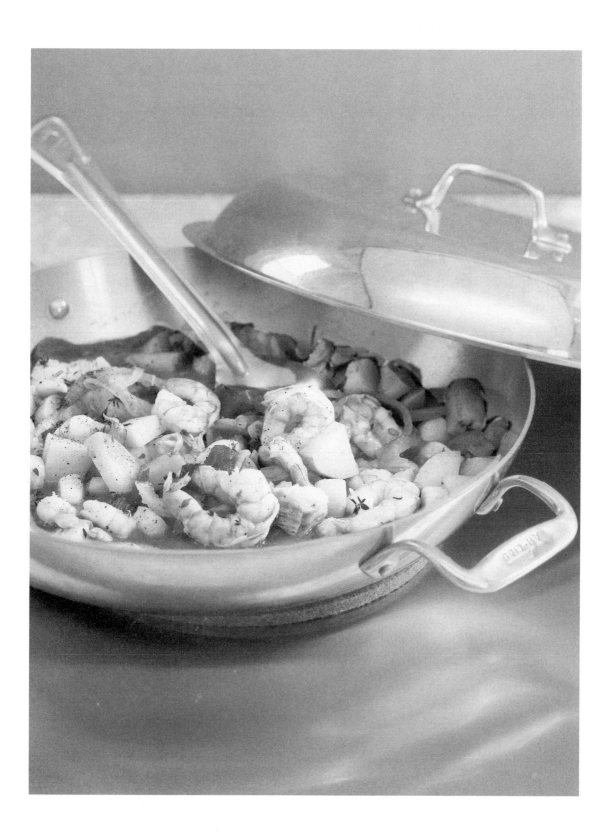

Salads

SIDE SALADS

Tomato, Cucumber, and Mint Salad

SERVES 4

NOTHING BEATS THIS SALAD on a hot summer day. The deep, sweet flavor of the tomatoes is shown off by herbs, red onion, and lime juice, while the cucumbers add great crunch.

4 tomatoes, chopped	2 tablespoons finely chopped red onion
2 cucumbers, peeled and chopped	1 tablespoon olive oil
1 cup chopped fresh mint	$\frac{1}{8}$ teaspoon salt
1 cup chopped fresh parsley	Black pepper to taste
Juice of 2 limes	

Combine all the ingredients in a large bowl. Toss gently and serve.

PREP TIME: 15 minutes　**TOTAL TIME:** 15 minutes

PER SERVING, ABOUT: Calories: 83 Protein: 3 g Carbohydrate: 12 g Dietary Fiber: 3 g
Sugars: 5 g Total Fat: 4 g Saturated Fat: 1 g Cholesterol: 0 mg Calcium: 68 mg Sodium: 165 mg

Sweet and Spicy Cabbage Salad

SERVES 4

RAW CABBAGE IS A great source of vitamin C and, like other cruciferous vegetables, contains potent cancer-fighting phytonutrients. Feel free to adjust the spice to your tastes.

3 cups shredded cabbage

2 oranges, peeled and sectioned (see page 346)

1 tablespoon sesame oil

½ teaspoon cayenne or fresh hot peppers to taste

¼ teaspoon salt

Black pepper to taste

Toss all the ingredients together in a large bowl. Let sit at room temperature for at least 5 minutes or in the refrigerator for up to 24 hours before serving.

PREP TIME: 10 minutes   **TOTAL TIME:** 10 minutes

PER SERVING, ABOUT: Calories: 74 Protein: 1 g Carbohydrate: 11 g Dietary Fiber: 3 g
Sugars: 8 g Total Fat: 4 g Saturated Fat: 1 g Cholesterol: 0 mg Calcium: 47 mg Sodium: 82 mg

Greens with Grapes

SERVES 4

THE CONTRAST OF THE sweetness of the grapes and balsamic vinegar with the bitterness of the greens makes a memorable salad.

1 cup seedless red grapes, cut in half

3 cups bitter greens, such as radicchio, escarole, frisée, watercress, or dandelion greens, or a mix of these, well washed

1 tablespoon chopped red onion

2 tablespoons balsamic vinegar

1 tablespoon olive oil

⅛ teaspoon salt

Black pepper to taste

Place the grapes, greens, and onion in a large bowl. Dress with the vinegar, oil, salt, and pepper. Toss gently and serve.

PREP TIME: 5 minutes   **TOTAL TIME:** 5 minutes

PER SERVING, ABOUT: Calories: 73 Protein: 1 g Carbohydrate: 10 g Dietary Fiber: 1 g
Sugars: 8 g Total Fat: 4 g Saturated Fat: 1 g Cholesterol: 0 mg Calcium: 13 mg Sodium: 82 mg

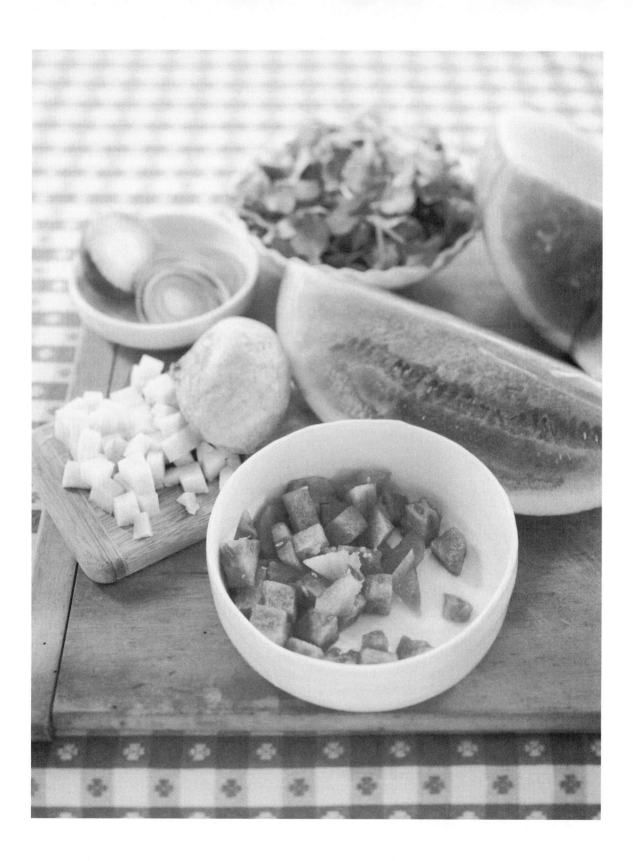

Watermelon with Jicama and Arugula

SERVES 4

SPICY ARUGULA IS WELL matched with sweet watermelon and crunchy jicama in this unique salad.

4 cups arugula

1 cup diced jicama

1 cup diced watermelon

1 tablespoon minced red onion

⅛ teaspoon salt

Black pepper to taste

24 sprays Wish-Bone Balsamic Breeze Spritzer

1. Combine the arugula, jicama, watermelon, red onion, salt, and pepper in a large bowl.

2. Spray with dressing, toss gently, and serve.

PREP TIME: 10 minutes   **TOTAL TIME:** 10 minutes

PER SERVING, ABOUT: Calories: 39 Protein: 1 g Carbohydrate: 7 g Dietary Fiber: 2 g Sugars: 3 g Total Fat: 0 g Saturated Fat: 0 g Cholesterol: 0 mg Calcium: 39 mg Sodium: 131 mg

Fennel Salad with Creamy Avocado

SERVES 4

THE CREAMINESS OF THE avocado is a great contrast to the crispy fennel.

1 avocado, skin and pit removed

1 tablespoon diced onion

2 tablespoons lemon juice

1 tablespoon olive oil

⅛ teaspoon salt

Black pepper to taste

2 cups very thinly sliced fennel

Combine the avocado, onion, lemon juice, oil, salt, and pepper in a food processor until smooth, about 1 minute. Toss the avocado dressing with the fennel and serve.

PREP TIME: 5 minutes   **TOTAL TIME:** 5 minutes

PER SERVING, ABOUT: Calories: 122 Protein: 2 g Carbohydrate: 9 g Dietary Fiber: 5 g Sugars: 1 g Total Fat: 10 g Saturated Fat: 1 g Cholesterol: 0 mg Calcium: 38 mg Sodium: 110 mg

Cucumber and Honeydew Salad

SERVES 4

THIS JUICY SALAD MAKES a great start to a meal; eating low-calorie, water-rich foods like this dish as your first course has been shown to reduce the number of calories you consume at a meal. This salad tastes best if the cucumber and honeydew pieces are approximately the same size so you get the sweetness of the honeydew and the crunch of the cucumber in the same bite.

2 cups peeled, sliced, and cubed
　 cucumber

2 cups cubed honeydew

2 tablespoons finely chopped red onion

3 tablespoons red wine vinegar

1 tablespoon olive oil

⅛ teaspoon salt

Black pepper to taste

Toss all the ingredients together and serve or keep in the refrigerator for up to 4 hours before serving.

PREP TIME: 10 minutes　**TOTAL TIME:** 10 minutes

PER SERVING, ABOUT: Calories: 74 Protein: 1 g Carbohydrate: 11 g Dietary Fiber: 1 g
Sugars: 8 g Total Fat: 4 g Saturated Fat: 1 g Cholesterol: 0 mg Calcium: 18 mg Sodium: 90 mg

Peach and Grilled Onion Salad

SERVES 4

THE COMBINATION OF SWEET fruit and cooked onion turns everyday salad greens into an exciting dish. Try this in summer when peaches are at their best. You could also substitute ripe pears for the peaches when peaches are not available.

Vegetable oil cooking spray

1 onion, sliced

2 peaches, sliced

2 tablespoons sherry vinegar

1 tablespoon olive oil

4 cups hearty lettuce, such as frisée, escarole, or romaine, well washed

⅛ teaspoon salt

Black pepper to taste

1. Heat a heavy-bottomed skillet over medium heat and coat with cooking spray. Add the onion and cook until browned, about 5 minutes.

2. Turn off the heat and add the peaches, vinegar, and oil. Stir gently to combine.

3. Put the greens in a large bowl and dress with the warm peaches and onion. Season with salt and pepper and serve.

PREP TIME: 5 minutes   **TOTAL TIME:** 12 minutes

PER SERVING, ABOUT: Calories: 70 Protein: 1 g Carbohydrate: 9 g Dietary Fiber: 2 g
Sugars: 5 g Total Fat: 4 g Saturated Fat: 1 g Cholesterol: 0 mg Calcium: 27 mg Sodium: 81 mg

Grape and Avocado Salad

SERVES 4

THIS SWEET AND SAVORY salad will make you think of grapes in a new way. It's good any time of year especially in the fall and early winter when California grapes are available and delicious.

1 cup seedless green grapes, halved

1 avocado, skin and pit removed, flesh diced

1 cup celery, sliced

1 cup chopped fresh Italian parsley

2 tablespoons cider vinegar

1 tablespoon olive oil

$1/8$ teaspoon salt

Black pepper to taste

1. Combine the grapes, avocado, celery, and parsley in a medium bowl.

2. Dress with the vinegar, oil, salt, and pepper and serve.

PREP TIME: 5 minutes   TOTAL TIME: 5 minutes

PER SERVING, ABOUT: Calories: 113 Protein: 1 g Carbohydrate: 9 g Dietary Fiber: 4 g Sugars: 5 g Total Fat: 9 g Saturated Fat: 1 g Cholesterol: 0 mg Calcium: 41 mg Sodium: 109 mg

---

GREAT GRAPES

You may have noticed that grapes are frequently used in the recipes and meal plans and, sometimes, in very unique or interesting ways. I'm a big grape fan, and that's why I have partnered with the California Table Grape commission (they represent the American-grown grapes that appear in your supermarket from May through December). Grapes have the same compound—resveratrol, a phytonutrient that promotes heart health and fights cancer—that has made red wine so famous. Of course, it's best to get resveratrol from whole fruit, and make wine an occasional treat. Also, the whole fruit is much more satisfying and lower in calories than either wine or grape juice.

Papaya and Avocado Salad

SERVES 4

PAPAYA, LOADED WITH VITAMIN C and sprinkled with B vitamins, is a great option in the winter when fresh fruit is often limited to apples and pears. This salad is good with any variety of ripe papaya available, especially the Caribbean large red papaya, which is absolutely delicious. You can also substitute mango for papaya.

2 cups cubed papaya

1 avocado, skin and pit removed, flesh cut into cubes

1 cup sliced celery

1 tablespoon fresh lime juice

1 tablespoon sesame oil

¼ teaspoon minced ginger

⅛ teaspoon salt

Combine all the ingredients in a medium bowl. Let sit at room temperature for at least 10 minutes before serving, or make in advance and store tightly covered in the refrigerator for up to an hour.

PREP TIME: 5 minutes **TOTAL TIME:** 15 minutes

PER SERVING, ABOUT: Calories: 132 Protein: 1 g Carbohydrate: 12 g Dietary Fiber: 5 g Sugars: 5 g Total Fat: 10 g Saturated Fat: 1 g Cholesterol: 0 mg Calcium: 33 mg Sodium: 98 mg

MAIN DISH SALADS

Scallops with Jicama and Oranges

SERVES 4

THIS FRESH-TASTING DISH IS perfect for either lunch or dinner.

2 cups peeled and cubed jicama

2 oranges, peeled and sectioned (see page 346)

¼ teaspoon salt (⅛ for salad, ⅛ for scallops)

Juice of 1 lime

½ cup cilantro

Vegetable oil cooking spray

1 pound (12 to 16) sea scallops, each sliced in half horizontally

Black pepper to taste

1. Heat a large heavy-bottomed skillet over medium heat.

2. Combine the jicama, oranges, ⅛ teaspoon salt, lime juice, and cilantro in a large bowl.

3. Spray the skillet with cooking spray and place the scallops in the pan. As soon as you put in the last scallop, flip the first scallop (if you would prefer to work slowly, cook half of the scallops at a time). As soon as you flip the last scallop, remove the first scallop to a clean plate. The scallops should be cooked only 30 seconds on each side. Season the scallops with ⅛ teaspoon salt and pepper.

4. Add the scallops to the jicama mixture, toss, and serve.

    PREP TIME: 18 minutes   TOTAL TIME: 20 minutes

PER SERVING, ABOUT: Calories: 160 Protein: 20 g Carbohydrate: 17 g Dietary Fiber: 5 g Sugars: 7 g Total Fat: 1 g Saturated Fat: 0 g Cholesterol: 37 mg Calcium: 67 mg Sodium: 334 mg

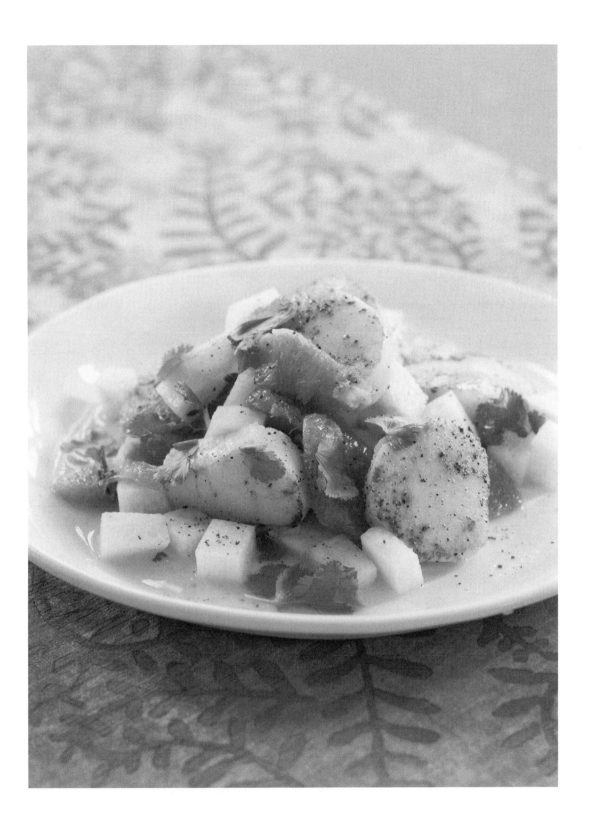

Shrimp, Avocado, and Sesame Seed Salad

SERVES 4

YOU'LL LOVE THIS SIMPLE shrimp salad: quick and easy enough for a meal on the fly but elegant enough to serve for a special occasion.

1 pound shrimp, cooked and shelled

4 cups very thinly sliced cabbage

1 avocado, skin and pit removed, flesh sliced

2 tablespoons sesame seeds

1 tablespoon sesame oil

1 tablespoon rice wine vinegar

1 tablespoon pickled ginger, very thinly sliced (available at some grocery stores and most Asian markets), optional

¼ teaspoon salt

Black pepper to taste

Combine all the ingredients in a large bowl. Let sit for 5 minutes at room temperature or up to 1 hour refrigerated before serving.

PREP TIME: 10 minutes   TOTAL TIME: 10 minutes

PER SERVING, ABOUT: Calories: 266 Protein: 26 g Carbohydrate: 10 g Dietary Fiber: 5 g Sugars: 3 g Total Fat: 14 g Saturated Fat: 2 g Cholesterol: 172 mg Calcium: 99 mg Sodium: 331 mg

Tuna Cake Salad

SERVES 4

TINY TUNA CAKES SERVED with greens is a fresh spin on tuna salad. Canned light tuna, which is high in protein and omega-3 fatty acids, has very low levels of mercury compared to other varieties of tuna.

Vegetable oil cooking spray

12 ounces chunk light tuna in water, such as StarKist, drained

2 tablespoons finely chopped onion

2 crispbreads, such as Wasa (any variety with the Best Life seal), crushed

1/2 cup Better'n Eggs, or 2 whole eggs

4 cups salad greens

25 sprays Wish-Bone Balsamic Breeze Salad Spritzer, or 2 teaspoons olive oil, 1 tablespoon balsamic vinegar, and 1/4 teaspoon salt

Black pepper to taste

1. Heat a heavy-bottomed skillet over medium heat and coat with cooking spray.

2. Mix together the tuna, onion, crispbreads, and eggs in a medium bowl. Form into 16 small cakes, each approximately 1 inch in diameter.

3. Cook the cakes in the skillet until browned, about 3 minutes per side.

4. Place the greens in a large bowl and toss with the dressing and pepper. Divide the greens among 4 plates, top each with 4 tuna cakes, and serve.

PREP TIME: 14 minutes   TOTAL TIME: 20 minutes

PER SERVING, ABOUT (analyzed using Better'n Eggs and Wish-Bone Spritzer):
Calories: 163 Protein: 25 g Carbohydrate: 8 g Dietary Fiber: 3 g Sugars: 1 g Total Fat: 3 g Saturated Fat: 1 g Cholesterol: 36 mg Calcium: 112 mg Sodium: 242 mg

Trout with Cabbage and Black-Eyed Peas

SERVES 4

CRUNCHY CABBAGE, RICH-TASTING BLACK-EYED PEAS and a mustard dressing with a hint of sweetness make this a standout salad.

4 tablespoons mustard (with no more than 60 mg sodium per teaspoon)

2 tablespoons cider vinegar

2 tablespoons olive oil

1 tablespoon honey

⅛ teaspoon salt

Black pepper to taste

1 cup raw shredded beets

4 cups shredded cabbage

¼ cup chopped red onion

2 cups canned no-salt-added black-eyed peas, drained and rinsed, or cooked (see page 345)

Vegetable oil cooking spray

1 pound trout, skin removed and cut into 4 portions, about 4 ounces each

1. Heat a heavy-bottomed skillet over medium heat.

2. Combine the mustard, vinegar, oil, honey, salt, and pepper in a small bowl.

3. Combine the beets, cabbage, red onions, and black-eyed peas in a large bowl. Toss with the mustard sauce.

4. Coat the skillet with cooking spray. Cook the trout for 2 minutes. Flip and cook for an additional 2 minutes.

5. Divide the cabbage mixture among 4 plates, top each with a piece of trout, and serve.

PREP TIME: 10 minutes   **TOTAL TIME:** 15 minutes

PER SERVING, ABOUT: Calories: 390 Protein: 32 g Carbohydrate: 35 g Dietary Fiber: 9 g Sugars: 13 g Total Fat: 14 g Saturated Fat: 3 g Cholesterol: 67 mg Calcium: 141 mg Sodium: 309 mg

Rotisserie Chicken Salad with Oranges and Pistachios

SERVES 4

TIRED OF HAVING ROTISSERIE chicken with the standard sides? Try this fuss-free recipe, which is both flavorful and unique.

2 ½ pounds rotisserie chicken, skin removed, meat peeled from bone and roughly chopped (yields 3 to 3½ cups chopped chicken meat)

2 oranges, peeled and sectioned (see page 346)

1 tablespoon finely chopped red onion

1 tablespoon olive oil

1 tablespoon sherry vinegar

⅛ teaspoon salt

Black pepper to taste

4 cups romaine, chopped

¼ cup pistachios, toasted and roughly chopped (see page 346)

1. Combine the chicken, oranges, red onion, oil, vinegar, salt, and pepper in a large bowl. Set aside for 5 to 10 minutes.

2. Add the greens and pistachios and toss gently.

3. Divide among 4 plates and serve.

PREP TIME: 15 minutes   TOTAL TIME: 15 minutes

PER SERVING, ABOUT: Calories: 315 Protein: 36 g Carbohydrate: 12 g Dietary Fiber: 3 g Sugars: 7 g Total Fat: 14 g Saturated Fat: 3 g Cholesterol: 101 mg Calcium: 67 mg Sodium: 433 mg

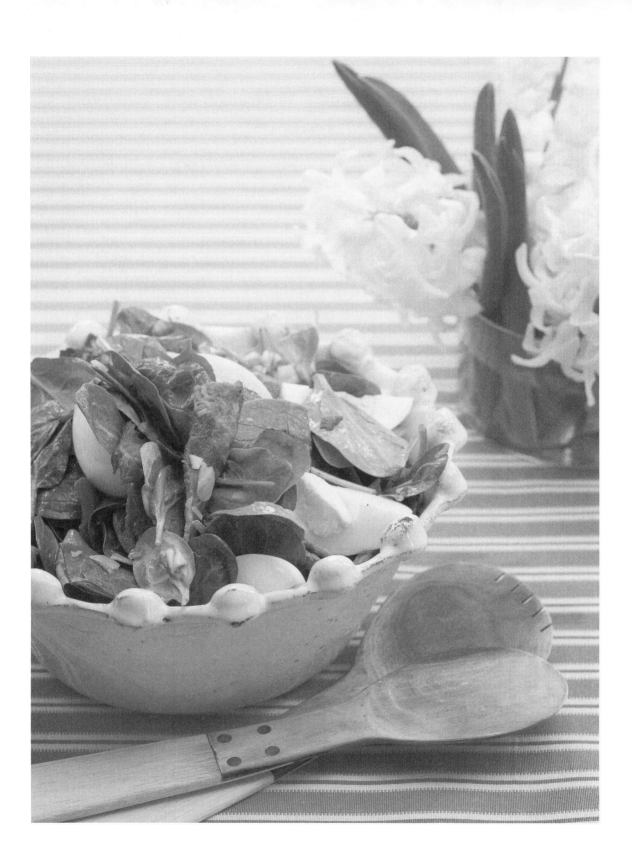

Spinach Salad with Turkey Bacon

SERVES 4

THIS RECIPE IS A lighter version of the traditional favorite.

4 cups spinach, well washed

8 hard-boiled eggs, chopped

6 slices turkey bacon, cut in half lengthwise and then across into ½-inch slices

1 tablespoon diced red onion

1 tablespoon red wine vinegar

1½ teaspoons olive oil

30 sprays Wish-Bone Red Wine Mist Vinaigrette, or 2 tablespoons olive oil and 1 tablespoon red wine vinegar

Black pepper to taste

1. Heat a heavy-bottomed skillet over medium heat.

2. Combine the spinach and hard-boiled eggs in a large bowl.

3. Cook the bacon in the skillet for 5 minutes, stirring regularly. Add the red onion, vinegar, and oil. Cook for 1 minute.

4. Add the bacon-onion mixture, either warm or at room temperature, dressing, and pepper to the spinach. Gently toss and serve.

PREP TIME: 5 minutes   **TOTAL TIME:** 20 minutes

PER SERVING, ABOUT: Calories: 236 Protein: 17 g Carbohydrate: 3 g Dietary Fiber: 1 g Sugars: 1 g Total Fat: 17 g Saturated Fat: 5 g Cholesterol: 436 mg Calcium: 82 mg Sodium: 515 mg

Duck Salad

SERVES 4

ENJOY THE CLASSIC COMBINATION of duck and oranges in this simple, elegant salad.

12 ounces duck breast, skin removed
(Note: if buying breasts with skin,
the skin weighs almost as much as
the meat)

Vegetable oil cooking spray

1 cup shredded carrot

1 cup chopped celery

2 oranges, peeled and sectioned (see
page 346)

2 tablespoons roughly chopped almonds

4 cups mixed greens

2 tablespoons orange juice

2 tablespoons rice wine vinegar

1 tablespoon sesame oil

¼ teaspoon salt

Black pepper to taste

1. Heat a heavy-bottomed skillet over medium heat. Coat the duck with cooking spray. Place in the skillet and cook for 3 minutes. Flip and cook for an additional 3 minutes. Remove from the skillet and let rest for at least 5 minutes.

2. Combine the carrot, celery, oranges, almonds, and greens in a large bowl.

3. Combine the orange juice, vinegar, oil, salt, and pepper in a small bowl.

4. Slice the duck against the grain and add to the salad mixture. Lightly toss with the dressing and serve immediately.

PREP TIME: 10 minutes   TOTAL TIME: 25 minutes

PER SERVING, ABOUT: Calories: 221 Protein: 20 g Carbohydrate: 15 g Dietary Fiber: 4 g
Sugars: 9 g Total Fat: 10 g Saturated Fat: 2 g Cholesterol: 66 mg Calcium: 87 mg Sodium: 250 mg

Steak and Kohlrabi Salad

SERVES 4

KOHLRABI, A MEMBER OF the cabbage family, is not only delicious but it's also full of vitamin C and potassium. If you can't find kohlrabi, you can use green cabbage.

MARINADE

2 tablespoons rice wine vinegar

1 tablespoon sesame oil

1 teaspoon minced fresh ginger

2 teaspoons minced fresh garlic

STEAK

1 pound flank steak, pierced repeatedly with a fork and sliced against the grain into ¼-inch slices

Vegetable oil cooking spray

1 onion, sliced

¼ teaspoon salt (⅛ for meat after cooking, ⅛ for kohlrabi mixture)

3 cups peeled and shredded kohlrabi

4 teaspoons rice wine vinegar (with no more than 250 mg sodium per tablespoon)

2 teaspoons sesame oil

Black pepper to taste

6 cups salad greens

1. Mix the marinade ingredients together in a medium bowl. Pour the marinade onto a large plate and place the steak in the marinade. If the steak is not completely covered with marinade, turn it after 10 minutes and let sit for another 5 minutes.

2. Heat a large skillet over medium heat. Coat the skillet with cooking spray. Cook the onion until translucent, about 3 minutes.

4. Remove the steak from the marinade and add to the skillet. Cook until just browned, about 3 minutes, stirring often. Remove from the heat and season with ⅛ teaspoon salt.

5. Combine the kohlrabi, vinegar, oil, remaining ⅛ teaspoon salt, and pepper in a large bowl.

6. Add the steak to the kohlrabi mixture.

7. Just before serving, add the greens, toss lightly, and serve immediately.

PREP TIME: 20 minutes   **TOTAL TIME:** 30 minutes

PER SERVING, ABOUT: Calories: 264 Protein: 28 g Carbohydrate: 17 g Dietary Fiber: 6 g
Sugars: 8 g Total Fat: 10 g Saturated Fat: 3 g Cholesterol: 48 mg Calcium: 118 mg Sodium: 338 mg

Summer Steak Salad

SERVES 4

THIS RECIPE PAIRS TENDER steak with a tangy salad made of crisp and flavorful summer vegetables. Once you try this dish, it just might become your meal of choice for a picnic or barbecue.

2 tomatoes, chopped	⅛ teaspoon salt
½ cucumber, thinly sliced	Black pepper to taste
4 radishes, sliced	12 ounces skirt steak
2 tablespoons diced red onion	Vegetable oil cooking spray
4 tablespoons sherry vinegar	4 cups spinach, well washed
2 tablespoons olive oil	

1. Combine the tomatoes, cucumber, radishes, red onion, vinegar, oil, salt, and pepper in a medium bowl. Let sit at room temperature for up to an hour or in the refrigerator for up to 12 hours, or use immediately.

2. Heat a large heavy-bottomed skillet over medium heat. Coat the steak with cooking spray. Cook the steak in the skillet until browned, about 2 minutes. Turn the steak and cook for an additional 2 minutes.

3. Remove the steak from the pan and let rest for at least 5 minutes. Slice thinly against the grain. Toss the steak and spinach with the tomato-cucumber salad and serve.

PREP TIME: 10 minutes   **TOTAL TIME:** 20 minutes

PER SERVING, ABOUT: Calories: 229 Protein: 18 g Carbohydrate: 6 g Dietary Fiber: 2 g Sugars: 3 g Total Fat: 15 g Saturated Fat: 4 g Cholesterol: 42 mg Calcium: 53 mg Sodium: 163 mg

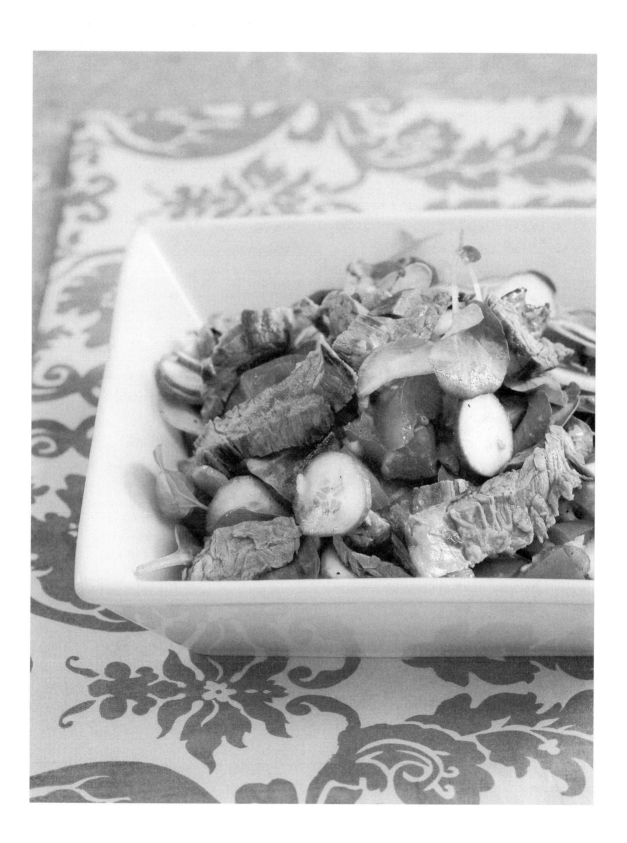

Buffalo with Chilled Roasted Greens

SERVES 4

THIS DISH IS FANTASTIC with the slight bitterness of radicchio or with the milder flavor of roasted cabbage. If you can't find buffalo, a beef skirt steak will work well.

2 heads radicchio, each cut into 8 wedges, or 1 head red cabbage, individual leaves removed

Vegetable oil cooking spray

2 tablespoons balsamic vinegar

1 tablespoon olive oil

½ cup pine nuts

½ cup dark or golden raisins

⅛ teaspoon salt

Black pepper to taste

1 pound buffalo skirt steak

1. Preheat the oven to 375°F.

2. Place the greens on a sheet pan and coat with cooking spray. Roast until the edges are browned, about 10 minutes. Remove from the oven, place in a large bowl, and toss with the vinegar, oil, pine nuts, raisins, salt, and pepper.

3. Turn the oven to broil. Place the steak in a roasting pan and broil for 3 minutes. Flip over and cook for 2 more minutes. Remove from the oven and test with a meat thermometer; if it reads 130°F, place the meat on a cutting board. If the temperature is lower, return to the oven for an additional 1 to 3 minutes before retesting the temperature.

4. Let the steak rest for 5 minutes. Slice thinly against the grain.

5. Add the steak to the greens, toss, and serve.

    PREP TIME: 5 minutes   **TOTAL TIME:** 25 minutes

PER SERVING, ABOUT: Calories: 325 Protein: 28 g Carbohydrate: 20 g Dietary Fiber: 2 g Sugars: 13 g Total Fat: 17 g Saturated Fat: 2 g Cholesterol: 0 mg Calcium: 23 mg Sodium: 132 mg

LABEL LOOKOUT! USDA ORGANIC

This seal means that at least 95 percent of the ingredients in the product have met the USDA's national organic standards, which touch on every step of the growing, processing, shipping, and handling of the product. For instance, crops with the USDA organic seal are grown without most conventional pesticides, petroleum-based fertilizers, or sewage sludge-based fertilizers (which is fertilizer from, yes, the sewage system that has been treated and is legal to use). Animals raised organically eat organic feed, get no antibiotics or growth hormones, and are housed and cared for according to strict standards. These are just a few of the many stringent regulations. The USDA licenses certifying agencies all over the world to inspect and ensure that the product meets the standards; you may also see the certifier's name on the label.

Lamb Salad with Cucumber and Yogurt

SERVES 4

YOGURT IS A HEALTHFUL replacement for sour cream or mayonnaise because it is lower in calories and rich in calcium.

1 cup fresh cilantro

1 cup fresh parsley

1 tablespoon olive oil

1/4 teaspoon turmeric

1/2 teaspoon cumin (1/4 for marinade, 1/4 for salad)

1/8 teaspoon cayenne

1/2 cup fresh lemon juice

1/4 cup rice wine vinegar

1 pound lamb loin, sliced into 1-inch cubes

1 cucumber, peeled and sliced

1/4 red onion, sliced

1/4 cup pine nuts

1/4 cup golden raisins

1 cup nonfat yogurt

1 tablespoon white vinegar

1/4 cup fresh mint, finely sliced

1/8 teaspoon salt

Black pepper to taste

4 cups romaine, chopped

1. Combine the cilantro, parsley, oil, turmeric, 1/4 teaspoon cumin, cayenne, lemon juice, and rice wine vinegar in a food processor and puree until smooth, about 1 minute.

2. Put the herb marinade mixture in a plastic bag and add the lamb. Seal the bag and mix it around to make sure that the lamb is coated with the marinade. Marinate the lamb at room temperature for 15 minutes or for up to 1 day in the refrigerator.

3. Preheat the oven to 375°F. Heat a large heavy-bottomed ovenproof skillet over medium heat. Cook the lamb in the skillet until just browned on all sides, about 2 minutes per side. Put the lamb in the oven until it is cooked to medium rare, about 5 minutes. Remove from the heat.

4. Combine the cucumber, red onion, nuts, raisins, yogurt, white vinegar, mint, 1/4 teaspoon cumin, salt, and pepper in a large bowl. Toss until evenly dressed. Add the lamb and gently toss. Serve over a bed of romaine.

PREP TIME: 25 minutes   TOTAL TIME: 35 minutes

PER SERVING, ABOUT: Calories: 351 Protein: 31 g Carbohydrate: 23 g Dietary Fiber: 3 g Sugars: 9 g Total Fat: 16 g Saturated Fat: 4 g Cholesterol: 74 mg Calcium: 208 mg Sodium: 224 mg

Taco Salad

SERVES 4

THIS SALAD IS EASY to love: the dressing is creamy and flavorful because of the reduced-fat sour cream and avocados, the black beans and Cheddar cheese add richness, and the chips provide a truly satisfying crunch.

2 avocados, skin and pits removed, flesh mashed with the back of a fork

½ cup reduced-fat sour cream

1½ teaspoons chili powder

¼ cup plus 2 tablespoons salsa, not black bean (with no more than 150 mg sodium per 2 tablespoons)

Juice of 1 large lime or juice of 1½ regular limes

6 cups chopped romaine

3 large tomatoes, chopped

1 cucumber, peeled and sliced into ¼-inch rounds

2¼ cups canned low-sodium black beans, such as Goya, drained and rinsed, or cooked (see page 345)

1½ cups baked corn chips

¼ cup plus 2 tablespoons reduced-fat shredded Cheddar

1. Combine the avocados, sour cream, chili powder, salsa, and lime juice in a medium bowl.

2. Combine the romaine, tomatoes, cucumber, black beans, corn chips, and Cheddar in a large bowl.

3. Toss the lettuce mixture gently with the avocado mixture and serve.

PREP TIME: 15 minutes   TOTAL TIME: 15 minutes

PER SERVING, ABOUT: Calories: 420 Protein: 18 g Carbohydrate: 54 g Dietary Fiber: 18 g Sugars: 8 g Total Fat: 17 g Saturated Fat: 5 g Cholesterol: 17 mg Calcium: 221 mg Sodium: 264 mg

Sandwiches, Wraps, and Crispbreads

Grilled Tofu, Lettuce, and Tomato

SERVES 4

MOVE OVER, BLT. THIS healthier version—a TLT—benefits from tofu, which is high in protein, low in fat, and cholesterol free. This remake will become a favorite of both kids and adults!

1 pound firm tofu, sliced in half
    horizontally

3 tablespoons ketchup

3 tablespoons water

¼ cup cider vinegar

1 tablespoon chili powder

1 tablespoon minced onion

1 clove garlic, crushed

1 tablespoon molasses

Black pepper to taste

Vegetable oil cooking spray

8 slices whole grain bread

4 tablespoons mayonnaise (with no more
    than 50 calories per tablespoon), such
    as Hellmann's Canola Cholesterol Free

4 leaves romaine

4 thick slices tomato

4 thick slices onion

1. Place a paper towel on a plate and put the tofu on top. Cover with another paper towel and place a heavy pot on top of the tofu. Leave the tofu pressing while preparing the other ingredients (for at least 5 minutes and up to 1 hour) to get rid of water.

2. Heat a heavy-bottomed skillet over medium heat.

3. Mix the ketchup, water, vinegar, chili powder, minced onion, garlic, molasses, and pepper in a medium bowl.

4. Remove the tofu and marinate in the ketchup mixture for at least 10 minutes or up to 12 hours. Refrigerate if marinating for more than 1 hour.

5. Coat the skillet with cooking spray and cook the tofu in a single layer until browned, about 5 minutes. Flip and cook until the other side is browned, about 5 minutes. (You may need to do this in a couple of batches, depending on the size of your pan.) Tofu can be stored in the refrigerator at this point for making sandwiches within the next 24 hours.

6. Toast the bread, spread each slice with mayonnaise, and layer on the tofu, lettuce, tomato, onion, and the second slice of toast. Serve.

PREP TIME: 20 minutes   **TOTAL TIME:** 30 minutes

PER SERVING, ABOUT: Calories: 334 Protein: 18 g Carbohydrate: 37 g Dietary Fiber: 7 g Sugars: 7 g Total Fat: 13 g Saturated Fat: 1 g Cholesterol: 0 mg Calcium: 205 mg Sodium: 559 mg

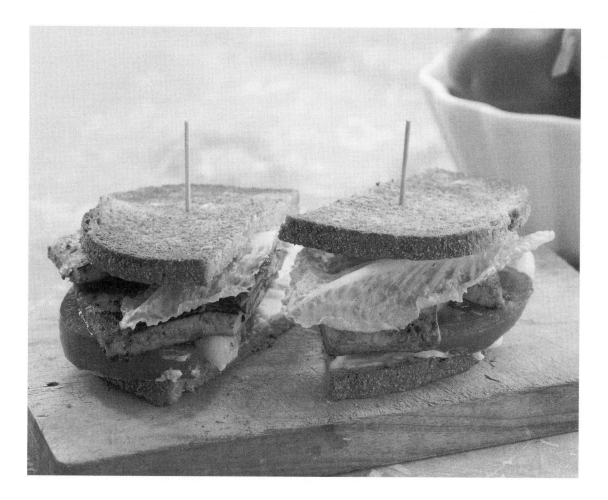

Refried Bean Wrap

SERVES 4

THIS WRAP WORKS GREAT as a meal at home or to go. It is easy to pack this burrito to be reheated or eaten at room temperature.

Vegetable oil cooking spray

1 onion, chopped

2 cups canned no-salt-added pinto beans, drained and rinsed, or cooked (see page 345)

2 tablespoons water

1 cup fresh corn, cut off the cob, or frozen, defrosted at room temperature

3 ounces reduced-fat Cheddar, shredded (about ¾ cup)

½ cup salsa, not black bean (with no more than 150 mg sodium per 2 tablespoons)

2 cups spinach, well washed

4 whole wheat tortillas

1 avocado, skin and pit removed, flesh sliced

1. Heat a heavy-bottomed skillet over medium heat.

2. Spray the hot skillet with cooking spray, add the onion, and cook, stirring often, until the onion is translucent, about 5 minutes.

3. Add the beans and water. Mash the beans with the back of a fork or a potato masher while cooking in the pan; also use a spatula to turn the beans so they cook and brown but do not stick and burn at the bottom of the pan. Cook for about 5 minutes. (If the beans seem dry add another tablespoon or two of water.) Mix in the corn, cheese, salsa, and spinach and cook for another 2 minutes.

4. To assemble, place the tortillas on individual plates, spread one-quarter of the bean mixture on each tortilla, add the avocado, roll, and serve.

PREP TIME: 10 minutes TOTAL TIME: 25 minutes

PER SERVING, ABOUT: Calories: 421 Protein: 21 g Carbohydrate: 63 g Dietary Fiber: 17 g
Sugars: 2 g Total Fat: 11 g Saturated Fat: 3 g Cholesterol: 12 mg Calcium: 276 mg Sodium: 531 mg

Portobello Sandwiches with White Beans and Roasted Garlic

SERVES 4

REPLACE DELI MEATS WITH a nutrient-packed portobello. The meaty texture of this mushroom makes it a perfect substitute for fattier ingredients.

4 portobello mushrooms

Vegetable oil cooking spray

⅛ teaspoon salt

6 cloves roasted garlic (see page 344)

1 cup canned no-salt-added white beans, drained and rinsed, or cooked (see page 345)

1 tablespoon olive oil

2 teaspoons fresh rosemary

4 whole wheat English muffins, such as Pepperidge Farm

4 leaves romaine

1. Preheat the oven to 375°F. Coat each portobello with cooking spray and place on a sheet pan. Cook for 5 minutes, flip, and cook for 5 more minutes. Remove from the oven and season with salt.

2. Combine the roasted garlic, beans, oil, and rosemary in a food processor and process for 1 minute.

3. Slice and toast the English muffins. Spread the muffin bottoms with the white bean spread, top each with 1 mushroom, 1 romaine leaf, and a muffin top. Serve.

PREP TIME: 10 minutes　**TOTAL TIME:** 20 minutes

PER SERVING, ABOUT: Calories: 260 Protein: 12 g Carbohydrate: 45 g Dietary Fiber: 12 g
Sugars: 2 g Total Fat: 6 g Saturated Fat: 1 g Cholesterol: 0 mg Calcium: 119 mg Sodium: 253 mg

Crispbread Open–Faced Sandwich with Sardines and Sweet Pepper

SERVES 2

THIS QUICK AND FLAVORFUL sandwich calls for sardines, which have stellar credentials: they're rich in omega-3s, environmentally sustainable, very low in mercury, and affordable.

½ sweet red pepper, finely chopped

1 can (3.5 ounces) sardines packed in olive oil, drained

2 teaspoons fresh lemon juice

2 tablespoons chopped parsley

2 tablespoons finely chopped red onion

4 crispbreads, such as Wasa (any variety with the Best Life seal)

In a medium bowl combine the pepper, sardines, lemon juice, parsley, and red onion until well mixed. Place the salad on crackers. Serve.

PREP TIME: 5 minutes   **TOTAL TIME:** 5 minutes

PER SERVING, ABOUT: Calories: 184 Protein: 14 g Carbohydrate: 21 g Dietary Fiber: 6 g
Sugars: 2 g Total Fat: 6 g Saturated Fat: 1 g Cholesterol: 65 mg Calcium: 197 mg Sodium: 412 mg

Crab Salad Roll

SERVES 4

IT IS HARD TO go wrong with good quality crabmeat gently seasoned with fresh ingredients.

16 ounces crabmeat, jumbo lump if possible

½ teaspoon mustard powder

⅛ teaspoon paprika

3 stalks celery, finely chopped

1½ tablespoons fresh lemon juice

2 tablespoons light mayonnaise, such as Hellmann's

Black pepper to taste

4 whole wheat 100-calorie wraps, tortillas or flatbreads, such as Multi-Grain Flatout Flatbreads

1. Gently combine the crabmeat taking care not to break up the lumps of meat, mustard powder, paprika, celery, lemon juice, mayonnaise, and pepper in a large bowl.

2. Divide the crab mixture evenly among the flatbreads and roll lengthwise, cut in half, and serve.

   PREP TIME: 5 minutes   **TOTAL TIME:** 5 minutes

PER SERVING, ABOUT: Calories: 228 Protein: 30 g Carbohydrate: 19 g Dietary Fiber: 8 g
Sugars: 2 g Total Fat: 7 g Saturated Fat: 1 g Cholesterol: 89 mg Calcium: 264 mg Sodium: 591 mg

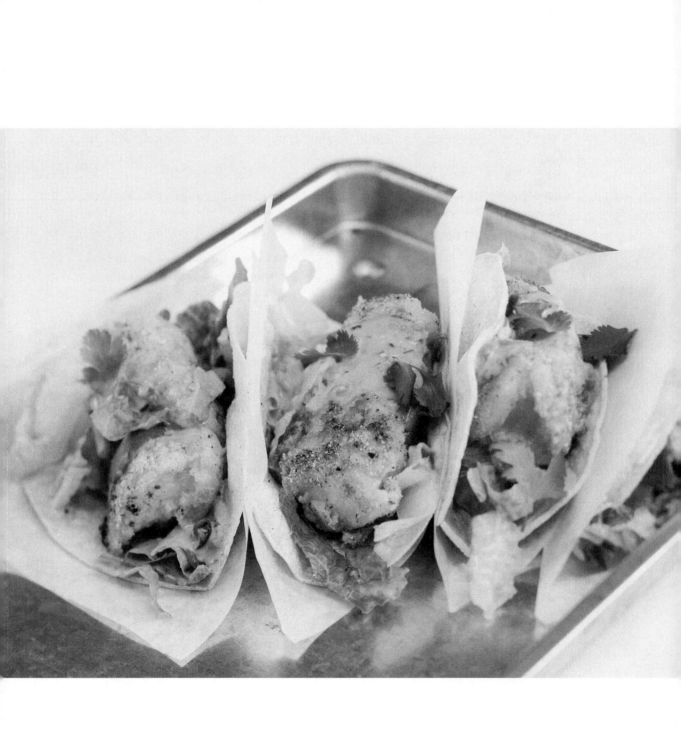

Fish Taco

SERVES 4

GET A TASTE OF Latin America with this healthful fish taco.

4 corn tortillas

½ cup salsa (with no more than 150 mg sodium per 2 tablespoons)

1 tablespoon mayonnaise (with no more than 50 calories per tablespoon), such as Hellmann's Canola Cholesterol Free

2 egg whites, or ⅓ cup AllWhites

½ cup cornmeal, preferably whole grain

1 pound cod or mahimahi fillets, cut into 4 pieces, about 4 ounces each

Vegetable oil cooking spray

1 lime

⅛ teaspoon salt

2 cups chopped romaine

2 tablespoons fresh cilantro

1. Preheat the oven to 350°F. Wrap the tortillas in foil and heat in the oven for 10 minutes.

2. Combine the salsa and mayonnaise in a small bowl and set aside.

3. Heat a large heavy-bottomed skillet over medium heat.

4. Pour the egg whites and cornmeal onto separate plates.

5. Dip each piece of fish in the eggs, then coat with the cornmeal. Place on a clean, dry plate until all the pieces of fish are coated.

6. Lightly coat the hot skillet with cooking spray and place the fish in the pan. Cook the fish on each side until browned and just done inside, 3 to 5 minutes, depending on the thickness of the fish. Remove from the pan and place on a new clean dinner plate. Squeeze lime over fish and season with salt.

7. To assemble, place the tortillas on dinner plates and spread each with 1 teaspoon of the salsa mixture. On one-half of each tortilla, layer the fish, romaine, cilantro, and drizzle the remaining salsa mixture on top. Fold the tortilla in half and serve.

PREP TIME: 5 minutes   **TOTAL TIME:** 20 minutes

PER SERVING, ABOUT: Calories: 265 Protein: 26 g Carbohydrate: 29 g Dietary Fiber: 4 g Sugars: 2 g Total Fat: 5 g Saturated Fat: 0 g Cholesterol: 49 mg Calcium: 67 mg Sodium: 340 mg

Fish Cake

SERVES 4

THIS HEARTY SANDWICH WILL appeal to all. If possible, use a Pacific cod, which is both healthful and environmentally conscious.

1 pound cod fillets

Vegetable oil cooking spray

1 heaping cup canned no-salt-added white beans, drained and rinsed, or cooked (see page 345)

4 crispbreads, such as Wasa (any variety with the Best Life seal), crushed

½ cup fresh Italian parsley

2 cloves garlic, minced

¼ cup Better'n Eggs, or 1 whole egg

⅛ teaspoon salt

4 whole wheat English muffins

2½ tablespoons mustard (preferably with no more than 50 mg sodium per teaspoon, such as Gulden's)

4 leaves romaine

1. Preheat the oven to 375°F. Coat the cod with cooking spray and place in an ovenproof pan. Bake until cooked through, about 10 minutes.

2. Combine the cod, beans, crispbreads, parsley, garlic, eggs, and salt in a food processor until just combined, about 1 minute.

3. Heat a heavy-bottomed ovenproof skillet over medium heat. Form the cod mixture into 4 cakes. Coat the skillet with cooking spray and place the cakes in the pan. Cook until brown on one side, about 5 minutes. Flip the cakes and place in the oven for 10 minutes.

4. Split the English muffins and toast.

5. To assemble, spread each muffin top with mustard. Place 1 fish cake and 1 leaf of romaine on each muffin. Cover with a muffin top and serve.

PREP TIME: 10 minutes   TOTAL TIME: 35 minutes

PER SERVING, ABOUT (analyzed using Better'n Eggs): Calories: 375 Protein: 36 g Carbohydrate: 53 g Dietary Fiber: 13 g Sugars: 0 g Total Fat: 4 g Saturated Fat: 1 g Cholesterol: 49 mg Calcium: 150 mg Sodium: 471 mg

Flank Steak and Balsamic Onion Sandwich

SERVES 4

THIS SIMPLE STEAK AND onion sandwich is a nutritious option because it calls for a lean cut of beef.

1 onion, thinly sliced

Vegetable oil cooking spray

1 tablespoon balsamic vinegar

⅛ teaspoon salt

12 ounces flank steak, pierced repeatedly with a fork before cooking

4 whole wheat sandwich buns (about 115 calories each)

4 tablespoons grainy mustard

4 leaves romaine

1. Heat two heavy-bottomed skillets over medium heat. Coat the onions with cooking spray and cook in the skillet for 5 minutes. Add the vinegar and salt and continue cooking for 5 more minutes.

2. Cut the steak horizontally to make two thin steaks that are the same diameter as the original steak. Pound with a rolling pin for 1 minute.

3. Coat the steak with cooking spray and cook for 2 minutes in the second skillet. Turn the steak and cook for an additional 2 minutes. Check to see if the meat is just slightly pink in the center by gently slicing through the middle of it with a sharp knife. If not, return to the skillet for an additional minute or two.

4. Let the meat rest on a cutting board for 5 minutes, and then slice against the grain as thinly as possible.

5. Slice each bun and spread each bun top with mustard. Divide the beef and onion into 4 equal portions and place the beef, onion, and lettuce on the bottom bun, cover with the top bun, and serve.

PREP TIME: 5 minutes   **TOTAL TIME:** 15 minutes

PER SERVING, ABOUT: Calories: 271 Protein: 22 g Carbohydrate: 25 g Dietary Fiber: 3 g Sugars: 2 g Total Fat: 9 g Saturated Fat: 3 g Cholesterol: 49 mg Calcium: 64 mg Sodium: 490 mg

Entrées

MEAT

Buffalo with Blackberries

SERVES 4

BUFFALO ISN'T AVAILABLE EVERYWHERE, but if you can get it, it's an extremely lean and healthy red meat choice. Even if it's not sold near you, you could always order it online. You can also substitute beef rib eye for the buffalo in this recipe.

2 cups fresh blackberries, or frozen, defrosted at room temperature

2 tablespoons minced red onion

2 tablespoons balsamic vinegar

1 tablespoon extra virgin olive oil

1/8 teaspoon salt

Black pepper to taste

1 pound buffalo ribeye, cut into 4 steaks, about 4 ounces each, at room temperature

Vegetable oil cooking spray

1. Combine the blackberries, onion, vinegar, oil, salt, and pepper in a medium bowl.

2. Heat a large heavy-bottomed skillet over medium heat.

3. Coat the meat with cooking spray and cook in the skillet for 3 minutes. Flip the meat and cook for an additional 3 minutes, or until the internal temperature reaches 130°F. The time will vary, depending on the thickness of the meat. Buffalo meat is extremely lean; cooking it on the rare to medium-rare side will ensure that it's most tender.

4. Place the individual steaks on plates and top with the blackberry mixture. Serve.

PREP TIME: 10 minutes   TOTAL TIME: 16 minutes

PER SERVING, ABOUT: Calories: 183 Protein: 25 g Carbohydrate: 9 g Dietary Fiber: 4 g Sugars: 5 g Total Fat: 5 g Saturated Fat: 1 g Cholesterol: 0 mg Calcium: 28 mg Sodium: 124 mg

CHOICE CUTS

You might be surprised to discover just how fat laden some of your favorite meats are. Take a 4-ounce hamburger: it weighs in with 24 g of fat (that's nearly 5 teaspoons). And 9 of those fat grams are from cholesterol-raising saturated fat—more than half your daily limit if you're eating 1,600 calories per day. If you make an easy swap, for instance, having a piece of beef tenderloin instead, you can cut your intake of fat and saturated fat by more than 65 percent.

Other cuts that can help you keep your fat intake in check include:

Beef: Flank steak; T-bone; any cut with the word loin in it, such as sirloin, top loin, or tenderloin; any cut with the word round in it, such as top round or eye of round; ground beef that's at least 90 percent lean (lean ground beef is best used in chilis or casseroles)

Buffalo: Ribeye; shoulder; top round; top sirloin

Lamb: Arm chop; leg shank; leg sirloin; leg top round; loin chop

Pork: Center loin chop; lean ham; loin rib chop; shoulder blade steak; sirloin roast; tenderloin; top loin chop; top loin roast

Veal: Blade or arm; cutlet; rib loin chop

Flank Steak with Potatoes and Garlic

SERVES 4

IN THE MOOD FOR steak and potatoes? Try this version. If you can find organic beef, all the better (see page 85).

2 cups grated potatoes

⅛ teaspoon salt

Black pepper to taste

4 cloves roasted garlic (see page 344)

2 tablespoons balsamic vinegar

1 tablespoon olive oil

Vegetable oil cooking spray

12 ounces flank steak, pierced repeatedly with a fork

1. Heat an ovenproof 9-inch heavy-bottomed skillet over medium heat. Heat another larger skillet over medium heat and preheat the oven to 375°F.

2. Combine the potatoes, salt, and pepper in a medium bowl and let sit for 5 minutes.

3. Combine the roasted garlic, vinegar, and oil in a food processor and puree until smooth, about 1 minute. Set aside.

4. Generously coat the 9-inch skillet with cooking spray. Spread the potatoes out in the skillet to cover the entire bottom of the pan. Cook until browned on one side, about 5 minutes. Flip the potatoes and bake in the oven for 10 minutes.

5. Coat the larger skillet with cooking spray. Cook the flank steak until browned on one side, about 3 minutes. Flip and cook until browned on the other side, about 3 more minutes.

6. Remove the steak from the pan and let rest for 5 minutes. Slice thinly against the grain.

7. Serve the potatoes topped with steak and garnish the steak with the garlic-balsamic sauce.

PREP TIME: 10 minutes   TOTAL TIME: 30 minutes

PER SERVING, ABOUT: Calories: 274 Protein: 22 g Carbohydrate: 26 g Dietary Fiber: 3 g Sugars: 3 g Total Fat: 9 g Saturated Fat: 3 g Cholesterol: 36 mg Calcium: 47 mg Sodium: 133 mg

Beef with Tomatoes and Olives Over Pasta

SERVES 4

BEEF MOVES OUT OF the starring role in this dish, but it still adds loads of flavor and nutrients. You'll get plenty of protein from both the meat and the Barilla PLUS pasta.

1 onion, sliced

Vegetable oil cooking spray

8 ounces beef top round, cut into ½-inch cubes

¼ cup dry white wine

½ cup water

1½ cups chopped fresh tomatoes, or canned no-salt-added diced tomatoes

⅓ cup pitted olives

2 tablespoons fresh chopped basil

¼ teaspoon salt (⅛ for beef, ⅛ for pasta)

¼ cup nonfat yogurt

7 ounces (about ½ package) Barilla PLUS rotini

1 tablespoon olive oil

1. Preheat the oven to 375°F.

2. Heat a heavy-bottomed ovenproof skillet over medium heat.

3. Spray the onion with cooking spray and cook the onion in the skillet for 5 minutes. Add the beef and cook until browned, about 10 minutes, stirring.

4. Add the wine, water, tomatoes, and olives to the skillet. Bring to a boil and cover. Put in the oven for 1 hour. Remove the skillet from the oven and stir in the basil, ⅛ teaspoon salt, and yogurt.

5. Cook the pasta according to the package directions. Toss with the oil and ⅛ teaspoon salt.

6. Mix the pasta with the beef and serve.

   PREP TIME: 10 minutes   **TOTAL TIME:** 1 hour 30 minutes

PER SERVING, ABOUT: Calories: 379 Protein: 24 g Carbohydrate: 45 g Dietary Fiber: 5 g Sugars: 9 g Total Fat: 9 g Saturated Fat: 3 g Cholesterol: 38 mg Calcium: 92 mg Sodium: 318 mg

Baked Pork Tenderloin

SERVES 4

THE MARRIAGE OF THE marinade ingredients with the lean and flavorful tenderloin makes for a memorable dish. You can serve it with any whole grain side, such as whole wheat couscous or brown rice.

4 cloves garlic, minced

1 tablespoon olive oil

2 tablespoons chili powder

2 tablespoons dark brown sugar

1 teaspoon ground cumin

1 teaspoon dried oregano

½ teaspoon cinnamon

½ teaspoon unsweetened cocoa powder, such as Hershey's Natural Cocoa

¼ teaspoon salt

1 pound pork tenderloin

1. Combine the garlic, oil, chili powder, sugar, cumin, oregano, cinnamon, cocoa, and salt in a food processor and process until it becomes a paste, about 2 minutes.

2. Rub the pork with the mixture and allow to marinate at room temperature for 1 hour or in the refrigerator for up to 24 hours.

3. Preheat the oven to 375°F.

4. Place in a baking pan and bake for 20 to 25 minutes, or until the internal temperature reaches 140°F. (The temperature will rise while it is resting.) Let rest for at least 10 minutes before slicing. Slice into ½-inch-thick slices and serve.

PREP TIME: 1 hour 10 minutes   TOTAL TIME: 1 hour 40 minutes

PER SERVING, ABOUT: Calories: 204 Protein: 25 g Carbohydrate: 8 g Dietary Fiber: 2 g Sugars: 5 g Total Fat: 8 g Saturated Fat: 2 g Cholesterol: 74 mg Calcium: 41 mg Sodium: 243 mg

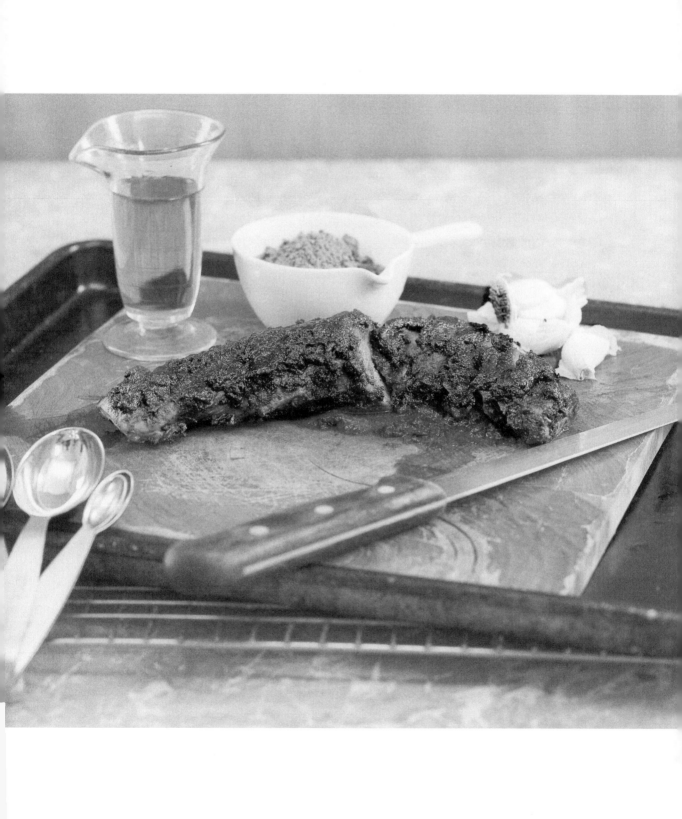

Pork Chops with Apples and Onion

SERVES 4

THE PAIRING OF PORK and apples is a classic for a good reason: the sweetness of the apples brings out the juicy, subtle flavor of the meat.

1 onion, sliced	1 teaspoon sage
Vegetable oil cooking spray	¼ teaspoon salt (⅛ for relish, ⅛ for meat)
2 apples, peeled, cored, and sliced	Black pepper to taste
1 tablespoon cider vinegar	4 pork chops, bone in, about 4 ounces each

1. Place a medium saucepan over medium heat. Coat the onion with cooking spray and cook for 5 minutes. Add the apples, vinegar, and sage. Cook for 10 minutes, stirring often. Add ⅛ teaspoon salt, and pepper.

2. Heat a heavy-bottomed skillet over medium heat. Once the pan is hot, cook the pork chops for 2 minutes if thin, 5 if thick. Turn the pork over and cook for an additional 2 to 4 minutes, depending on the thickness. The meat is done when it's still slightly pink in the middle.

3. Season the pork with ⅛ teaspoon salt and pepper. Top the pork with the apple relish and serve.

PREP TIME: 10 minutes   TOTAL TIME: 25 minutes

PER SERVING, ABOUT: Calories: 208 Protein: 25 g Carbohydrate: 13 g Dietary Fiber: 2 g Sugars: 8 g Total Fat: 6 g Saturated Fat: 2 g Cholesterol: 71 mg Calcium: 37 mg Sodium: 222 mg

Sloppy Joes

SERVES 4

THIS FAMILIAR DISH CAN be a smart choice with a few small changes that cut calories but none of the flavor or satisfaction.

Vegetable oil cooking spray

1 onion, finely chopped

1 large sweet pepper, seeded and finely chopped

12 ounces 95 percent lean ground beef

1¼ cups chopped fresh tomatoes, or canned no-salt-added tomatoes

1 cup canned no-salt-added kidney beans, drained and rinsed, or cooked, mashed with the back of a fork (page 345)

4 tablespoons tomato paste

4 tablespoons cider vinegar

⅛ teaspoon cloves

¼ teaspoon cinnamon

½ teaspoon brown sugar

¼ teaspoon salt

Black pepper to taste

4 whole wheat hamburger rolls (with about 170 calories each)

1. Heat a large skillet over medium heat and coat with cooking spray. Add the onion and sweet pepper. Cook for 3 minutes, stirring.

2. Crumble in the ground beef and cook until browned; keep breaking it apart with a spoon for about 4 minutes.

3. Stir in the tomatoes, beans, tomato paste, vinegar, cloves, cinnamon, sugar, salt, and pepper. Cook for an additional 4 minutes.

4. Divide the mixture evenly between the 4 rolls and serve.

PREP TIME: 10 minutes   **TOTAL TIME:** 25 minutes

PER SERVING, ABOUT: Calories: 415 Protein: 34 g Carbohydrate: 60 g Dietary Fiber: 14 g Sugars: 5 g Total Fat: 6 g Saturated Fat: 2 g Cholesterol: 52 mg Calcium: 72 mg Sodium: 451 mg

Cottage Pie

SERVES 4

WHO SAYS YOU CAN'T have comfort food if you're trying to eat healthfully? This dish, which uses nutritious ingredients, is truly soothing. You can enjoy the tasty ground beef filling topped with a mashed potato crust without feeling an ounce of guilt!

POTATOES

2 medium potatoes, skin on

2 teaspoons olive oil

¼ teaspoon salt

BEEF

Vegetable oil cooking spray

2 large carrots, peeled and finely chopped

1 onion, chopped

1 pound 95 percent lean ground beef

4 cups spinach, well washed

To make the potatoes:

1. Place the potatoes in a pot and cover with water. Bring to a boil and cook until the potatoes are tender, about 20 minutes.

2. Drain the potatoes well. Add the oil and salt and mash with a wooden spoon until smooth, some lumps can remain.

While the potatoes are cooking, prepare the beef mixture:

3. Preheat the oven to 375°F. Heat a heavy-bottomed skillet over medium heat.

4. Lightly coat the skillet with cooking spray. Add the carrots and onion and cook until slightly browned, about 4 minutes, stirring often.

5. Add the beef and cook until browned, about 5 minutes.

6. Turn off the heat and stir the spinach into the beef mixture.

To assemble:

7. In a 9-inch pan or 4 individual 4- or 5-inch ramekins, place the beef mixture and cover with the mashed potatoes.

8. Bake in the oven for 10 minutes if using warm ingredients. (If you assemble the pies and refrigerate, then reheat in a 375°F oven until warm throughout, about 20 minutes.)

9. After baking the pies, turn the oven to broil until the tops of the potatoes are browned, about 5 minutes. Serve.

PREP TIME: 10 minutes   **TOTAL TIME:** 45 minutes

PER SERVING, ABOUT: Calories: 282 Protein: 27 g Carbohydrate: 24 g Dietary Fiber: 5 g
Sugars: 4 g Total Fat: 8 g Saturated Fat: 3 g Cholesterol: 69 mg Calcium: 68 mg Sodium: 276 mg

LABEL LOOKOUT! CERTIFIED HUMANE

This seal certifies that the animals that produce egg, dairy, meat, or poultry products were raised in a humane manner—that is, they lived in a safe and clean environment without overcrowding, ate healthful food, received no antibiotics or hormones, were treated gently, and were slaughtered in a humane fashion. Certified Humane does not mean that the product is USDA Organic, although some standards overlap. Many products carry both seals.

CERTIFIED HUMANE RAISED & HANDLED

* Meets the Humane Farm Animal Care Program standards, which include nutritious diet without antibiotics, or hormones, animals raised with shelter, resting areas, sufficient space and the ability to engage in natural behaviors.

Baked Eggplant and Ground Beef

SERVES 4

THIS SATISFYING LAYERED BAKED dish can be made ahead of time and reheated for dinner. It is good for a group or can be frozen in airtight containers in individual portions.

4 cups thinly sliced eggplant

1 onion, thinly sliced

2 cloves roasted garlic, minced (see page 344)

Vegetable oil cooking spray

12 ounces lean (90%) ground beef

1 tablespoon fresh oregano

½ teaspoon cinnamon

½ teaspoon cumin

⅛ teaspoon salt

Black pepper to taste

1 cup Quick Tomato Sauce (page 340), or prepared sauce, such as Barilla Marinara

½ cup water

1. Preheat the oven to 375°F. Heat a large heavy-bottomed skillet over medium heat.

2. Coat the eggplant, onion, and roasted garlic with cooking spray. Place on a sheet pan and cook in the oven for 15 minutes.

3. Coat the hot skillet with cooking spray. Cook the beef in the skillet, stirring often, until browned, about 5 minutes. Stir in the oregano, cinnamon, cumin, salt, and pepper.

4. Coat a square 9-inch pan with cooking spray. Pour in ½ cup tomato sauce and top with ½ eggplant mixture, ½ beef mixture, the remaining ½ eggplant mixture, and the beef mixture. Pour in the remaining ½ cup tomato sauce. Pour water around the edges of the pan.

5. Cook in the oven for 40 minutes and serve.

PREP TIME: 20 minutes   TOTAL TIME: 1 hour, 15 minutes

PER SERVING, ABOUT: Calories: 296 Protein: 20 g Carbohydrate: 25 g Dietary Fiber: 7 g Sugars: 13 g Total Fat: 14 g Saturated Fat: 4 g Cholesterol: 55 mg Calcium: 71 mg Sodium: 308 mg

Lamb Chops with Balsamic Roasted Garlic Puree

SERVES 4

THE FLAVORS OF LEMON, roasted garlic, and balsamic vinegar enhance the succulent lamb chops. To ensure that the meat is tender, cook to medium rare. This dish is easy enough to prepare for a weeknight dinner but special enough for a big event or party.

4 cloves roasted garlic (see page 344)

Zest and juice of 1 lemon

1 tablespoon balsamic vinegar

1 large onion, sliced

2 cloves garlic, finely chopped

1 tablespoon olive oil

4 lamb chops, 5 ounces each including bone

Vegetable oil cooking spray

1/8 teaspoon salt

1. Combine the roasted garlic, lemon zest, and vinegar in a food processor and puree until smooth, about 2 minutes. Set aside.

2. Turn the oven to broil.

3. On a plate, mix the lemon juice, onion, garlic, and oil. Place the lamb in a single layer on the plate for 5 minutes. Turn the lamb over to marinate the other side for 5 minutes.

4. Coat a sheet pan with cooking spray and place the lamb on the pan. Remove the onion and garlic from the marinade and place on top of the lamb. Broil for 2 minutes. Flip the lamb over and broil for an additional 2 minutes. The lamb should be medium-rare at this point; if you wish to cook it more, return to the broiler until done to your liking.

5. Season lamb with salt and serve each lamb chop with a spoonful of garlic puree.

PREP TIME: 15 minutes   TOTAL TIME: 20 minutes

PER SERVING, ABOUT: Calories: 183 Protein: 15 g Carbohydrate: 7 g Dietary Fiber: 1 g Sugars: 3 g Total Fat: 10 g Saturated Fat: 3 g Cholesterol: 47 mg Calcium: 28 mg Sodium: 240 mg

Rib Eye Steak with Onion Relish

SERVES 4

STEAK AND ONIONS ARE often served together and this recipe makes it easy to see why. The sweet and sour onion relish works as a condiment that makes an already delicious cut of meat taste even better.

Vegetable oil cooking spray

1 onion, sliced

1 stalk celery, chopped

½ red pepper, seeded and chopped

⅓ cup cider vinegar

2 tablespoons water

1 tablespoon brown sugar

¼ teaspoon salt (⅛ for relish, ⅛ for steak)

1 pound ribeye steak, all fat trimmed, at room temperature

Black pepper to taste

1. Heat a medium heavy-bottomed pot over medium heat.

2. Coat the pot with cooking spray. Add the onion, celery, and red pepper and cook until browned, about 7 minutes.

3. Add the vinegar, water, sugar, and ⅛ teaspoon salt and cook over medium heat for 10 minutes.

4. Heat a large heavy-bottomed skillet over medium heat.

5. Cook the steak in the skillet until browned, about 4 minutes. Flip the steak and cook the other side until browned, 3 to 4 more minutes. Test the meat with a meat thermometer and remove when 130°F for medium-rare (remember meat will continue to cook once removed from the heat) or 140°F for medium.

6. Season the steaks with the remaining ⅛ teaspoon salt and pepper. Serve with the onion relish.

PREP TIME: 15 minutes   **TOTAL TIME:** 35 minutes

PER SERVING, ABOUT: Calories: 214 Protein: 22 g Carbohydrate: 11 g Dietary Fiber: 1 g
Sugars: 8 g Total Fat: 9 g Saturated Fat: 3 g Cholesterol: 60 mg Calcium: 39 mg Sodium: 232 mg

POULTRY

Duck with Plums

SERVES 4

SWEET-TART FRESH PLUMS BALANCE the richness of duck. Cooking the duck without skin or fat gives a healthful twist to this elegant dish.

2 ripe plums, pitted and sliced as thinly as possible

1 tablespoon finely chopped red onion

2 tablespoons balsamic vinegar

1 tablespoon olive oil

⅛ teaspoon salt

Black pepper to taste

Vegetable oil cooking spray

12 ounces lean duck breast, cut into 4 pieces, about 3 ounces each, skin and fat removed (Note: The fat and skin weigh nearly as much as the lean meat, so when buying duck, you may have to buy 24 ounces of breast to get 12 ounces of lean meat.)

1. Preheat the oven to 375°F. Heat a heavy-bottomed ovenproof skillet over medium heat.

2. Combine the plums, onion, vinegar, oil, salt, and pepper in a medium bowl. Set aside.

3. Coat the skillet with cooking spray and place the duck with the side where the skin was facing down. Cook until browned, about 2 minutes.

4. Flip the duck and place the skillet in the oven. The duck will taste best if cooked to medium rare and still pink inside, about 3 minutes. Cook longer if you desire more well-done meat.

5. Serve topped with the plum mixture.

PREP TIME: 10 minutes　TOTAL TIME: 15 minutes

PER SERVING, ABOUT: Calories: 160　Protein: 17 g　Carbohydrate: 5 g　Dietary Fiber: 1 g
Sugars: 5 g　Total Fat: 7 g　Saturated Fat: 2 g　Cholesterol: 66 mg　Calcium: 7 mg　Sodium: 123 mg

Chicken with Spring Onions and Mashed Spring Vegetables

SERVES 4

THE DELICATE FLAVORS OF spring vegetables complement juicy pan roasted chicken. If possible, use organic free range chicken breasts to ensure the best flavor.

2 cups fresh or frozen peas

2 cups fresh or frozen snow peas

2 cups Italian parsley

¼ teaspoon salt (⅛ for puree, ⅛ for chicken)

Black pepper to taste

Vegetable oil cooking spray

4 large green onions (scallions), sliced in half lengthwise

1 pound skinless boneless chicken breasts, about 4 ounces each

1. Fill a medium pot three-quarters full of water and bring to a boil. Cook the peas and snow peas for 1 minute and drain.

2. Puree the peas, snow peas, parsley, ⅛ teaspoon salt, and pepper in a food processor until smooth, about 2 minutes. Set aside.

3. Heat a large heavy-bottomed ovenproof skillet over medium heat. Preheat the oven to 375°F.

4. Coat the skillet with cooking spray and place the green onions in the skillet side by side. Place each chicken breast on top of 2 green onions. Once the onions soften, wrap them around the chicken breasts.

5. Cook until the chicken is browned, about 5 minutes. Flip the chicken and cook until browned, about 4 more minutes.

6. Place the skillet in the oven and cook until the chicken is just done, about 7 minutes. The chicken is done when it is just barely pink in the middle; it will continue to cook after you remove it from the pan.

7. Divide the vegetable puree among 4 plates. Season the chicken with the remaining ⅛ teaspoon salt, place on top of the puree, and serve.

PREP TIME: 5 minutes   **TOTAL TIME:** 30 minutes

PER SERVING, ABOUT: Calories: 218 Protein: 32 g Carbohydrate: 16 g Dietary Fiber: 6 g Sugars: 5 g Total Fat: 3 g Saturated Fat: 0 g Cholesterol: 66 mg Calcium: 93 mg Sodium: 242 mg

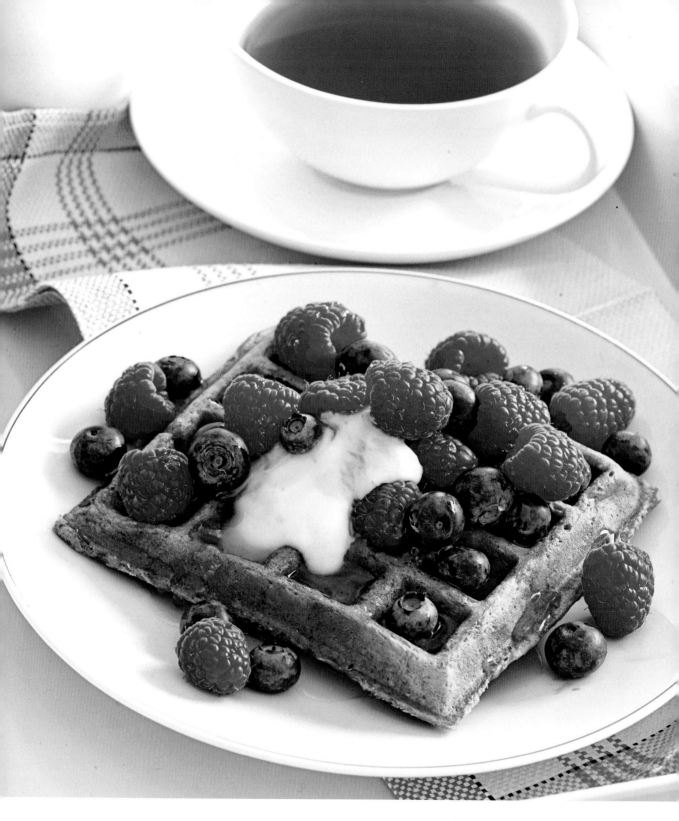

Ginger Waffles (PAGE 23)

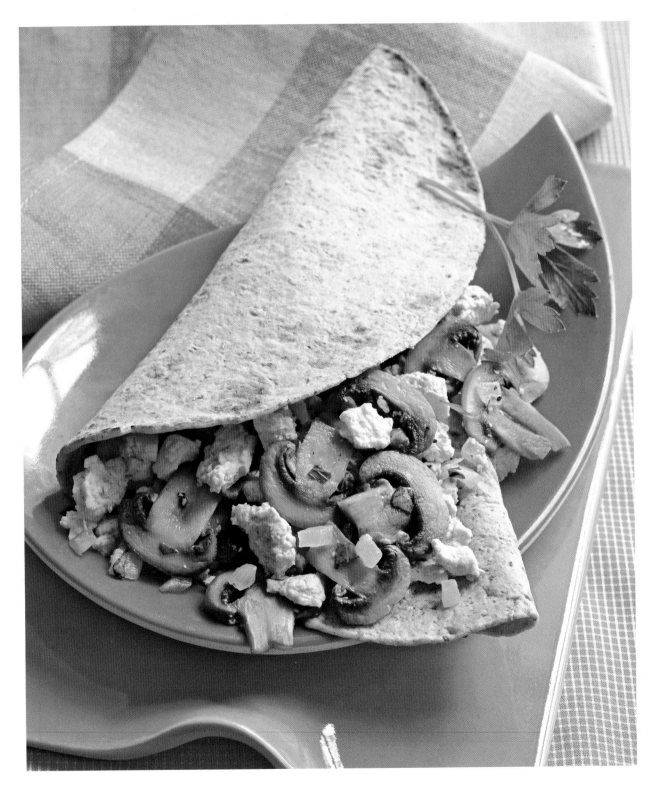

Tofu Mushroom Scramble on Whole Wheat Tortilla (PAGE 27)

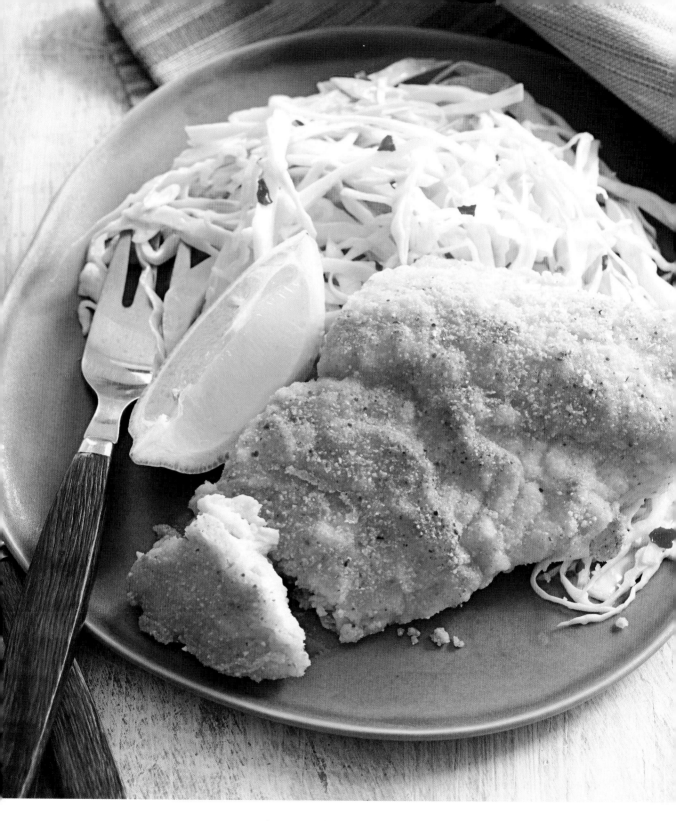

Cornmeal-Crusted Catfish with Spicy Slaw (PAGE 145)

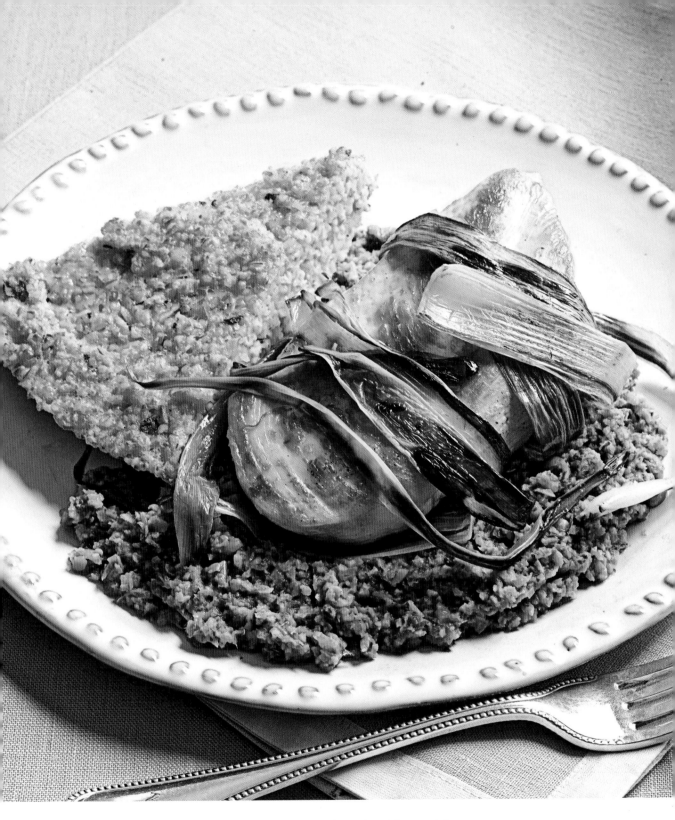

Chicken with Spring Onions and Mashed Spring Vegetables (PAGE 116)

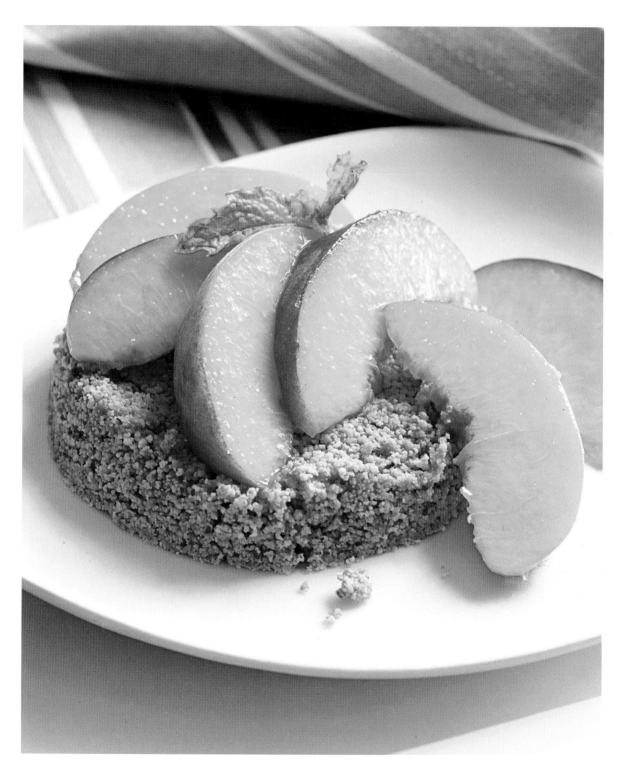

Uncooked Stone Fruit Tart (PAGE 205)

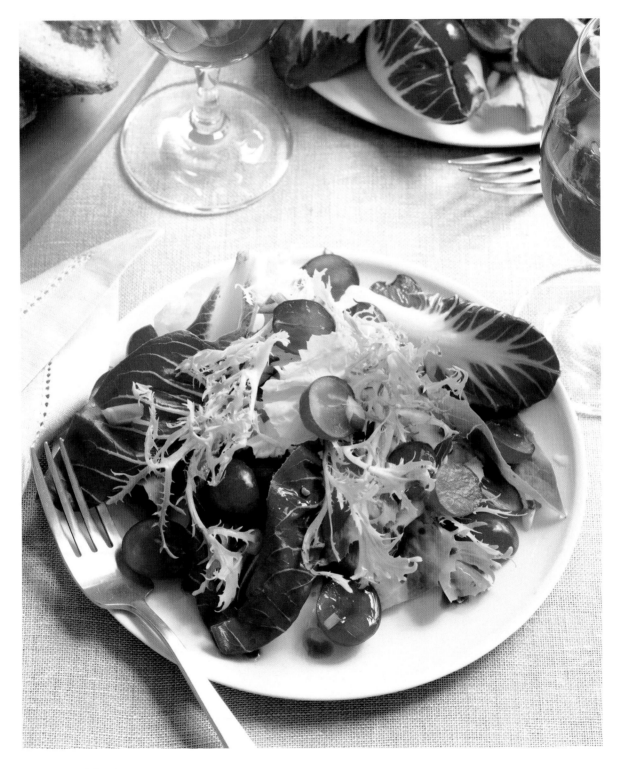

Greens with Grapes (PAGE 65)

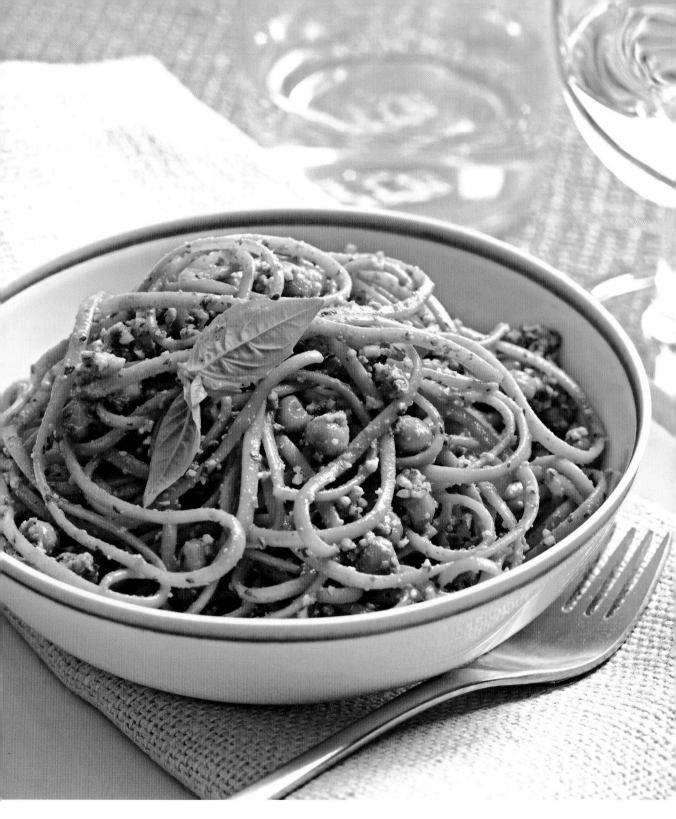

Angel Hair Pasta with Walnuts and Peas (PAGE 148)

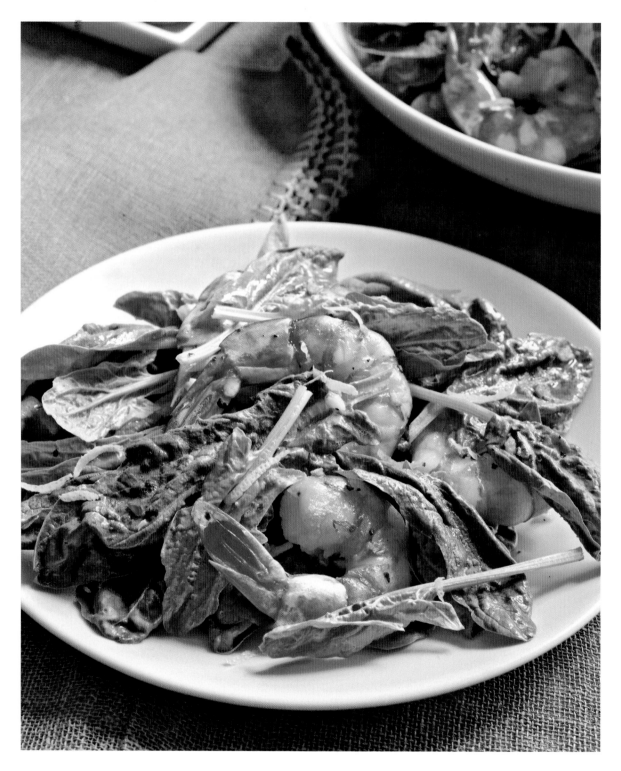

Pan-Roasted Shrimp with Lemon, Garlic, and Spinach (PAGE 135)

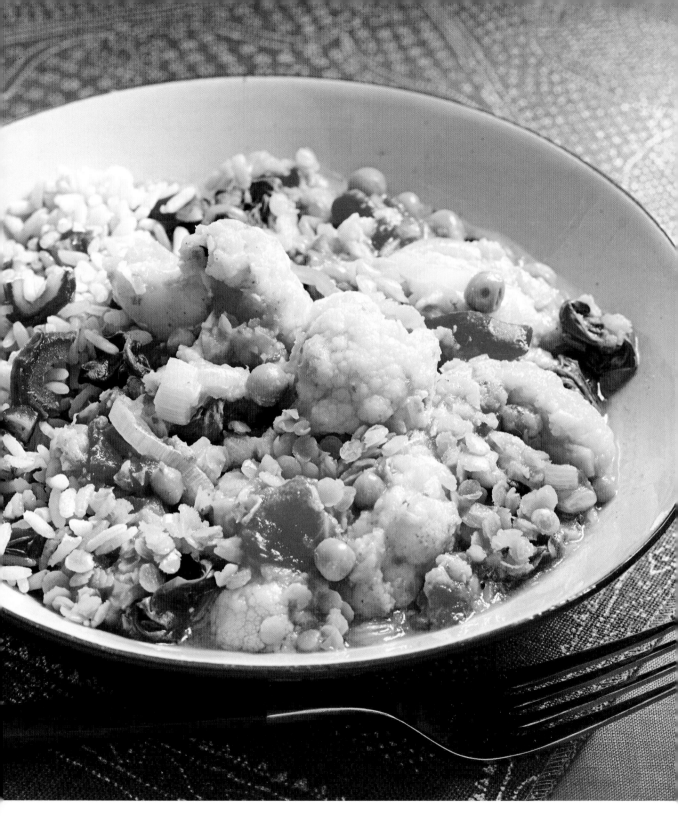

Cauliflower Curry with Red Lentils (PAGE 155)

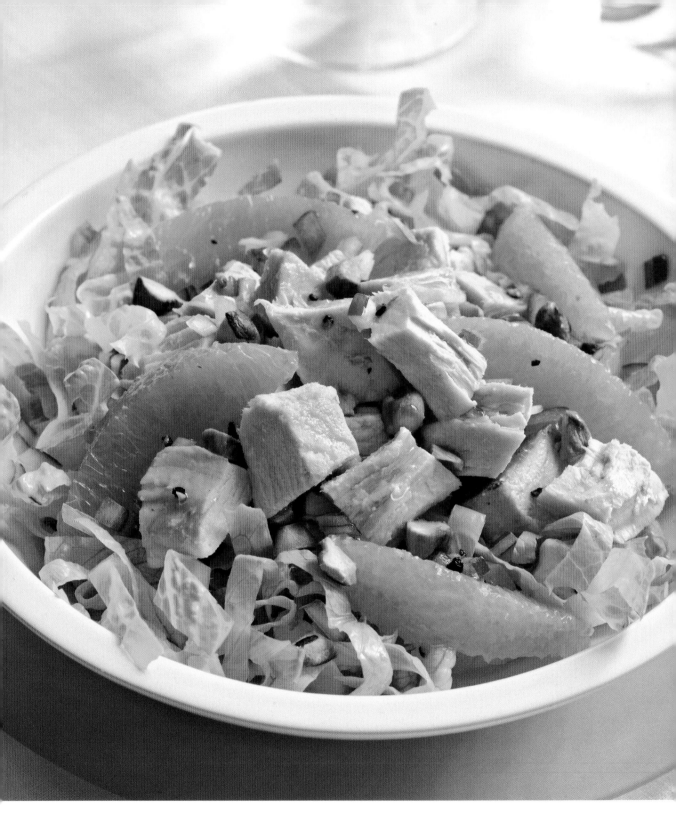

Rotisserie Chicken Salad with Oranges and Pistachios (PAGE 77)

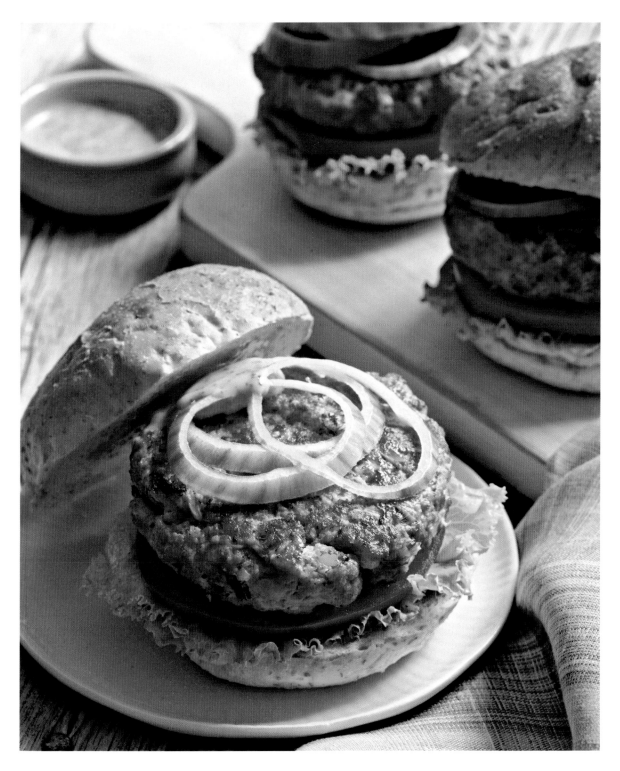

Turkey Burger (PAGE 128)

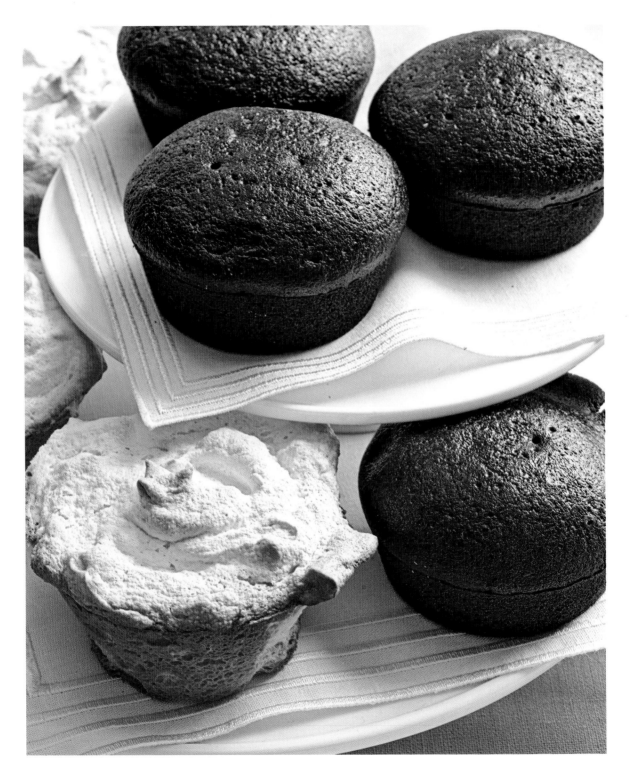

Angel Food Cake and Chocolate Cake (PAGES 219 AND 217)

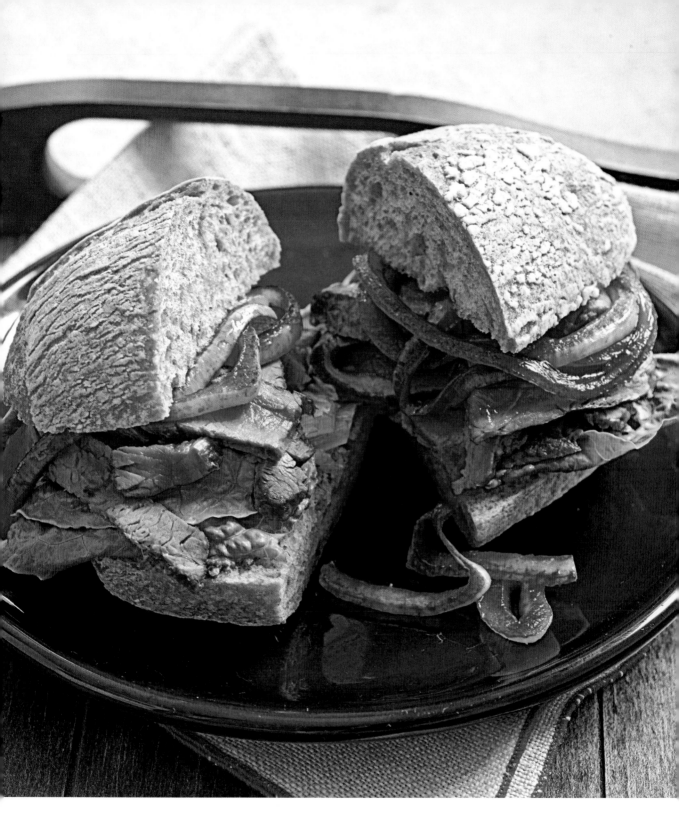

Flank Steak and Balsamic Onion Sandwich (PAGE 99)

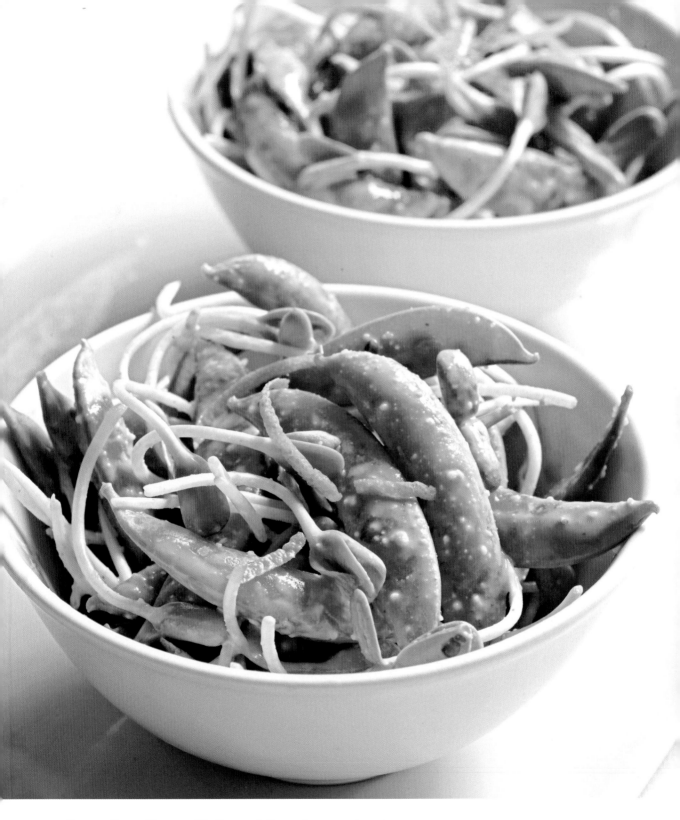

Sugar Snap Peas with Peanut Dressing (PAGE 188)

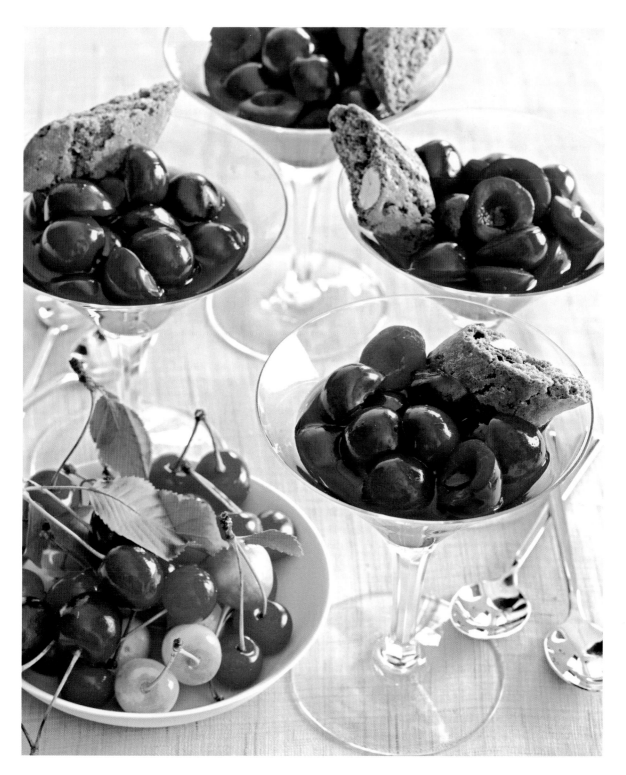

Marinated Cherries with Chocolate Biscotti (PAGE 204)

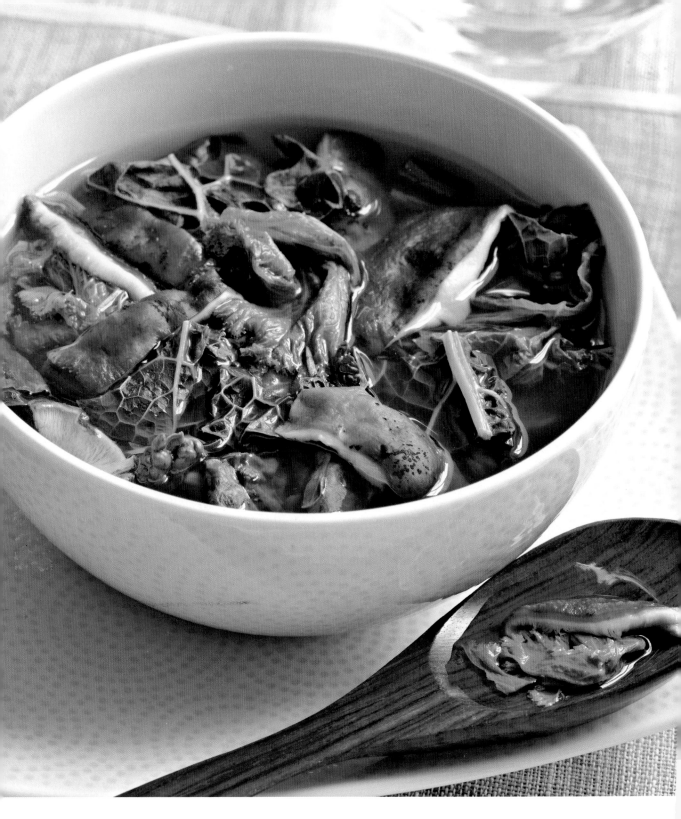

Shiitake Mushroom and Greens Soup (PAGE 39)

PICKS FOR PANS

While I don't shy away from using olive oil or any of the other healthy fats included in this book, I do try to keep the amounts in check because even healthy fats are high in calories. Therefore, it's important to choose a pan that's relatively stick-free when you're sautéing, searing, or pan grilling. Teflon used to be the first choice, but now there are worries that it may release harmful chemicals at high heat—not to mention, many nonstick pans tend to chip. Thomas Griffiths, a certified master chef and associate dean at the Culinary Institute of America in Hyde Park, New York, offers tips for choosing the perfect pan:

- Choose thicker and more heavy-bottomed skillets or sauté pans for even heat distribution. This means fewer hot and cool spots on the pan, which could burn food in spots and undercook in others. Thin pans increase the likelihood that food will stick and burn.

- Go for iron or stainless pans. They both conduct heat evenly and retain it for a long time. Cast iron becomes seasoned over time, which makes food even less likely to stick, plus it's inexpensive and can take a lot of abuse. With stainless pans, you'll have more choices than with cast iron. Before buying, pick up and compare stainless pans; go for the one that feels most comfortable and solid, especially where the handle connects to the pan.

- Save money with aluminum pans, which are more affordable than stainless. As long as you find a thick-bottomed pan, you should be all set, although you won't get quite the performance of stainless or cast iron. And note that aluminum pans do tend to pit over time.

- Take care with enamel pans. Enamel coated cast-iron pans are good because they're heavy and food won't stick as much, but be sure not to use metal utensils; they chip the enamel.

- Splurge on copper, which is an excellent heat conductor. These pricier pans make for gorgeous-looking cookware—that is, if you've got the time to polish it.

Once you have got the right pan, Griffiths has the following tips for minimizing sticking, which we use throughout this book:

- Use *some* oil. Pour a small amount into your pan, or, at the very least, rub the meat, poultry, or seafood in oil before cooking.

- Preheat the pan. This is called "conditioning." You want the pan to be very hot *before* you add the oil. If you've already oiled your food, wait to put the food into the pan until the pan is hot. When cooking a piece of meat, poultry, or fish, cook on both sides, then let it rest for about five minutes so juices recirculate throughout. If you have a very thick piece, don't burn it—after cooking on both sides, finish cooking it in the oven until it's cooked through.

- Learn from experience. Each pan is different, so a little trial and error is involved in discovering which pans work best for, say, searing fish, and which are better for flipping pancakes.

Sweet Potato with Turkey Hash

SERVES 4

LOOK FOR GREAT TASTING sweet potatoes at your local farmers' market from late summer to midwinter. They make all the difference in this comforting, cool-weather dish. If you don't have leftover turkey, you'll find instructions for cooking a turkey tenderloin on the following page.

4 medium sweet potatoes

14 ounces coarsely chopped cooked turkey

1 onion, finely chopped

2 sweet peppers, seeded and chopped

3 stalks celery, chopped

2 cups chopped button mushrooms

1 cup chopped fresh parsley

6 tablespoons (¼ cup plus 2 tablespoons) fat-free milk

1 egg, beaten

2 cloves garlic, minced

1 teaspoon curry powder

½ teaspoon paprika

Heaping ⅛ teaspoon salt

Vegetable oil cooking spray

1. Preheat the oven to 375°F.

2. Stab the potatoes about 4 times each with a fork.

3. Place the potatoes on a sheet pan and cook until tender, about 50 minutes.

4. Mix the turkey, onion, peppers, celery, mushrooms, parsley, milk, egg, garlic, curry powder, paprika, and salt together in a bowl and let stand for 30 minutes.

5. Heat a heavy-bottomed ovenproof skillet over medium heat. Coat the skillet with cooking spray and cook the turkey mixture for 15 minutes.

6. Remove the sweet potatoes from the oven and set aside.

7. Turn the oven to broil and place the skillet under the broiler until the turkey mixture is golden brown, about 5 minutes.

8. Cut the potatoes in half and fill with the turkey mixture. Serve immediately.

To cook turkey tenderloin:

1. Preheat the oven to 375°F.

2. Heat a medium ovenproof sauté pan over medium heat.

3. Lightly coat the pan with cooking spray.

4. Place 18 ounces turkey tenderloin in the pan and cook on each side for 4 minutes.

5. Place the pan in the oven and cook for 15 minutes. Cool until room temperature.

PREP TIME: 10 minutes   **TOTAL TIME:** 1 hour 10 minutes

PER SERVING, ABOUT: Calories: 332 Protein: 33 g Carbohydrate: 35 g Dietary Fiber: 7 g
Sugars: 14 g Total Fat: 7 g Saturated Fat: 2 g Cholesterol: 122 mg Calcium: 151 mg Sodium: 461 mg

Roasted Turkey on Spinach with Cranberry Onion Relish

SERVES 4

WHY WAIT UNTIL THANKSGIVING to have a feast? Enjoy a holiday-type meal all year round with this recipe. Fresh cranberries freeze beautifully, or substitute chopped apples, pears, or peaches.

4 turkey legs, about 12 ounces each (yields about 4 ounces cooked turkey each)

Vegetable oil cooking spray

1 cup fresh cranberries

½ onion, sliced

1 tablespoon balsamic vinegar

¾ teaspoon sugar

¼ teaspoon salt (⅛ for cranberries, ⅛ for turkey)

Black pepper to taste

1 tablespoon chopped fresh thyme, or 1 teaspoon dried

1 tablespoon chopped fresh sage, or 1 teaspoon dried

1 tablespoon chopped fresh Italian parsley

4 cups spinach, well washed

30 sprays Wish-Bone Salad Spritzer Balsamic Breeze, or 2 teaspoons olive oil and 1 tablespoon balsamic vinegar

1. Preheat the oven to 375°F. Heat a heavy-bottomed ovenproof skillet over medium-high heat.

2. Coat the turkey with cooking spray.

3. Cook the turkey in the skillet until browned, approximately 6 minutes per side.

4. Place the skillet in the oven for about 15 minutes, until the pink just disappears and the interior temperature is 160°F. The turkey will continue cooking after it is removed from the oven. Let the turkey cool.

5. Heat the cranberries, onion, vinegar, sugar, and ⅛ teaspoon salt in a medium saucepan over medium heat. Cook until it becomes thick and saucy, about 15 minutes, stirring often.

6. Remove the skin from the turkey by gently pulling it away from the meat.

7. Rub the turkey legs with the remaining ⅛ teaspoon salt, pepper, thyme, sage, and parsley. Set aside.

8. To serve, place the spinach in a large bowl and toss with the dressing.

9. Divide the spinach among 4 plates and top each with a turkey leg. Garnish with one-quarter of the cranberry sauce and serve.

PREP TIME: 15 minutes   **TOTAL TIME:** 40 minutes

PER SERVING, ABOUT: Calories: 209 Protein: 35 g Carbohydrate: 7 g Dietary Fiber: 2 g
Sugars: 3 g Total Fat: 4 g Saturated Fat: 1 g Cholesterol: 116 mg Calcium: 71 mg Sodium: 250 mg

Roasted Chicken Breasts with Herbs on Collard Greens

SERVES 4

THIS IS A SIGNIFICANTLY more healthful version of fried chicken and collard greens. Enjoy it any time you'd like!

³/₄ cup whole wheat bread crumbs, tightly packed

¹/₂ onion, chopped

1 teaspoon chopped fresh thyme, or ¹/₂ teaspoon dried

1 teaspoon chopped fresh rosemary, or ¹/₂ teaspoon dried

1 teaspoon mustard powder

4 cloves garlic, finely chopped (2 for bread crumbs, 2 for greens)

¹/₄ teaspoon salt (¹/₈ for bread crumbs, ¹/₈ for greens)

Vegetable oil cooking spray

4 skinless boneless chicken breasts, about 4 ounces each

4 cups collard greens, well washed and julienned

2 tablespoons balsamic vinegar

Black pepper to taste

1. Preheat the oven to 375°F.

2. Heat a heavy-bottomed ovenproof skillet, large enough to comfortably fit the chicken breasts, over medium heat.

3. Combine the bread crumbs, onion, thyme, rosemary, mustard powder, 2 garlic cloves, and ¹/₈ teaspoon salt in a food processor for 1 minute.

4. Lightly coat the skillet with cooking spray and place the chicken breasts smooth side down. Cook until browned, about 3 minutes.

5. Remove the pan from the heat and turn the chicken over. Coat the browned side of the chicken with the bread crumb mixture.

6. Place the skillet in the oven and cook for 10 minutes.

7. Lightly coat the greens with the cooking spray.

8. Toss the greens with the remaining 2 garlic cloves and ¹/₈ teaspoon salt.

9. Place the greens on a sheet pan and cook in the oven for 10 minutes, tossing every 3 minutes. (You can cook the greens while the chicken cooks if there's enough room in the oven.)

10. Remove the greens and immediately toss with the vinegar and pepper.

11. To serve, divide the collard greens among 4 plates and top each with 1 chicken breast.

PREP TIME: 15 minutes **TOTAL TIME:** 30 minutes

PER SERVING, ABOUT: Calories: 215 Protein: 30 g Carbohydrate: 18 g Dietary Fiber: 3 g Sugars: 3 g Total Fat: 2 g Saturated Fat: 1 g Cholesterol: 66 mg Calcium: 100 mg Sodium: 259 mg

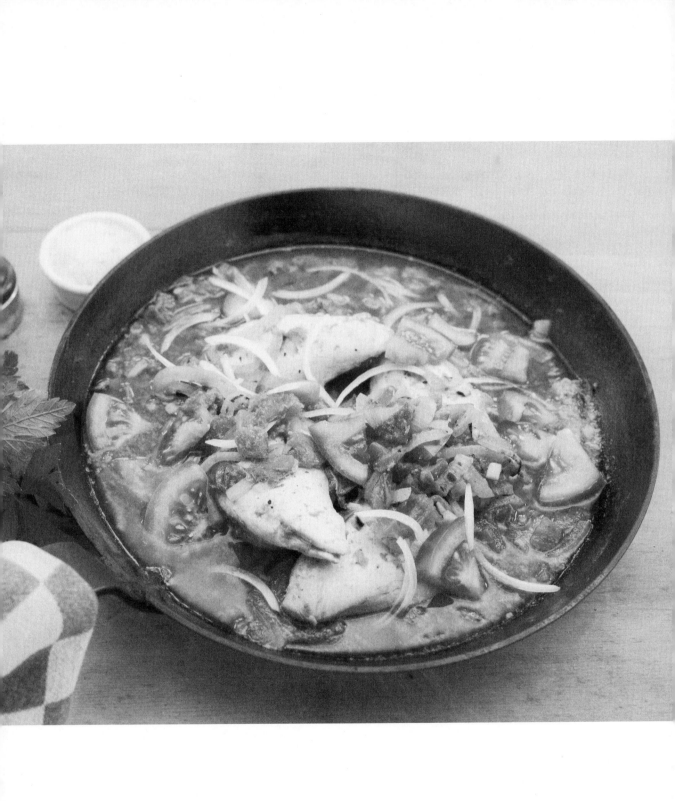

Chicken Poached in White Wine with Tomatoes

SERVES 4

WHO SAID EASY CAN'T be elegant, too? You can have this mouthwatering dish on the table in just 25 minutes.

Vegetable oil cooking spray

1 onion, sliced

2 cloves garlic, minced

2 tomatoes, seeded and diced

1 cup dry white wine

1 cup water

Pinch of cayenne, or more to taste

1 pound boneless skinless chicken breasts, cut into 4 portions, about 4 ounces each

1/8 teaspoon salt

1. Heat a large heavy-bottomed skillet over medium heat and coat with cooking spray.

2. Add the onion and cook for 5 minutes. Add the garlic and cook for an additional 5 minutes.

3. Add the tomatoes, wine, water, and cayenne and bring to a boil.

4. Add the chicken and cover with the tomato mixture. Bring to a boil. Reduce the heat to low and simmer for 5 minutes. Add salt and serve immediately.

PREP TIME: 5 minutes   TOTAL TIME: 30 minutes

PER SERVING, ABOUT: Calories: 169 Protein: 27 g Carbohydrate: 6 g Dietary Fiber: 1 g Sugars: 3 g Total Fat: 2 g Saturated Fat: 0 g Cholesterol: 66 mg Calcium: 30 mg Sodium: 152 mg

Chicken Breasts with Pumpkin Seeds

SERVES 4

THIS SATISFYING RECIPE IS influenced by a Mexican mole sauce; it includes pumpkin seeds, cocoa, and a variety of other spices. The complex, rich flavors of the sauce make your everyday chicken breast taste new and exciting. Although there are many ingredients involved in making this delicious sauce, the preparation is quite simple.

1 tablespoon chopped onion

4 cloves garlic, each cut in half

1 tomato, seeded and cut into 4 pieces

2 tablespoons raisins

1 tablespoon chili powder

Pinch of cloves

2 teaspoons unsweetened cocoa, such as
    Hershey's Natural Cocoa

½ cup hulled pumpkin seeds

1 teaspoon cinnamon

¼ teaspoon salt

4 skinless boneless chicken breasts, about
    4 ounces each

Vegetable oil cooking spray

1. Preheat the oven to 375°F.

2. Combine the onion, garlic, tomato, raisins, chili powder, cloves, cocoa, pumpkin seeds, cinnamon, and salt in a food processor and puree until smooth, about 1 minute.

3. Coat the chicken breasts with the pumpkin-seed mixture.

4. Coat a large heavy-bottomed pan with cooking spray and place the chicken in the pan.

5. Cook in the oven until the chicken is just cooked through, about 15 minutes, and serve.

    PREP TIME: 10 minutes   **TOTAL TIME:** 25 minutes

PER SERVING, ABOUT: Calories: 307 Protein: 37 g Carbohydrate: 12 g Dietary Fiber: 3 g
Sugars: 4 g Total Fat: 14 g Saturated Fat: 3 g Cholesterol: 66 mg Calcium: 50 mg Sodium: 246 mg

Sweet-and-Sour Stuffed Chicken

SERVES 4

YOU CAN WHIP THIS dish up over the weekend when you have more time, and enjoy it all week long. It's worth the effort

1 large onion, minced

1 apple, cored and shredded

⅓ cup dried apricots, finely chopped

⅓ cup dark raisins

⅓ cup pitted prunes, finely chopped

2 cloves garlic, minced

1 teaspoon extra virgin olive oil

1 tablespoon chopped fresh sage

1 teaspoon ground cinnamon

⅛ teaspoon salt

¼ teaspoon freshly ground black pepper

1 whole chicken, about 1¾ pounds

½ cup freshly squeezed orange juice

1. Preheat the oven to 375°F.

2. Mix together the onion, apple, apricots, raisins, prunes, garlic, oil, sage, cinnamon, salt, and pepper in a medium bowl.

3. To remove the skin from the chicken, place the chicken with the back facing up and cut through the skin. Using a paper towel to help you grip, peel the skin off the chicken. Wash the chicken in cold water and then pat dry.

4. Stuff the chicken with the fruit mixture.

5. Place the chicken, breast side down, in a medium roasting pan and pour in the orange juice. Cover the chicken and bake, basting every 15 minutes until the meat easily separates from the bone, about 1½ hours. Serve.

PREP TIME: 20 minutes   **TOTAL TIME:** 1 hour 50 minutes

PER SERVING, ABOUT: Calories: 355 Protein: 37 g Carbohydrate: 39 g Dietary Fiber: 4 g Sugars: 26 g Total Fat: 7 g Saturated Fat: 2 g Cholesterol: 115 mg Calcium: 70 mg Sodium: 204 mg

Turkey Burger

SERVES 4

SATISFY A HANKERING FOR a hamburger with this lower-calorie option. It's just as flavorful, but more diet friendly.

1 pound ground turkey breast

¼ onion, shredded, on the large holes of a hand grater or in a food processor

¼ cup finely chopped green onion (scallion)

2 slices whole wheat bread, toasted and processed in a food processor for 1 minute to make bread crumbs

¼ cup Better'n Eggs, or 1 egg, beaten

2 cloves garlic, finely chopped

⅛ teaspoon ground mustard

Black pepper to taste

Vegetable oil cooking spray

4 whole wheat hamburger buns (with about 115 calories each)

1 tablespoon mustard

8 leaves romaine

8 thick slices tomato

4 slices red onion

1. Thoroughly mix the turkey, onion, green onion, bread crumbs, egg, garlic, mustard, and pepper to taste in a large bowl. Form the mixture into 4 patties.

2. Heat a large heavy-bottomed skillet over medium heat.

3. Lightly coat the pan with cooking spray and place the patties in the pan. Cook until the pink just disappears in the center, about 4 minutes on each side, or until a thermometer inserted into the center of the burger reads 160°F.

4. Slice the buns. Spread each top with mustard. Place the lettuce, tomato, onion, and a burger on the bottom bun and cover with the top. Serve.

PREP TIME: 10 minutes　**TOTAL TIME:** 20 minutes

PER SERVING, ABOUT: Calories: 367 Protein: 29 g Carbohydrate: 36 g Dietary Fiber: 6 g Sugars: 3 g Total Fat: 13 g Saturated Fat: 3 g Cholesterol: 143 mg Calcium: 118 mg Sodium: 487 mg

SEAFOOD

Wild Salmon with Sweet Corn and Tomatoes

SERVES 4

FORGET ABOUT HAMBURGERS AND hot dogs. This is *the* dish to make in the summer, when Alaskan wild salmon is available. Pair the fish with sweet corn and tomatoes from the farmers' market for a fresh, satisfying meal.

Vegetable oil cooking spray

3 onions, sliced

6 teaspoons fresh thyme, or 3 teaspoons dried

3 cups fresh corn, cut off the cob, or frozen, defrosted at room temperature

6 tomatoes, each cut into 8 pieces

³/₄ cup fresh basil, ripped or roughly chopped

³/₈ teaspoon salt (¹/₈ heaping teaspoon for corn mixture, ¹/₈ heaping teaspoon for salmon)

1¹/₄ pounds Pacific wild salmon, cut into 4 pieces, about 5 ounces each

1. Heat a large heavy-bottomed skillet over medium heat. Coat with cooking spray, add the onions, and cook until translucent, about 5 minutes. Add the thyme and corn and cook for 3 minutes. Add the tomatoes and basil, toss with the heaping ¹/₈ teaspoon salt, and remove the mixture from the skillet.

2. Rinse the skillet and reheat over medium heat. Coat with cooking spray and place the salmon in the pan. Cook until slightly brown, about 3 minutes. Flip the salmon and cook the other side until just cooked through, about 3 minutes. Check the middle of the fillet; it is done when there is just a drop of bright orange remaining.

3. Season the salmon with the remaining heaping ¹/₈ teaspoon salt. Spoon the corn-tomato mixture onto individual plates, place the salmon on top, and serve.

PREP TIME: 10 minutes   TOTAL TIME: 25 minutes

PER SERVING, ABOUT: Calories: 390 Protein: 35 g Carbohydrate: 45 g Dietary Fiber: 7 g
Sugars: 13 g Total Fat: 10 g Saturated Fat: 2 g Cholesterol: 78 mg Calcium: 59 mg Sodium: 298 mg

BRING HOME A HEALTHY CATCH

When it comes to foods, there is perhaps none as hotly debated as fish. Although it's one of the healthiest sources of protein (it's low in saturated fat and rich in healthy fat), it's also a troubling source of contaminants, such as mercury, which is harmful to the nervous system, and PCBs, carcinogens that come from industrial pollution. Not to mention that certain fishing practices are downright damaging—drastically diminishing the fish supply, killing dolphins and other marine life, and disturbing the ocean, river, and lake ecology. It's enough to turn you off of fish completely. But you can still include it in your diet if you choose carefully. As long as you vary your picks, opting for species that are eco-friendly, low in contaminants, and preferably high in omega-3s, you can enjoy fish twice a week (this is what the American Heart Association recommends).

Finding a fish that meets these criteria can be tough, but not impossible. For instance, all of the fish in these recipes are low in contaminants and ecologically sustainable. Plus, many recipes feature omega-3-rich fish, such as trout, salmon, sardines, and canned light tuna. Other omega-3-rich fish that are low in mercury are: Arctic char, herring, mackerel (except for king mackerel), and sablefish. Omega-3s have been shown to protect the joints, brain, and heart, as well as a developing fetus. (Another way to get these fats, of course, is through fish oil supplements.) Plant-based omega-3s from walnuts, flaxseeds, and other sources are also healthful, but not as potent and effective as fish oils.

Information on fish changes regularly, so to stay on top of fish safety, check out my Web site, www.thebestlife.com, for periodic updates, and go to the Web sites of Blue Ocean Institute (www.blueocean.org), Monterey Bay Aquarium (www.mbayaq.org), Environmental Defense Fund (www.edf.org), and the Food and Drug Administration (www.fda.gov).

Poached Wild Salmon with Zucchini and Mustard

SERVES 4

WILD SALMON, WHICH IS available fresh from the spring through September, is one of the best foods for your body; it is loaded with heart-healthy omega-3 fatty acids and essential vitamins and minerals. Try this simple poaching technique that highlights the naturally flavorful fish.

Vegetable oil cooking spray

2 onions, sliced

1 pound zucchini, sliced

2 tablespoons grainy mustard

2 tablespoons olive oil

¼ teaspoon salt

1 tablespoon finely chopped chives

1 cup dry white wine

1 cup water

1 pound wild salmon, cut into 4 pieces, about 4 ounces each

Juice of 2 lemons

1. Heat a large heavy-bottomed skillet over medium heat. Coat with cooking spray, add the onions, and cook until translucent, about 5 minutes.

2. Add the zucchini and cook for 5 minutes, stirring constantly. Remove the onions and zucchini from the pan and place in a medium mixing bowl. Toss with mustard, oil, salt, and chives. Set aside.

3. In a large frying pan, bring the wine and water to a boil. Reduce the heat to low and simmer. Add the salmon, cover, and cook until the fish is just cooked through, 3 to 5 minutes, depending on thickness. Make a small cut and peek in the middle of the fillet; make sure that most of the deep orange color is gone. Take care not to overcook as the fish will continue cooking even after it is removed from the pan.

4. Remove the salmon immediately from the cooking liquid and put on individual plates. Squeeze the lemon juice on the fish. Serve with zucchini.

PREP TIME: 10 minutes **TOTAL TIME:** 25 minutes

PER SERVING, ABOUT: Calories: 287 Protein: 25 g Carbohydrate: 12 g Dietary Fiber: 2 g Sugars: 5 g Total Fat: 15 g Saturated Fat: 2 g Cholesterol: 62 mg Calcium: 55 mg Sodium: 307 mg

Rockfish Steamed with Ginger, Garlic, Green Onions, and Sesame

SERVES 4

THIS RECIPE, WHICH USES rockfish, a mildly sweet fish with a flaky firm texture, is simple but elegant. Rockfish is a wild fish that is both healthful and sustainable.

Vegetable oil cooking spray

8 outermost cabbage leaves from Savoy or Napa varieties, if possible

1 tablespoon minced ginger

2 cloves garlic, chopped

4 green onions (scallions), sliced in half lengthwise

½ tablespoon dark or cold-pressed light sesame oil

1 pound rockfish, skin removed, cut into 4 pieces, about 4 ounces each

2 tablespoons sesame seeds

2 tablespoons water

⅛ teaspoon salt

1. Preheat the oven to 375°F.

2. Coat a 12-inch ovenproof skillet or 9 x 13-inch baking dish with cooking spray. Cover the bottom of the skillet or dish with 4 cabbage leaves.

3. In a medium bowl, toss the ginger, garlic, and green onions with the oil.

4. Place 4 onion halves on top of the cabbage leaves, and place the fish on top of the onions. Cover with the remaining 4 onion halves and the remaining ginger-garlic mixture. Sprinkle on the sesame seeds. Place the remaining 4 cabbage leaves on top. Add the water to the skillet.

5. Tightly cover the skillet with foil and cook until the fish easily flakes, about 12 minutes. Lift the cabbage, season the fish with salt, replace the cabbage, and serve.

PREP TIME: 10 minutes   TOTAL TIME: 25 minutes

PER SERVING, ABOUT: Calories: 192 Protein: 23 g Carbohydrate: 4 g Dietary Fiber: 1 g Sugars: 1 g Total Fat: 9 g Saturated Fat: 2 g Cholesterol: 40 mg Calcium: 58 mg Sodium: 162 mg

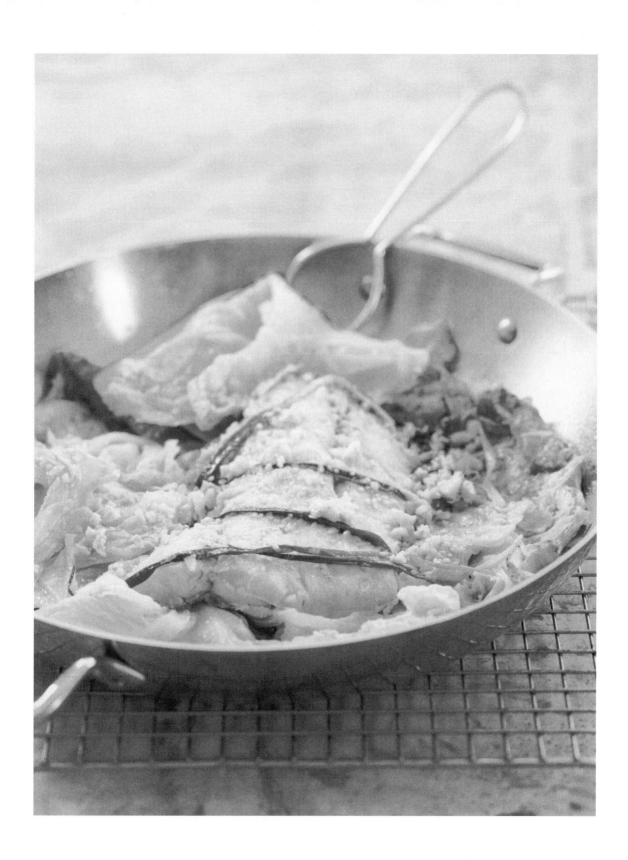

Tilapia with Carrot Ginger Puree

SERVES 4

YOU CAN FEEL GOOD about cooking with tilapia: it's one of the more ecologically sustainable fish raised right in the United States. It's a good way to convert anyone who's not a big fish fan because it's mild tasting yet juicy.

4 large carrots, peeled and chopped	1 tablespoon olive oil
1 teaspoon minced fresh ginger	1/4 teaspoon salt (1/8 for carrots, 1/8 for fish)
1 teaspoon minced fresh garlic	Vegetable oil cooking spray
1/2 cup water	1 pound tilapia fillets, cut into 4 portions, 4 ounces each

1. Preheat the oven to 375°F.

2. Place the carrots, ginger, and garlic in a medium pan and cover with water. Bring to a boil and cook until the carrots are tender, about 10 minutes.

3. Heat a large heavy-bottomed skillet over medium heat.

4. Puree the carrot mixture, 1/2 cup water, oil, and 1/8 teaspoon salt in a food processor until smooth, about 1 minute. Set the puree aside.

5. Coat the hot skillet with cooking spray. Cook the fish until browned, about 2 minutes. Turn and cook for an additional 2 minutes. Tilapia is a delicate fish, so take care not to overcook.

6. Remove the fish from the pan, season with the remaining 1/8 teaspoon salt, and place fillets on individual plates. Top with the puree and serve.

PREP TIME: 15 minutes   **TOTAL TIME:** 31 minutes

PER SERVING, ABOUT: Calories: 170 Protein: 24 g Carbohydrate: 7 g Dietary Fiber: 2 g
Sugars: 3 g Total Fat: 6 g Saturated Fat: 1 g Cholesterol: 57 mg Calcium: 37 mg Sodium: 254 mg

Pan-Roasted Shrimp with Lemon, Garlic, and Spinach

SERVES 4

LOOKING FOR A FAST recipe that tastes like you've been slaving over a stove all day long? Try this dish! Pair it with a side of whole grain pasta, brown rice, or other whole grain.

4 cups spinach, well washed	Juice of 1 lemon
4 cloves garlic, minced	1 tablespoon extra virgin olive oil
Vegetable oil cooking spray	⅛ teaspoon salt
1 pound raw shrimp, shelled and deveined	Black pepper to taste

1. Place the spinach in a large bowl. Set aside.

2. Heat a large heavy-bottomed skillet over medium-low heat.

3. Coat the garlic with cooking spray and cook in the skillet until slightly browned, about 3 minutes.

4. Coat the shrimp with cooking spray.

5. Increase the heat to medium and add the shrimp, cooking on each side for 2 minutes.

6. Put the shrimp in the bowl with the spinach and toss with lemon juice, oil, salt, and pepper. Serve.

PREP TIME: 3 minutes   TOTAL TIME: 10 minutes

PER SERVING, ABOUT: Calories: 173 Protein: 24 g Carbohydrate: 5 g Dietary Fiber: 1 g
Sugars: 1 g Total Fat: 7 g Saturated Fat: 1 g Cholesterol: 172 mg Calcium: 98 mg Sodium: 265 mg

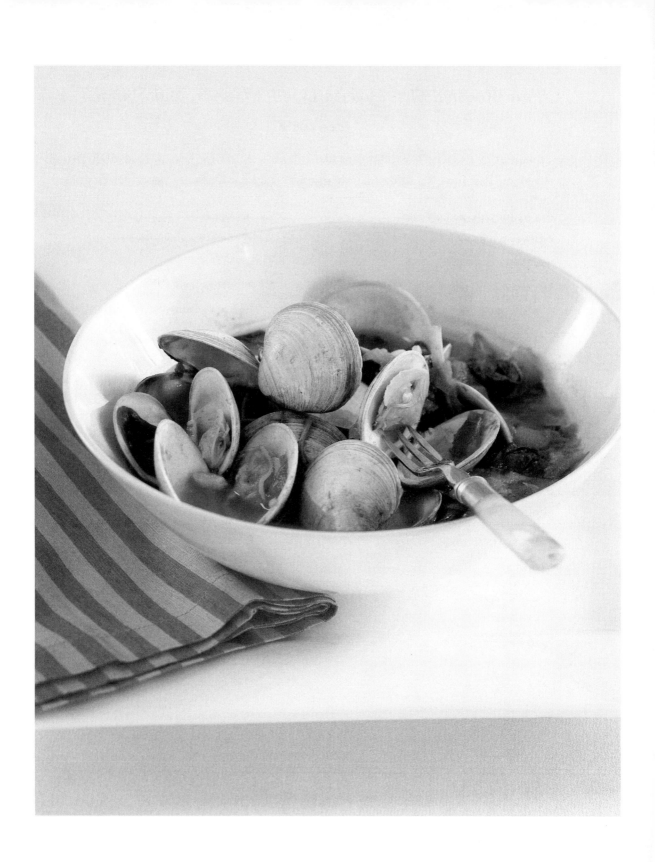

Clams Steamed with Turkey Bacon, Tomatoes, and Spinach

SERVES 4

CLAMS ARE A GREAT seafood choice because they are environmentally sustainable and contain few or no contaminants. They're also an excellent source of vitamin B12 and iron.

48 small, 36 medium, or 24 large clams

2 slices turkey bacon, chopped

1 medium onion, chopped

4 cloves garlic, minced

1/8 teaspoon dried red pepper flakes, or
   more to taste

4 cups diced fresh tomatoes, or canned
   no-salt-added diced tomatoes

1 cup dry white wine

4 cups spinach, well washed

1. Soak the clams in cold water for 20 minutes. Discard any open clams.

2. Heat a large heavy-bottomed stockpot over medium heat. Cook the bacon in the pot for 5 minutes, stirring occasionally. Add the onion, garlic, and red pepper flakes and cook for 5 minutes, stirring occasionally. Add the tomatoes and cook for 5 minutes, stirring occasionally.

3. Add the wine and clams and bring to a boil. Cover and cook, stirring occasionally, until the clams just open wide, about 6 minutes. Discard the clams that do not open. Stir in the spinach and cook until wilted, about 1 minute. Serve.

PREP TIME: 25 minutes   **TOTAL TIME:** 35 minutes

PER SERVING, ABOUT: Calories: 192 Protein: 18 g Carbohydrate: 17 g Dietary Fiber: 3 g
Sugars: 8 g Total Fat: 3 g Saturated Fat: 1 g Cholesterol: 42 mg Calcium: 118 mg Sodium: 227 mg

Mussels with White Wine and Garlic

SERVES 4

THIS CROWD-PLEASER IS ABSOLUTELY delicious *and* fun to eat! The dish looks dramatic and the process of getting the mussels out of their shells makes you work (just a little) for your food. Serve with slices of crusty whole wheat bread.

4 pounds mussels	2 cups dry white wine
8 cloves garlic, minced	

1. Right before you are ready to cook the mussels, fill a sink half full of cold water. Add the mussels and mix them around. If there is anything stuck to the mussel shells, remove. Discard any open mussels.

2. Put the garlic and white wine in a large pot. Add the mussels and cover. Cook over high heat until you can see steam forcing its way out from under the lid. Shake the pot to help the mussels cook evenly, and cook for an additional 5 minutes. Check to see if the mussels have opened. If not, return the lid immediately and cook for another 3 minutes.

3. Using a slotted spoon, remove the mussels and put them into individual serving bowls. Discard any mussels that did not open.

4. Bring the liquid the mussels were cooked in to a boil and cook for 1 minute.

5. Pour the liquid over the mussels and serve immediately.

PREP TIME: 10 minutes   **TOTAL TIME:** 20 minutes

PER SERVING, ABOUT: Calories: 150 Protein: 14 g Carbohydrate: 7 g Dietary Fiber: 0 g
Sugars: 0 g Total Fat: 3 g Saturated Fat: 0 g Cholesterol: 32 mg Calcium: 39 mg Sodium: 328 mg

Shrimp Curry

SERVES 4

SERVE THIS EXOTIC, RICH-TASTING dish over brown rice or whole wheat couscous.

Vegetable oil cooking spray

1 onion, chopped

½ teaspoon cayenne, or more to taste

2 cloves garlic, finely chopped

2 tablespoons curry powder

½ teaspoon powdered ginger

2 cups chopped fresh tomatoes, or canned
no-salt-added tomatoes

½ cup light coconut milk

3 cups water

1 pound shrimp, shelled and deveined

⅛ teaspoon salt

Black pepper to taste

1. Heat a large heavy-bottomed stockpot over medium heat and coat the pot with cooking spray.

2. Cook the onion until translucent, about 5 minutes. Add the cayenne, garlic, curry powder, and ginger and cook for an additional 2 minutes, stirring constantly.

3. Add the tomatoes, coconut milk, and water and bring to a boil. Reduce to a simmer for 10 minutes.

4. Add the shrimp. Bring to a boil again and cook for an additional 1 minute. Season with salt and pepper. Serve.

PREP TIME: 7 minutes   TOTAL TIME: 30 minutes

PER SERVING, ABOUT: Calories: 183 Protein: 25 g Carbohydrate: 10 g Dietary Fiber: 2 g
Sugars: 3 g Total Fat: 5 g Saturated Fat: 2 g Cholesterol: 172 mg Calcium: 94 mg Sodium: 258 mg

Pecan–Crusted Trout with Peaches

SERVES 4

THE COMBINATION OF TROUT with pecans and peaches puts this dish in the category of southern comfort. If possible, use U.S. farm-raised rainbow trout, which is delicious, sustainable, and free of contaminants.

1 cup thinly sliced peaches	1/2 cup AllWhites, or 3 egg whites
2 tablespoons minced onion	1/2 cup ground pecans
1/2 teaspoon oregano	1/4 cup cornmeal, preferably whole grain
1 tablespoon sherry vinegar	1 pound trout fillets, cut into 4 pieces, about 4 ounces each
1/2 teaspoon olive oil	Vegetable oil cooking spray
1/8 teaspoon salt	
Black pepper to taste	

1. Heat a large heavy-bottomed skillet over medium heat.

2. In a medium bowl, combine the peaches, onion, oregano, vinegar, oil, salt, and pepper. Set aside.

3. Place the egg whites on a large plate. Mix the pecans and cornmeal on another large plate.

4. Take each piece of trout and coat with the egg whites, then the pecan mixture. Place the dipped pieces of trout on a clean plate.

5. Coat the skillet with cooking spray and place the trout in the pan. If there is not enough room to cook the trout comfortably in a single layer, cook in two batches. Cook until the crust is browned, about 3 minutes. Flip the trout and cook for an additional 3 minutes.

6. Serve the trout topped with the peach mixture.

PREP TIME: 10 minutes   TOTAL TIME: 20 minutes

PER SERVING, ABOUT: Calories: 289 Protein: 25 g Carbohydrate: 13 g Dietary Fiber: 3 g Sugars: 5 g Total Fat: 16 g Saturated Fat: 2 g Cholesterol: 94 mg Calcium: 38 mg Sodium: 192 mg

Roasted Rockfish with Clementines

SERVES 4

THE FLAVORS OF THE fish and citrus in this recipe complement each other wonderfully. If clementines are not available, use oranges.

1 pound rockfish, cut into 4 pieces, about
    4 ounces each

4 clementines, zested, peeled, and broken
    into individual sections

1 tablespoon olive oil

Vegetable oil cooking spray

1 cup chopped green onions (scallions)

⅛ teaspoon salt

1. Heat a large heavy-bottomed skillet over medium heat.

2. Rub the fish with the clementine zest. In a medium bowl, toss the clementine sections with oil.

3. Coat the skillet with cooking spray. Add the green onions and cook for 3 minutes, stirring often. Add the fish, skin side down, and cook until the skin is browned, about 3 minutes. Flip the fish, add the clementines, and cook for about 2 more minutes, until the fish just begins to flake but the center is still translucent. The fish will continue to cook even after it is removed from the pan.

4. Season the fish with salt and garnish with clementines and green onions.

PREP TIME: 5 minutes **TOTAL TIME:** 15 minutes

PER SERVING, ABOUT: Calories: 204 Protein: 24 g Carbohydrate: 16 g Dietary Fiber: 4 g
Sugars: 9 g Total Fat: 6 g Saturated Fat: 1 g Cholesterol: 40 mg Calcium: 105 mg Sodium: 158 mg

Sole in Celery and Turnip Broth

SERVES 4

THE DELICATE TASTE AND texture of the fish is highlighted by the accompanying vegetables, which are used both in the poaching broth and as a cold relish. You can also make this dish with flounder fillets.

3 cups water

1 onion, finely chopped

2 cups finely chopped celery (1 for broth, 1 for garnish)

2 cups finely chopped turnips (1 for broth, 1 for garnish)

$1/4$ teaspoon peppercorns

1 tablespoon chopped fresh rosemary

2 tablespoons white vinegar

Zest and juice of 1 lemon

1 tablespoon olive oil

$1/4$ cup chopped fresh Italian parsley

$1/8$ teaspoon salt

1 pound sole fillets, cut into 4 pieces, about 4 ounces each

Vegetable oil cooking spray

1. Bring the water, onion, 1 cup celery, 1 cup turnips, peppercorns, rosemary, and vinegar to a boil in a large skillet. Reduce the heat to a simmer and cook for 10 minutes.

2. Combine the remaining 1 cup celery and 1 cup turnips with the lemon zest and juice, oil, parsley, and salt in a medium bowl. Set aside.

3. Put the sole in a single layer in the skillet and bring the liquid to a boil. Cover the skillet and turn off the heat. Let the sole sit, covered, until just cooked, 2 to 5 minutes, depending on the thickness of the fish.

4. Remove the sole from the broth and place on individual plates. Spoon 1 tablespoon broth on top of each portion of fish, and top with the cold celery and turnip mixture. Serve.

PREP TIME: 10 minutes   TOTAL TIME: 35 minutes

PER SERVING, ABOUT: Calories: 179 Protein: 23 g Carbohydrate: 11 g Dietary Fiber: 2 g
Sugars: 6 g Total Fat: 5 g Saturated Fat: 1 g Cholesterol: 54 mg Calcium: 66 mg Sodium: 219 mg

Broiled Mahimahi with Grapes and Leeks

SERVES 4

THE UNEXPECTED COMBINATION OF grapes and leeks is outstanding with mahimahi, a sustainable and healthful seafood choice with a steaklike texture.

1 pound mahimahi fillets, cut into 4 pieces, about 4 ounces each

1 cup seedless green grapes

1 cup finely sliced leeks, well washed

Vegetable oil cooking spray

⅛ teaspoon salt

1 lemon, cut into 4 pieces

½ teaspoon lemon zest

1. Turn the oven to broil.

2. Place the mahimahi, grapes, and leeks on a sheet pan and coat with cooking spray.

3. Place the pan under the broiler for 3 minutes. Flip the mahimahi and return to broil for 2 more minutes.

4. Remove from the oven. Season with salt, squeeze the lemon juice on the mahimahi, garnish with zest, and serve.

PREP TIME: 5 minutes   **TOTAL TIME:** 10 minutes

PER SERVING, ABOUT: Calories: 221 Protein: 21 g Carbohydrate: 8 g Dietary Fiber: 1 g Sugars: 6 g Total Fat: 11 g Saturated Fat: 4 g Cholesterol: 57 mg Calcium: 35 mg Sodium: 150 mg

Cod with Broiled Grapefruit and Avocado Butter

SERVES 4

THIS DISH IS A snap to prepare, but sophisticated enough to wow your guests. The creamy avocado mellows out the citrusy grapefruit and adds healthy fat. If you'd like, you can substitute mahimahi in place of the cod.

1 avocado, peeled and pit removed

1 tablespoon chives

1 tablespoon olive oil

1 pound cod fillet, cut into 4 pieces, about 4 ounces each

2 grapefruits, peeled, sections removed from pith (see page 346)

Vegetable oil cooking spray

⅛ teaspoon salt

1. Heat the oven to broil.

2. Combine the avocado, chives, and oil in a food processor and puree until smooth, about 1 minute. Set aside.

3. Coat the cod and grapefruit with cooking spray. Place on a sheet pan and put under the broiler for 2 minutes (this cooking time is for fish about 1½ inches thick; adjust the cooking time accordingly for different thicknesses of fish). Flip the cod and broil for 1 minute. Check to see if the cod is cooked to your liking. If necessary, return to the oven and broil for an additional 1 to 2 minutes.

4. Remove the cod and grapefruit and place on a platter. Season with salt and serve with the avocado mixture on top.

PREP TIME: 10 minutes   **TOTAL TIME:** 15 minutes

PER SERVING, ABOUT: Calories: 232 Protein: 22 g Carbohydrate: 16 g Dietary Fiber: 4 g
Sugars: 9 g Total Fat: 10 g Saturated Fat: 1 g Cholesterol: 49 mg Calcium: 50 mg Sodium: 137 mg

Cornmeal–Crusted Catfish with Spicy Slaw

SERVES 4

THIS LIGHTENED-UP VERSION OF a classic fried fish recipe offers all the flavor with significantly less fat. U.S. farm-raised catfish is sustainable and a very safe seafood choice.

Vegetable oil cooking spray

4 cups shredded cabbage, a mix of red and green

¼ cup sherry vinegar

¼ teaspoon hot pepper flakes, or more to taste

¼ cup mayonnaise (with no more than 50 calories per tablespoon), such as Hellmann's Canola Cholesterol Free

¼ teaspoon salt

1 pound catfish fillets, cut into 4 pieces, about 4 ounces each

¼ cup Better'n Eggs

¼ cup cornmeal, preferably whole grain

1 lemon, cut into quarters

1. Heat a large heavy-bottomed skillet over medium heat and coat with cooking spray.

2. In a medium bowl, combine the cabbage, vinegar, pepper flakes, mayonnaise, and salt. Use immediately or store in the refrigerator for up to 12 hours before serving.

3. Dip individual pieces of fish into the eggs and then the cornmeal.

4. Place the fish in a pan in a single layer (cook in two batches if the pan is too small). Cook until brown, about 3 minutes.

5. Turn the fish and cook until just cooked through, about 3 more minutes.

6. Place the fish on individual plates, top with the cabbage and a squeeze of lemon, and serve.

PREP TIME: 10 minutes   TOTAL TIME: 20 minutes

PER SERVING, ABOUT: Calories: 218 Protein: 22 g Carbohydrate: 13 g Dietary Fiber: 3 g Sugars: 3 g Total Fat: 8 g Saturated Fat: 1 g Cholesterol: 66 mg Calcium: 53 mg Sodium: 326 mg

VEGETARIAN

Roasted Summer Vegetable Parmesan

SERVES 4

THIS HEARTY DISH MAKES good use of the summer bounty. Round out the meal with a large fruit salad topped with vanilla yogurt.

1 ½ pounds eggplant, sliced

1 large green zucchini or yellow summer squash, sliced

1 large onion, sliced

4 cloves garlic, chopped

1 large red pepper, seeded and sliced

Vegetable oil cooking spray

9 crispbreads such as Wasa Multi Grain (or any variety with the Best Life seal), crushed

3 tomatoes, thinly sliced

1½ cups shredded part-skim mozzarella cheese

¾ cup marinara sauce, such as Barilla, mixed with ¾ cup water

¾ cup Parmesan

1. Preheat the oven to 375°F.

2. Place the eggplant, zucchini, onion, garlic, and red pepper on two sheet pans and coat with cooking spray. Cook in the oven for 15 minutes. Take the pans out of the oven and combine the vegetables on one sheet pan and toss together. Set aside.

3. Coat a 13 x 9-inch pan with cooking spray.

4. Place half of the crispbread crumbs on the bottom of the pan. Cover with half of the vegetable mixture, sliced tomatoes, mozzarella cheese, the remaining half of the vegetable mixture, and marinara sauce.

5. Mix the remaining crispbread crumbs and Parmesan and sprinkle on top of the casserole.

6. Bake for 40 minutes. Serve.

PREP TIME: 20 minutes **TOTAL TIME:** 1 hour

PER SERVING, ABOUT: Calories: 391 Protein: 25 g Carbohydrate: 51 g Dietary Fiber: 14 g Sugars: 13 g Total Fat: 12 g Saturated Fat: 6 g Cholesterol: 31 mg Calcium: 472 mg Sodium: 738 mg

---

LABEL LOOKOUT! BIODYNAMIC

Foods carrying this label not only meet the USDA organic requirements (see page 85) but they are also produced according to the "biodynamic" method. One of the guiding principles: the farm must be as self-sufficient and nonpolluting as possible. For instance, wastes generated from the farm are recycled to create fertilizer; the farm may produce its own animal feed; and water is recycled through the farm. Many products, including vegetables, grains, dairy, and wine, carry the seal. Although the standards are on par in many ways, not all companies carrying the Demeter biodynamic seal sport the USDA Organic seal simply because the producers haven't gone through the USDA certification process.

Angel Hair Pasta with Walnuts and Peas

SERVES 4

QUELL A PASTA CRAVING with this vegetarian dish, which provides high-quality protein thanks to Barilla PLUS. Walnuts also contribute some protein and healthy omega-3 fats as well.

1 cup walnuts

6 cloves roasted garlic (see page 344), or more to taste

½ cup basil, ripped into small pieces

⅓ cup water

7 ounces (½ package) Barilla PLUS thin spaghetti, cooked according to package instructions

2 cups fresh peas, or frozen, defrosted at room temperature

⅛ teaspoon salt

Black pepper to taste

Red pepper flakes to taste (optional)

1. Combine the walnuts, garlic, basil, and water in a food processor for 1 minute.

2. Toss the walnut mixture with the hot cooked pasta, peas, salt, pepper, and red pepper flakes, if desired, and serve.

PREP TIME: 10 minutes   **TOTAL TIME:** 10 minutes

PER SERVING, ABOUT: Calories: 442 Protein: 15 g Carbohydrate: 53 g Dietary Fiber: 11 g Sugars: 7 g Total Fat: 21 g Saturated Fat: 2 g Cholesterol: 0 mg Calcium: 63 mg Sodium: 296 mg

Thin Spaghetti with Sesame, Ginger, and Edamame

SERVES 4

THIS ONE-DISH MEAL, FLAVORED by fragrant ginger and rich-tasting sesame, is sure to satisfy.

8 ounces whole wheat or high-fiber thin spaghetti, such as Barilla Whole Grain

2¹⁄₂ cups shelled edamame (blanched fresh, or frozen)

2 cups shredded carrots

¹⁄₂ cup finely sliced green onions (scallions)

2 cups bean sprouts

¹⁄₂ teaspoon salt

4 teaspoons low-sodium soy sauce

1 tablespoon sesame oil

2 tablespoons tahini

4 teaspoons rice wine vinegar

¹⁄₂ cup chopped fresh cilantro

1 teaspoon finely chopped or grated fresh ginger

1 tablespoon honey

1. Cook the spaghetti according to the package directions. Run cold water over the pasta while draining from the cooking water.

2. Combine the pasta, edamame, carrots, green onions, and bean sprouts in a large bowl.

3. Process the salt, soy sauce, oil, tahini, vinegar, cilantro, ginger, and honey in a food processor until smooth, about 1 minute.

4. Toss the dressing with the spaghetti mixture and serve.

PREP TIME: 10 minutes   TOTAL TIME: 25 minutes

PER SERVING, ABOUT: Calories: 495 Protein: 28 g Carbohydrate: 72 g Dietary Fiber: 15 g Sugars: 17 g Total Fat: 14 g Saturated Fat: 2 g Cholesterol: 0 mg Calcium: 131 mg Sodium: 617 mg

Vegetable Cottage Pie

SERVES 4

THIS DELICIOUS VEGETARIAN VERSION of a meaty classic is certain to please all.

2 large potatoes, skin on

2 cups canned no-salt-added black-eyed
    peas, drained and rinsed, or cooked
    (see page 345)

Vegetable oil cooking spray

1 small eggplant (about 10 ounces) sliced
    into 1/4-inch-thick slices

2 medium carrots, peeled and finely
    chopped

1 onion, chopped

4 cloves garlic, minced

1 teaspoon minced fresh sage,
    or 1/2 teaspoon dried

1 teaspoon minced fresh rosemary,
    or 1/2 teaspoon dried

1/8 teaspoon cayenne

1/8 teaspoon paprika

4 cups spinach, well washed

2 tablespoons olive oil

1/4 teaspoon salt

1. Place the potatoes in a medium pot and cover with water. Bring to a boil and cook until the potatoes are tender, about 20 minutes.

2. Process the black-eyed peas in a food processor for 1 minute.

3. Heat a large heavy-bottomed skillet over medium-high heat.

4. Lightly coat the skillet with cooking spray. Add the eggplant, carrots, onion, garlic, sage, rosemary, cayenne, and paprika. Cook until slightly browned, about 15 minutes, stirring often.

5. Add the ground black-eyed peas, turn off the heat immediately, and stir in the spinach.

6. Drain the potatoes well and mash with a wooden spoon with the oil and salt until smooth; some lumps can remain.

7. To assemble, place the eggplant mixture in a 9-inch pan (or 4 individual 3-inch ramekins) and cover with mashed potatoes.

8. Bake for 10 minutes if using warm ingredients, or assemble the pies and refrigerate, then reheat in a 375°F oven until warm throughout, about 20 minutes.

9. Turn the oven to broil until the tops of the potatoes are browned, about 5 minutes. Serve.

PREP TIME: 10 minutes   **TOTAL TIME:** 55 minutes

PER SERVING, ABOUT: Calories: 359 Protein: 13 g Carbohydrate: 63 g Dietary Fiber: 17 g Sugars: 10 g Total Fat: 8 g Saturated Fat: 1 g Cholesterol: 0 mg Calcium: 113 mg Sodium: 212 mg

Mushroom Ragout Over Whole Grain Cake

SERVES 4

A RAGOUT IS A mixture of ingredients incorporated in a flavorful thick stew or sauce. This elegant dish works great with button mushrooms, or a variety of exotic mushrooms— cultivated ones such as shiitake or oyster mushrooms or wild ones such as chanterelle or morel mushrooms.

2 cups barley, wild rice, cracked wheat, or brown rice, cooked according to package instructions

1 pound tofu, pureed in a food processor for 1 minute

1 clove garlic, finely minced

1 teaspoon chopped fresh thyme

¼ teaspoon salt

Black pepper to taste

Vegetable oil cooking spray

1 onion, sliced

6 cups sliced mushrooms, any variety

1 cup dry red wine

2 cups thinly sliced Swiss chard leaves, well washed

1. Preheat the oven to 375°F. Heat a large heavy-bottomed skillet over medium heat.

2. Mix the barley, tofu, garlic, thyme, salt, and pepper in a large bowl. Spray a 9-inch pie plate or ovenproof skillet with cooking spray. Put the grain mixture in the plate and cook in the oven for 20 minutes.

3. Coat the hot skillet with cooking spray, add the onion and cook for 5 minutes. Lightly coat the mushrooms with cooking spray and cook in the skillet with the onions for 5 minutes, stirring often. Add the red wine and chard and bring to a boil. Reduce the heat to low and simmer for 10 minutes.

4. Cut the grain mixture into 4 pieces. Serve topped with the mushroom ragout.

PREP TIME: 15 minutes if grain is cooked   **TOTAL TIME:** 35 minutes

PER SERVING, ABOUT: Calories: 352 Protein: 24 g Carbohydrate: 36 g Dietary Fiber: 7 g Sugars: 4 g Total Fat: 11 g Saturated Fat: 2 g Cholesterol: 0 mg Calcium: 809 mg Sodium: 360 mg

Broccoli, White Bean, and Leek Tart

SERVES 4

VEGETARIANS AND MEAT EATERS alike will enjoy this dish. The white beans in this delicious, creamy-tasting tart provide protein with very little fat and no cholesterol. Round out the meal with bread dipped in olive oil, or brown rice or another grain tossed with toasted pine nuts or almonds (see page 346).

1½ cups water

¾ cup cornmeal, preferably whole grain

½ teaspoon salt (¼ for cornmeal, ¼ for broccoli)

Black pepper to taste

Vegetable oil cooking spray

3 cups canned no-salt-added white beans, drained and rinsed, or cooked (see page 345)

5 teaspoons olive oil

1½ tablespoons chopped fresh sage

2 small cloves garlic

6 cups broccoli florets

1½ cups leeks, very thinly sliced, well washed

1. Preheat the oven to 375°F.

2. Bring the water to a boil in a medium pot. Whisk in the cornmeal, reduce the heat to low, and simmer for 5 minutes, stirring often. Stir in ¼ teaspoon salt and pepper.

3. Coat a 9 x 13-inch baking pan with cooking spray. Pour the cornmeal mixture into the pan.

4. Puree the beans, oil, sage, and garlic in a food processor until smooth, about 1 minute.

5. Using a knife spread the bean mixture over the cornmeal.

6. Coat the broccoli and leeks with cooking spray and toss with ¼ teaspoon salt and pepper. Place the broccoli mixture on top of the beans and bake for 15 minutes. Serve.

PREP TIME: 10 minutes   TOTAL TIME: 35 minutes

PER SERVING, ABOUT: Calories: 265 Protein: 13 g Carbohydrate: 44 g Dietary Fiber: 10 g Sugars: 3 g Total Fat: 5 g Saturated Fat: 1 g Cholesterol: 0 mg Calcium: 146 mg Sodium: 185 mg

Whole Wheat Couscous with Roasted Winter Squash

SERVES 4

YOU CAN MAKE THIS recipe all year long; in winter, use acorn or butternut squash and in the spring or summer, you can use zucchini or yellow squash.

1 acorn squash, cut into 8 pieces, seeds removed

1 onion, peeled and cut into 4 pieces

Vegetable oil cooking spray

³/₄ cup water

1 tablespoon olive oil

¹/₂ cup whole wheat couscous

2 tablespoons dark or golden raisins

1 ¹/₂ cups canned no-salt-added chick peas, drained and rinsed, or cooked (see page 345)

¹/₄ cup chopped fresh mint

¹/₄ cup chopped fresh Italian parsley

2 tablespoons pine nuts

1. Preheat the oven to 375°F. Coat the squash and onion with cooking spray and bake on a sheet pan until the squash is soft, about 30 minutes.

2. Put the water and oil in a medium saucepan and bring to a boil. Stir in the couscous and raisins, cover, and remove from the heat. Keep covered for 5 minutes. Add the chickpeas, mint, and parsley.

3. Serve the couscous with the squash and onion and garnish with the pine nuts.

PREP TIME: 15 minutes   **TOTAL TIME:** 45 minutes

PER SERVING, ABOUT: Calories: 324 Protein: 11 g Carbohydrate: 54 g Dietary Fiber: 12 g Sugars: 7 g Total Fat: 9 g Saturated Fat: 1 g Cholesterol: 0 mg Calcium: 77 mg Sodium: 11 mg

Brown Rice with Pumpkin

SERVES 4

THIS HEARTY DISH MADE with brown rice is not as labor intensive as most risottos, but it's just as tasty.

Vegetable oil cooking spray

1 onion, sliced

1 cup short-grain brown rice

1 tablespoon olive oil

1 cup dry red wine

1/2 cup water

1 cup pumpkin, cooked and pureed (see page 348), or canned, such as Libby's Pure Pumpkin

1 cup canned no-salt-added white beans, drained and rinsed, or cooked (see page 345), and pureed in a food processor for 1 minute

1 teaspoon finely chopped fresh sage

2 cups spinach, well washed

1/4 teaspoon salt

4 tablespoons grated Parmesan

1. Heat a medium pot over medium heat. Coat with cooking spray and add the onion. Cook for 5 minutes. Add the rice and oil and cook for 2 minutes, stirring.

2. Add the wine and water. Bring to a boil, reduce the heat to low, and simmer, covered, for 20 minutes.

3. Add the pumpkin, beans, and sage and cook for 20 minutes, stirring often. Stir in the spinach and salt. Garnish with the Parmesan and serve.

PREP TIME: 13 minutes   **TOTAL TIME:** 1 hour 5 minutes

PER SERVING, ABOUT: Calories: 346 Protein: 11 g Carbohydrate: 57 g Dietary Fiber: 8 g Sugars: 3 g Total Fat: 7 g Saturated Fat: 2 g Cholesterol: 4 mg Calcium: 139 mg Sodium: 238 mg

Cauliflower Curry with Red Lentils

SERVES 4

THIS FLAVORFUL VEGETARIAN CURRY is full of vitamins, minerals, filling fiber, and protein.

Vegetable oil cooking spray

1 onion, sliced

1 teaspoon cumin

1 teaspoon mustard powder

1 tablespoon minced fresh ginger

2 cloves garlic, minced

1/4 teaspoon cayenne (optional)

2 cups chopped fresh tomatoes, or canned no-salt-added tomatoes

4 1/2 cups water

1 1/4 cups red lentils

1/2 teaspoon turmeric

1 teaspoon salt

Black pepper to taste

1 medium head cauliflower, cut into approximately 1-inch pieces

1 cup fresh or frozen peas

4 cups spinach, well washed

1. Heat a large heavy-bottomed stockpot over medium heat. Coat with cooking spray, add the onion, and cook until translucent, about 5 minutes. Add the cumin, mustard powder, ginger, garlic, and cayenne, if desired. Cook for 2 more minutes, stirring constantly.

2. Add the tomatoes, water, lentils, turmeric, salt, and pepper. Cook until the lentils are tender, about 20 minutes.

3. Add the cauliflower. Once the soup simmers, add the peas and spinach. Cook over low heat for about 2 more minutes. Serve.

PREP TIME: 15 minutes   **TOTAL TIME:** 50 minutes

PER SERVING, ABOUT: Calories: 324 Protein: 22 g Carbohydrate: 57 g Dietary Fiber: 14 g Sugars: 9 g Total Fat: 3 g Saturated Fat: 0 g Cholesterol: 0 mg Calcium: 121 mg Sodium: 225 mg

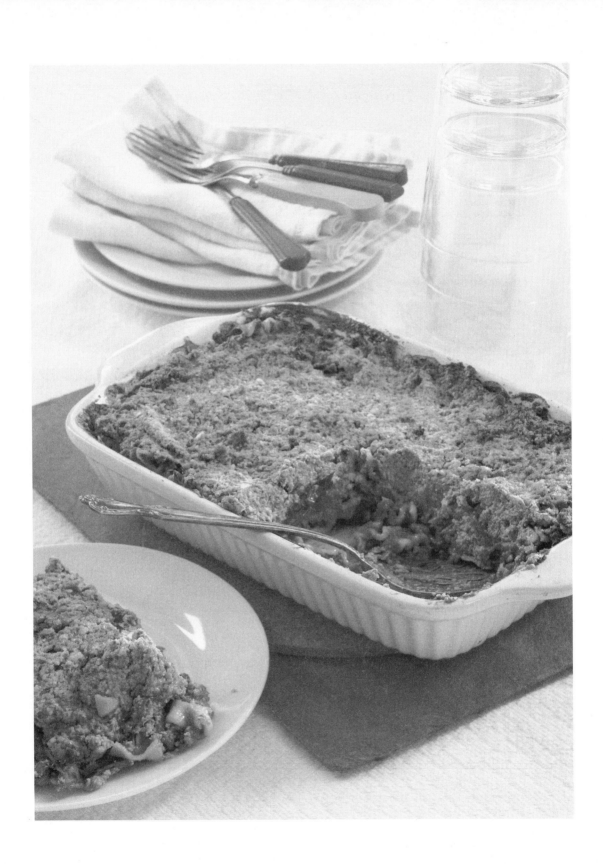

No-Cheese Vegetable Lasagna

SERVES 4

LASAGNA, WITHOUT CHEESE? YOU may be skeptical, but this dish is pure comfort food with less fat and cholesterol and fewer calories than your average lasagna—and you don't even need to precook the lasagna noodles. This is a great recipe to make ahead, store, and reheat before serving. You can also make this with rotini (see variation).

Vegetable oil cooking spray

½ cup almonds

½ cup walnuts

1 onion, thinly sliced

2 cloves garlic, minced

1 cup fresh basil leaves

⅛ teaspoon nutmeg

⅛ teaspoon salt

Black pepper to taste

½ cup water

1 cup marinara sauce, such as Barilla

4 ounces uncooked whole wheat lasagna noodles

2 cups spinach, well washed

2 cups fresh tomatoes, sliced and chopped, or canned no-salt-added diced tomatoes

1. Preheat the oven to 375°F. Coat a 9-inch square (or a 10 x 8-inch) pan with cooking spray.

2. Combine the almonds, walnuts, onion, garlic, basil, nutmeg, salt, pepper, and water in a food processor until smooth, about 1 minute.

3. Spread ½ cup of the marinara sauce on the bottom of the pan. Cover with pieces of uncooked noodles, 1 cup spinach, 1 cup tomatoes, and half of the nut mixture. Repeat the layers again. Bake for 50 minutes, until lightly browned. Serve.

VARIATION: For baked rotini, use 4 ounces fiber-enriched or high-fiber rotini, such as Barilla PLUS or Barilla Whole Grain. (Four ounces is about 1 heaping cup dry.) Cook pasta according to the package directions. In a large bowl combine all the ingredients except the marinara sauce. Cover the bottom of the pan with ½ cup marinara sauce, top with the pasta mixture, and finish with ½ cup marinara sauce spread over the pasta mixture. Bake for 40 minutes or until lightly browned. Serve.

PREP TIME: 15 minutes   **TOTAL TIME:** 1 hour 5 minutes

PER SERVING, ABOUT: Calories: 360 Protein: 13 g Carbohydrate: 37 g Dietary Fiber: 5 g Sugars: 4 g Total Fat: 21 g Saturated Fat: 2 g Cholesterol: 0 mg Calcium: 137 mg Sodium: 278 mg

Baked Beans on Grits

SERVES 4

THIS RECIPE IS THE perfect example of slimmed-down food that tastes as good as the full-fat version. Get ready to dig in.

3 cups cooking greens, such as collard greens, turnip greens, or kale, julienned

2 cups canned no-salt-added white beans, drained and rinsed, or cooked (see page 345)

2 carrots, peeled and sliced

1 apple, grated on the large holes of a grater

1 onion, finely chopped

¼ cup tomato paste

¼ cup molasses

2 teaspoons dry mustard

¼ teaspoon salt (⅛ for baked beans, ⅛ for corn grits)

Vegetable oil cooking spray

2 cups water

¾ cup corn grits

4 teaspoons extra virgin olive oil

1. Preheat the oven to 375°F.

2. Combine the greens, beans, carrots, apple, onion, tomato paste, molasses, mustard, and ⅛ teaspoon salt in a large bowl.

3. Coat an 8-inch square baking dish with cooking spray. Place the bean mixture in the baking dish.

4. Bake, covered, for 45 minutes.

5. Bring the water to a boil in a medium pot. Stir the grits, oil, and a heaping ⅛ teaspoon salt into the boiling water. Stir continuously, and cook until very thick, following the grits package directions.

6. Coat a 9-inch pie plate with cooking spray. Pour the grits onto the pie plate and let sit for about 10 minutes, until set. Slice into 4 pieces and serve topped with the baked bean mixture.

PREP TIME: 15 minutes   TOTAL TIME: 1 hour

PER SERVING, ABOUT: Calories: 364 Protein: 13 g Carbohydrate: 77 g Dietary Fiber: 10 g Sugars: 20 g Total Fat: 1 g Saturated Fat: 0 g Cholesterol: 0 mg Calcium: 196 mg Sodium: 200 mg

Side Dishes

GRAINS

Quinoa and Grapefruit

SERVES 4

THIS REFRESHING DISH, WHICH is both tart and sweet thanks to the grapefruit, delivers vitamin C and antioxidants.

³/₄ cup quinoa, rinsed

1 red or pink grapefruit, sectioned (see page 346)

2 tablespoons finely chopped green onions (scallions)

1 tablespoon olive oil

¹/₂ cup chopped fresh herbs, such as sorrel, Italian parsley, mint, or a mix of these

¹/₈ teaspoon salt

Black pepper to taste

24 sprays Wish-Bone Red Wine Vinaigrette Spritzer, or 2 tablespoons olive oil and 1 tablespoon red wine vinegar

1. Place the quinoa in a medium pot and cover with water. Bring to a boil and cook until the quinoa starts to get translucent around the edge, about 5 minutes. Drain the quinoa.

2. Combine the quinoa, grapefruit, green onions, oil, herbs, salt, and pepper in a medium bowl.

3. Add the dressing, toss gently, and serve.

   PREP TIME: 10 minutes   **TOTAL TIME:** 20 minutes

PER SERVING, ABOUT: Calories: 183 Protein: 5 g Carbohydrate: 28 g Dietary Fiber: 3 g Sugars: 5 g Total Fat: 5 g Saturated Fat: 1 g Cholesterol: 0 mg Calcium: 38 mg Sodium: 133 mg

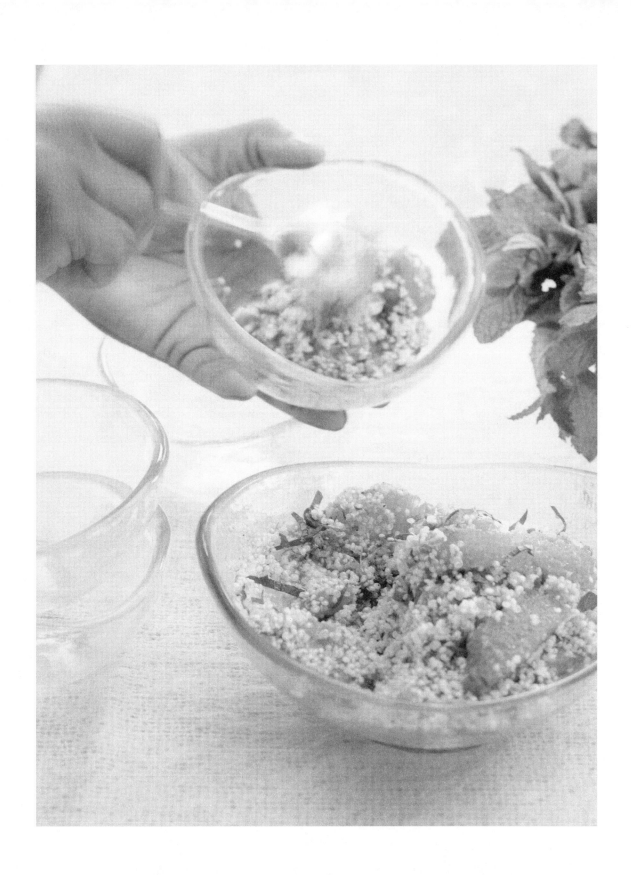

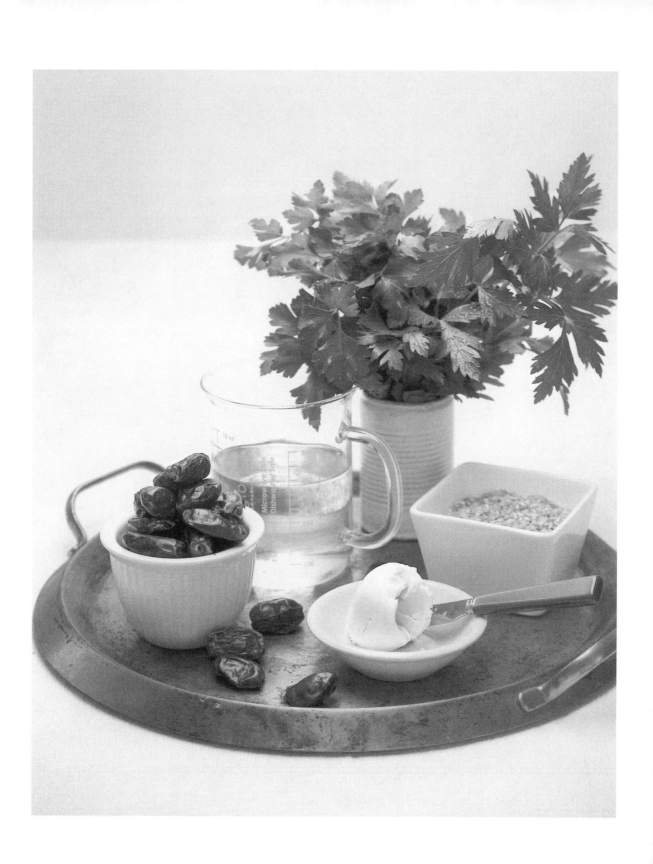

Brown Rice with Dates

SERVES 4

BROWN RICE TAKES 25 minutes longer to cook than white, but it's well worth the time because of its superior nutrition profile (more B vitamins, fiber, and phytonutrients). In this recipe, the sweetness of dates heightens the rich flavor of the rice.

1 cup brown rice

1½ cups water

4 dates, pits removed, and chopped

⅛ teaspoon salt

1 tablespoon healthy spread, such as Smart Balance Buttery Spread

¼ cup chopped fresh Italian parsley

Black pepper to taste

1. Place the rice, water, dates, salt, and spread in a medium pot. Bring to a boil. Stir and reduce the heat to low. Simmer, covered, for 30 minutes. Turn off the heat and leave covered for an additional 10 minutes.

2. Stir in the parsley and pepper. Serve.

   PREP TIME: 5 minutes   **TOTAL TIME:** 50 minutes

PER SERVING, ABOUT: Calories: 217 Protein: 4 g Carbohydrate: 43 g Dietary Fiber: 2 g Sugars: 5 g Total Fat: 4 g Saturated Fat: 1 g Cholesterol: 0 mg Calcium: 26 mg Sodium: 101 mg

Cracked Wheat with Golden Raisins and Pumpkin Seeds

SERVES 4

YOU'LL LOVE THIS SWEET and nutty-tasting side dish; it complements almost all poultry and seafood dishes.

1 cup cracked wheat

¼ cup golden raisins

¼ cup hulled pumpkin seeds

1 tablespoon olive oil

2 tablespoons finely chopped green onions (scallions)

⅛ teaspoon salt

Black pepper to taste

1. Place the cracked wheat and raisins in a medium pot and cover with water. Bring to a boil and drain immediately.

2. Place the cracked wheat in a bowl, toss with the pumpkin seeds, oil, green onions, salt, and pepper, and serve.

   PREP TIME: 10 minutes   **TOTAL TIME:** 15 minutes

PER SERVING, ABOUT: Calories: 219 Protein: 7 g Carbohydrate: 34 g Dietary Fiber: 5 g Sugars: 6 g Total Fat: 8 g Saturated Fat: 1 g Cholesterol: 0 mg Calcium: 22 mg Sodium: 77 mg

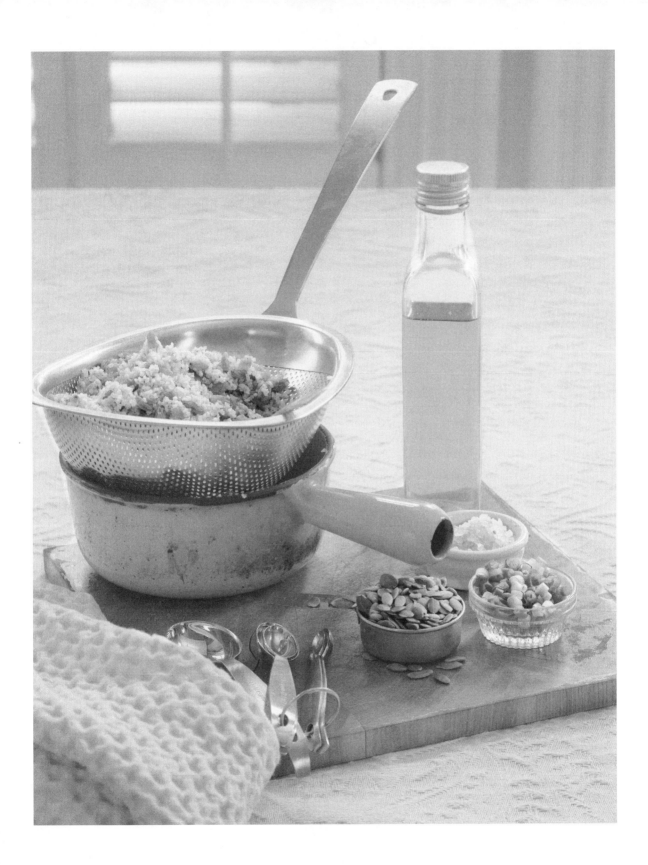

Barley and Mushrooms

SERVES 4

MUSHROOMS ARE LOADED WITH nutrients, such as heart-healthy copper and cancer-fighting selenium, and are also good sources of beneficial phytonutrients called polyphenols. The shiitake mushroom used in this recipe has a meaty texture and delicate earthy flavor that stands out in this dish.

³/₄ cup barley

1 tablespoon olive oil

¹/₂ onion, sliced

2 cups sliced shiitake mushrooms

1 teaspoon minced fresh sage

1 teaspoon minced fresh rosemary

2 tablespoons sherry vinegar

¹/₈ teaspoon salt

Black pepper to taste

1. Place the barley in a medium saucepan and cover with water. Bring to a boil. Reduce the heat to low and simmer. Cook until the barley is soft, about 15 minutes. Drain the barley, place in a bowl, and toss with oil. Set aside.

2. Heat a medium heavy-bottomed skillet over medium heat. Add the onion and mushrooms and cook, for about 5 minutes, stirring often. Add the sage and rosemary and continue cooking for an additional 5 minutes.

3. Combine the barley with the mushroom mixture. Add the vinegar, salt, and pepper and serve.

PREP TIME: 10 minutes   **TOTAL TIME:** 30 minutes

PER SERVING, ABOUT: Calories: 174 Protein: 6 g Carbohydrate: 30 g Dietary Fiber: 7 g Sugars: 2 g Total Fat: 4 g Saturated Fat: 1 g Cholesterol: 0 mg Calcium: 26 mg Sodium: 80 mg

Steel-Cut Oats "Polenta"

SERVES 4

OATS ARE NOT JUST for breakfast! With this delicious side dish, you'll score a healthy dose of B vitamins, calcium, protein, and fiber. You can also use old-fashioned oats, just cook according to the package directions.

1 cup steel-cut oats, such as Quaker	⅛ teaspoon salt
1 tablespoon olive oil	Black pepper to taste
1 tablespoon chopped fresh sage	Vegetable oil cooking spray

1. Cook the oats according to the package directions with the addition of oil and sage. When the oats are finished cooking, stir in the salt and pepper.

2. Coat a 9-inch pie plate with cooking spray. Pour the oats onto the plate and let sit until cool. Slice into 4 wedges.

3. Heat a medium heavy-bottomed skillet over medium heat. Coat the skillet with cooking spray, place oat cakes in skillet and cook until they are browned on each side, about 3 minutes per side. Serve.

PREP TIME: 5 minutes

TOTAL TIME: 30 minutes, depending on if you use quick or regular steel-cut oats

PER SERVING, ABOUT: Calories: 192 Protein: 6 g Carbohydrate: 27 g Dietary Fiber: 8 g Sugars: 0 g Total Fat: 6 g Saturated Fat: 1 g Cholesterol: 0 mg Calcium: 28 mg Sodium: 73 mg

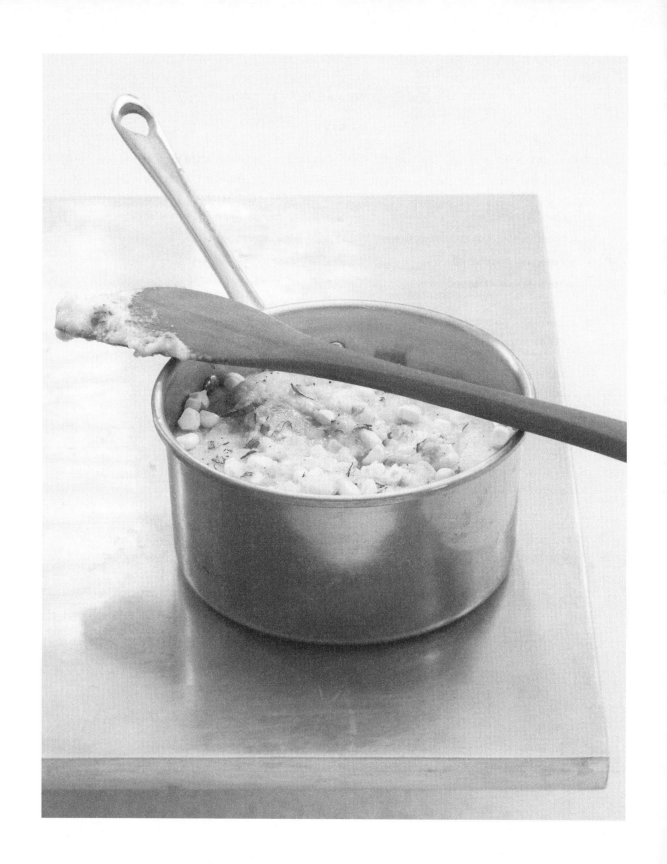

Corn Pudding

SERVES 4

THIS DISH LOOKS AND tastes creamy and indulgent, but it's a virtually fat-free rendition of the normally high-calorie side.

1 cup water

1 cup almond, soy, or fat-free milk

½ cup cornmeal, preferably whole grain

2 teaspoons chopped fresh sage

1 cup corn, cut off the cob, or frozen

⅛ teaspoon salt

Black pepper to taste

1. Bring the water and milk to a boil in a medium pot. Add the cornmeal, whisking the whole time you are adding it. Add the sage.

2. Reduce the heat to low and simmer for 5 minutes, stirring continuously. Add the corn, salt, and pepper. Serve.

PREP TIME: 5 minutes **TOTAL TIME:** 15 minutes

PER SERVING, ABOUT: Calories: 133 Protein: 5 g Carbohydrate: 27 g Dietary Fiber: 2 g
Sugars: 2 g Total Fat: 1 g Saturated Fat: 0 g Cholesterol: 1 mg Calcium: 95 mg Sodium: 116 mg

Wild Rice with Celery and Carrot

SERVES 4

WILD RICE HAS A unique, nutty, and delicious flavor. You can serve this dish hot, at room temperature, or as a cold salad.

1 cup uncooked wild rice	¼ teaspoon finely chopped fresh sage
2 cups cold water	1 tablespoon olive oil
1 stalk celery, chopped	⅛ teaspoon salt
1 carrot, peeled and chopped	Black pepper to taste

1. Rinse the rice with cold water.

2. Put the rice and cold water into a medium pot. Bring to a boil. Cook for 1 minute. Reduce the heat to low, cover, and cook for 30 minutes. When done, drain off any excess water using a strainer.

3. Stir in the celery, carrot, sage, oil, salt, and pepper. Serve.

PREP TIME: 5 minutes   **TOTAL TIME:** 40 minutes

PER SERVING, ABOUT: Calories: 181 Protein: 6 g Carbohydrate: 32 g Dietary Fiber: 3 g Sugars: 2 g Total Fat: 4 g Saturated Fat: 1 g Cholesterol: 0 mg Calcium: 18 mg Sodium: 94 mg

Olive Oil Roasted Potatoes

SERVES 4

THESE CRISPY ROASTED POTATOES seasoned with olive oil and fresh rosemary are a delicious way to prepare America's favorite vegetable.

3 cups sliced potatoes ($\frac{1}{2}$-inch cubes)	1 tablespoon fresh rosemary
2 tablespoons olive oil	$\frac{1}{8}$ teaspoon salt
4 cloves garlic	Black pepper to taste

1. Preheat the oven to 375°F with a sheet pan in the oven.

2. Toss all the ingredients together in a large bowl.

3. Once the oven and pan are hot, remove the pan from the oven, and quickly place the potato mixture on the pan.

4. Return the pan to the oven and cook until the potatoes are golden brown, about 15 minutes, stirring every 5 minutes. Serve.

PREP TIME: 5 minutes   **TOTAL TIME:** 20 minutes

PER SERVING, ABOUT: Calories: 154 Protein: 3 g Carbohydrate: 21 g Dietary Fiber: 2 g Sugars: 1 g Total Fat: 7 g Saturated Fat: 1 g Cholesterol: 0 mg Calcium: 22 mg Sodium: 79 mg

Whole Wheat Couscous Pilaf

SERVES 4

WHOLE WHEAT COUSCOUS IS an excellent and underutilized grain. It has all the benefits of a whole grain, is extremely quick to prepare, and is very versatile. If you can't find whole wheat couscous, you can use just about any whole grain, such as brown rice, cracked wheat, barley, or quinoa.

1½ cups water

1 cup whole wheat couscous

1 tablespoon olive oil

1 cup chopped fresh basil, parsley, and sorrel

⅛ teaspoon salt

1. Bring the water to a boil in a medium pot. Stir in the couscous, cover, remove from the heat, and let stand for 5 minutes.

2. Fluff the couscous with a fork while seasoning with oil, herbs, and salt. Serve hot, at room temperature, or cold.

PREP TIME: 5 minutes   **TOTAL TIME:** 15 minutes

PER SERVING, ABOUT: Calories: 296 Protein: 9 g Carbohydrate: 50 g Dietary Fiber: 9 g Sugars: 3 g Total Fat: 8 g Saturated Fat: 1 g Cholesterol: 0 mg Calcium: 58 mg Sodium: 87 mg

Couscous Tabbouleh

SERVES 4

THIS GRAIN SALAD IS especially delicious midsummer when tomatoes and mint are at their peak. The combination of tomatoes, mint, and parsley works in a familiar but fresh way with the addition of rice wine vinegar and whole wheat couscous. If you cannot find whole wheat couscous, you can prepare this dish with cracked wheat (the traditional ingredient for this dish), brown rice, or barley.

³/₄ cup water	1 cup chopped fresh Italian parsley
³/₄ cup whole wheat couscous	2 tablespoons chopped fresh mint
2 cups chopped tomatoes	2 tablespoons olive oil
2 tablespoons finely chopped chives	¹/₈ teaspoon salt
¹/₄ cup rice wine vinegar	Black pepper to taste

1. Bring the water to a boil in a medium pot. Stir in the couscous. Remove from the heat and cover for 5 minutes.

2. Put the couscous in a large bowl. Gently fluff with a fork. Toss in the tomatoes, chives, vinegar, parsley, mint, oil, salt, and pepper. Serve at room temperature or cold.

PREP TIME: 10 minutes   **TOTAL TIME:** 15 minutes

PER SERVING, ABOUT: Calories: 296 Protein: 9 g Carbohydrate: 50 g Dietary Fiber: 9 g Sugars: 3 g Total Fat: 8 g Saturated Fat: 1 g Cholesterol: 0 mg Calcium: 58 mg Sodium: 87 mg

VEGETABLES

Roasted Root Vegetables

SERVES 4

YOU PROBABLY DON'T EAT turnips and rutabagas very often, but after tasting this dish—a vastly more interesting version of French fries—these vegetables may become staples! As well they should; like broccoli, they are cruciferous vegetables full of potent anti-cancer compounds.

4 parsnips, peeled, cored, and chopped into long ¼-inch-thick strips

1 rutabaga, peeled and sliced into ¼-inch-thick pieces

2 medium turnips, peeled and sliced into ½-inch-thick pieces

2 medium carrots, peeled and sliced into long ½-inch-thick pieces

Vegetable oil cooking spray

2 teaspoons chopped fresh rosemary

⅛ teaspoon salt

Black pepper to taste

1. Preheat the oven to 375°F.

2. Lightly coat the vegetables with cooking spray and toss with the rosemary in a large bowl.

3. Place the vegetables on a sheet pan and place in the oven. Bake until browned, about 20 minutes, tossing regularly.

4. Remove from the oven and season with salt and pepper. Serve.

PREP TIME: 15 minutes   **TOTAL TIME:** 35 minutes

PER SERVING, ABOUT: Calories: 144 Protein: 3 g Carbohydrate: 34 g Dietary Fiber: 8 g Sugars: 11 g Total Fat: 1 g Saturated Fat: 0 g Cholesterol: 0 mg Calcium: 89 mg Sodium: 151 mg

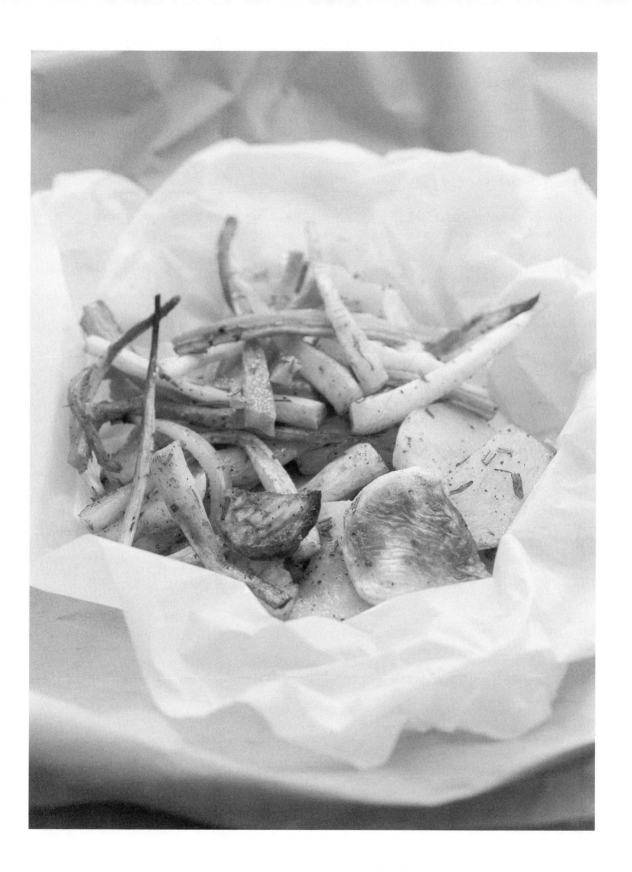

Roasted Beets with Horseradish

SERVES 4

THIS VERSION OF THE familiar combination of beets and horseradish is simple to prepare and full of flavor.

2 large beets, peeled, cut into ¼-inch-round slices, and halved

1 onion, chopped

Vegetable oil cooking spray

2 teaspoons fresh chopped thyme

1 teaspoon grated horseradish, or more to taste

⅛ teaspoon salt

Black pepper to taste

1. Preheat the oven to 375°F.

2. Heat a large heavy-bottomed ovenproof skillet over medium heat.

3. Lightly coat the beets and onion with cooking spray.

4. Add the beets and onion to the hot skillet and cook for 10 minutes, stirring often.

5. Add the thyme and place the skillet in the oven. Cook until tender, about 15 minutes.

6. Remove the skillet from the oven and toss the contents with horseradish, salt, and pepper. Serve.

PREP TIME: 5 minutes   **TOTAL TIME:** 30 minutes

PER SERVING, ABOUT: Calories: 46 Protein: 1 g Carbohydrate: 11 g Dietary Fiber: 2 g Sugars: 7 g Total Fat: 0 g Saturated Fat: 0 g Cholesterol: 0 mg Calcium: 27 mg Sodium: 112 mg

Mashed Celery Root

SERVES 4

THE FRESH FLAVOR AND rich mashed texture of celery root pair well with lots of different main dishes. Try this instead of mashed potatoes.

2 celery roots, peeled and chopped into 1-inch chunks

1 tablespoon olive oil

4 cloves roasted garlic (see page 344)

2 tablespoons chopped fresh parsley

Heaping ⅛ teaspoon salt

Black pepper to taste

1. Place the celery roots in a medium pot, cover with water, and bring to a boil. Cook until tender, about 25 minutes.

2. Drain the celery roots and place in a food processor with the oil, garlic, parsley, salt, and pepper. Puree and serve.

PREP TIME: 10 minutes   TOTAL TIME: 35 minutes

PER SERVING, ABOUT: Calories: 126 Protein: 3 g Carbohydrate: 21 g Dietary Fiber: 4 g
Sugars: 4 g Total Fat: 4 g Saturated Fat: 1 g Cholesterol: 0 mg Calcium: 101 mg Sodium: 301 mg

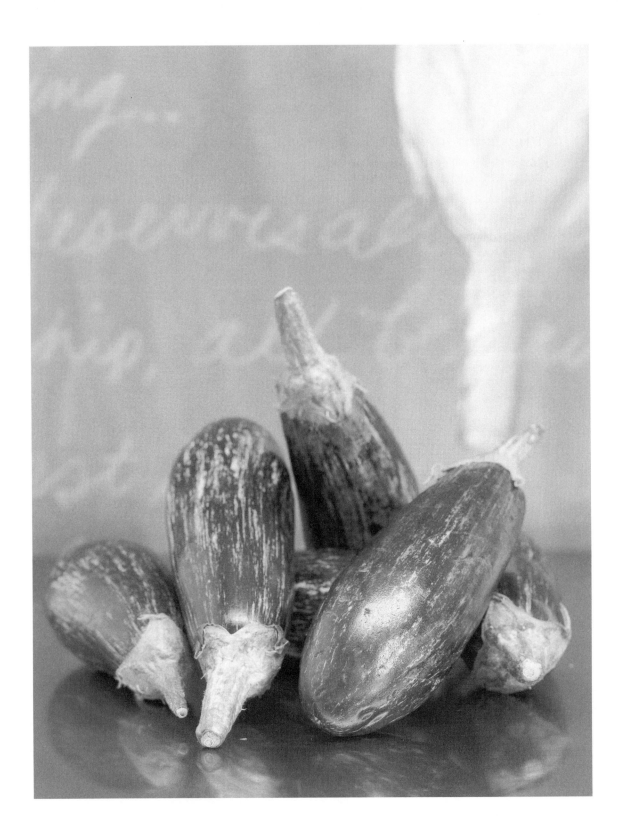

Roasted Eggplant

SERVES 4

IN THE SUMMER, MANY farmers' markets (as well as supermarkets throughout the year) carry a large selection of delicious eggplant varieties. This recipe is a great opportunity to experiment with different kinds, as it works well with all of them.

1½ pounds eggplant, sliced into ½-inch-thick pieces (cut large eggplants into rounds; if small, cut in half or in quarters lengthwise)

1 onion, sliced

8 cloves garlic, unpeeled

Vegetable oil cooking spray

¼ teaspoon salt

Black pepper to taste

1.   Preheat the oven to 375°F.

2.   Coat the eggplant, onion, and garlic with cooking spray.

3.   Place the vegetables on a baking sheet and roast until they are soft, about 15 minutes.

4.   Remove from the oven. Remove the garlic and set aside.

5.   Toss the eggplant and onion with salt and pepper.

6.   When the garlic is cool enough to touch, peel off the skin and the center core and add it to the eggplant. Serve.

PREP TIME: 10 minutes   **TOTAL TIME:** 25 minutes

PER SERVING, ABOUT: Calories: 62 Protein: 2 g Carbohydrate: 15 g Dietary Fiber: 6 g Sugars: 5 g Total Fat: 0 g Saturated Fat: 0 g Cholesterol: 0 mg Calcium: 32 mg Sodium: 151 mg

Roasted Broccoli with Balsamic Vinegar

SERVES 4

ROASTING BROCCOLI AT A high temperature results in a delicious side dish of one of the healthiest foods in existence. Broccoli is available throughout the year but if you get a chance, buy it in season (to find out when various produce is in season, see page 186) from your local farmers' market.

1 broccoli head, broken into approximately 1-inch florets

Vegetable oil cooking spray

4 cloves roasted garlic (see page 344)

⅛ teaspoon salt

2 tablespoons balsamic vinegar

1. Heat the oven to broil.

2. Coat the broccoli with cooking spray and place on a sheet pan. Cook in the oven for 4 minutes, stirring after 2 minutes. Toss the broccoli with the garlic, salt, and vinegar. Serve.

PREP TIME: 5 minutes   **TOTAL TIME:** 10 minutes

PER SERVING, ABOUT: Calories: 51 Protein: 3 g Carbohydrate: 10 g Dietary Fiber: 3 g Sugars: 3 g Total Fat: 0 g Saturated Fat: 0 g Cholesterol: 0 mg Calcium: 61 mg Sodium: 113 mg

Raw Garlicky Kale

SERVES 4

THIS IS A GREAT way to eat your greens! These simple ingredients combine to make a remarkable dish. It's such a favorite that you'll find it more than once in the meal plans.

2 tablespoons tahini

4 cloves roasted garlic (see page 344)

2 tablespoons cider vinegar

1 tablespoon water

⅛ teaspoon salt

Fresh hot red pepper to taste

4 cups raw kale, cut into extremely thin strips lengthwise, well washed

1. Combine the tahini, garlic, vinegar, water, salt, and hot pepper in a food processor and puree until smooth, about 1 minute.

2. Toss the kale and tahini dressing together. Serve immediately or refrigerate for several hours before serving.

PREP TIME: 10 minutes   TOTAL TIME: 10 minutes

PER SERVING, ABOUT: Calories: 87 Protein: 4 g Carbohydrate: 10 g Dietary Fiber: 2 g
Sugars: 0 g Total Fat: 5 g Saturated Fat: 1 g Cholesterol: 0 mg Calcium: 173 mg Sodium: 103 mg

Brussels Sprouts with Sesame Seeds

SERVES 4

MANY PEOPLE STEER CLEAR of Brussels sprouts because the veggie omits a sulfur smell if overcooked. But cook it right, as in this recipe, and you'll be rewarded with a crunchy, slightly nutty taste.

2 cups Brussels sprouts, cut in half	1 tablespoon sesame seeds
Vegetable oil cooking spray	1 teaspoon rice wine vinegar
1 teaspoon sesame oil	$\frac{1}{8}$ teaspoon salt

1. Heat a large heavy-bottomed skillet over medium heat.

2. Coat the Brussels sprouts with cooking spray. Place the sprouts cut side down in the skillet and cook until they just start to brown, about 3 minutes. If the sprouts are small, remove from the skillet; if they are large, turn over and cook the other side for 2 more minutes.

3. Put the sprouts in a large bowl and toss with the oil, sesame seeds, vinegar, and salt. Serve.

PREP TIME: 5 minutes   **TOTAL TIME:** 10 minutes

PER SERVING, ABOUT: Calories: 49 Protein: 2 g Carbohydrate: 5 g Dietary Fiber: 2 g
Sugars: 1 g Total Fat: 3 g Saturated Fat: 0 g Cholesterol: 0 mg Calcium: 22 mg Sodium: 85 mg

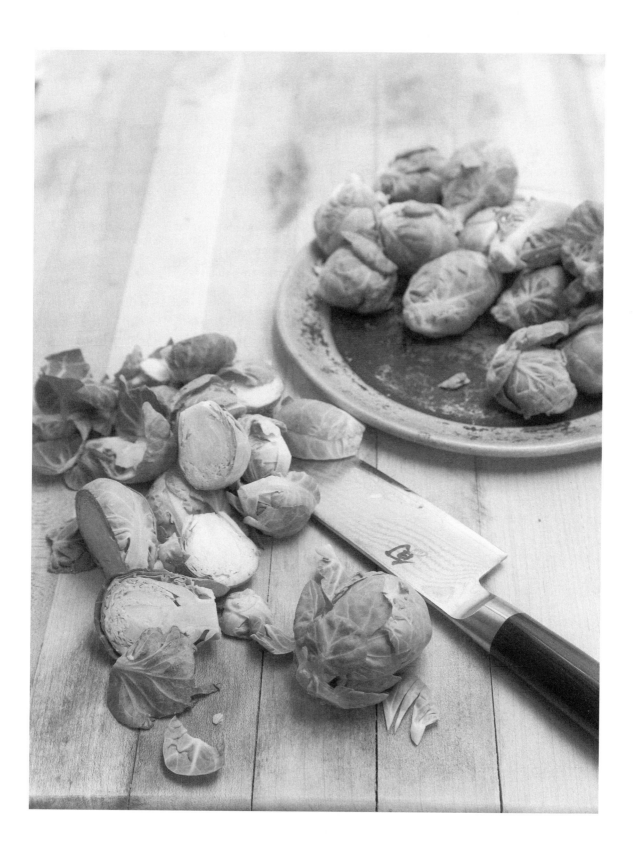

Okra, Corn, and Leek

SERVES 4

FRESH, SEASONAL OKRA IS a real treat! In fact, this recipe might even make you a convert if you think you don't like okra. Roasting the okra, as you do with this dish, produces a crisp vegetable instead of the slimy consistency you get when you slow-cook it.

1 leek, thinly sliced, well washed

Vegetable oil cooking spray

2 cups fresh okra, sliced in half lengthwise

½ cup fresh corn, cut off the cob, or frozen

⅛ teaspoon salt

Black pepper to taste

1. Heat a large heavy-bottomed skillet over medium-high heat.

2. Coat the leek with cooking spray and cook in the skillet for 5 minutes, stirring regularly.

3. Coat the okra with cooking spray, add to the skillet, and cook until the okra is browned, about 5 minutes, stirring regularly.

4. Add the corn and cook for an additional 3 minutes. Season with salt and pepper and serve.

PREP TIME: 7 minutes   **TOTAL TIME:** 20 minutes

PER SERVING, ABOUT: Calories: 56 Protein: 2 g Carbohydrate: 12 g Dietary Fiber: 3 g
Sugars: 2 g Total Fat: 1 g Saturated Fat: 0 g Cholesterol: 0 mg Calcium: 55 mg Sodium: 82 mg

Green Beans with Ginger and Garlic

SERVES 4

THIS IS A FANTASTIC way to prepare green beans. You can also try leaving out the ginger and adding fresh herbs, such as thyme.

Vegetable oil cooking spray

1 tablespoon minced fresh garlic

1 tablespoon minced fresh ginger

1 pound green beans, stem ends removed

Red pepper flakes to taste (optional)

⅛ teaspoon salt

1. Heat a large skillet over medium heat and coat with cooking spray. Add the garlic and ginger and cook for 3 minutes, stirring often.

2. Coat the green beans with cooking spray. Turn the heat up to high and add the green beans and red pepper flakes, if desired. Cook until the beans are slightly browned and slightly soft but still crunchy, 3 to 6 minutes, depending on the size of the beans, tossing continuously.

3. Remove the beans from the pan, season with salt, and serve.

PREP TIME: 5 minutes   **TOTAL TIME:** 15 minutes

PER SERVING, ABOUT: Calories: 40 Protein: 2 g Carbohydrate: 9 g Dietary Fiber: 4 g
Sugars: 2 g Total Fat: 0 g Saturated Fat: 0 g Cholesterol: 0 mg Calcium: 46 mg Sodium: 80 mg

WHAT'S IN SEASON?

People tell me that they *know* they should be eating more fruits and vegetables, but they just don't *like* them. Whenever I hear this, I have to wonder if they've ever had a really good tomato, peach, plum, carrot, or other produce picked that day, at peak ripeness? Buying seasonally, and even better, locally (which, by definition, is seasonal), can mean the difference between a fragrant, juicy, succulent peach and a dry, airy one. Even garlic and onions taste better when they're fresh.

Of course, it's not always possible to buy locally; farmers' markets are bare in the winter in colder climates, and some products, such as grapes, are rarely grown locally. (The closest to local are California grapes, which are around from May through December.) But during the spring through fall, if you're lucky enough to have a farmers' market in your area, or to grow your own produce, I can guarantee that your vegetable-hating days will be over! Another option: community supported agriculture (CSA); you pay a fee to a local farm and get regular deliveries of fruits and vegetables throughout the growing season. To find farmers' markets and CSAs in your area, go to www.localharvest.org. If there are none nearby, try your supermarket; it may have a local produce section.

Buying locally offers benefits beyond taste. Local produce is more nutritious because it's fresher; fruits and vegetables lose vitamins every day after they're picked. When produce is trucked across the country, it can be many days before it's delivered to your grocery store. Not to mention, all that shipping pollutes the air; buy locally and you'll help cut back on pollution.

Before heading to the farmers' market, take a look at some of the recipes in this book and make a shopping list. Dishes such as Tomato, Cucumber, and Mint Salad (page 64) will be fabulous in August and September when local tomatoes are ripest. And July and August, when peaches are peaking, would be a great time to try the Pecan-Crusted Trout with Peaches (page 140). You don't have to guess the best season for the Beef Stew with Winter Root Vegetables (page 55).

To help you figure out what's in season when, use the following chart. You'll notice that some veggies have more than one season—always a plus. This list will also help you figure out what's *not* in season; which explains why imported tomatoes are so expensive in the winter, or apples taste a little old in the summer. Note: This is just a starter list; feel free to poke around farmers' markets; you may discover produce you've never seen before.

SPRING (March, April, May)	**SUMMER** (June, July, Aug.)	**FALL** (Sept.,Oct.,Nov.)	**WINTER** (Dec., Jan., Feb.)
FRUITS			
Honeydew Melons, Oranges, Strawberries	Apricots, Blackberries, Blueberries, Cantaloupes, Cherries, Figs, Grapes, Honeydew Melons, Nectarines, Peaches, Plums, Raspberries, Strawberries, Watermelon	Apples, Cranberries, Grapes, Huckleberries, Pears, Persimmons, Pomegranates	Apples, Dates, Grapefruits, Oranges, Pears, Persimmons, Red Currants, Tangerines
VEGETABLES			
Artichokes, Asparagus, Broccoli, Collard Greens, Fennel, Fiddlehead Ferns, Morel Mushrooms, Mustard Greens, Snow Peas, Spinach, Sugar Snap Peas, Swiss Chard, Vidalia Onions, Watercress	Beets, Bell Peppers, Cucumbers, Eggplant, Garlic, Green Beans, Green Peas, Lima Beans, Okra, Radishes, Sweet Corn, Tomatoes, Zucchini	Acorn Squash, Bok Choy, Broccoli, Butternut Squash, Cauliflower, Celery Root, Garlic, Ginger, Mushrooms, Parsnips, Pumpkins, Rutabagas, Sweet Potatoes, Swiss Chard, Turnips	Bok Choy, Brussels Sprouts, Chestnuts, Kale, Leeks, Mushrooms, Parsnips, Rutabagas, Sweet Potatoes, Turnips, Winter Squash

Sugar Snap Peas with Peanut Dressing

SERVES 4

DELICIOUS RAW SUGAR SNAP PEAS are enhanced by a tasty dressing made of peanut butter. You'll find that the richness of the peanut butter combined with the freshness of a salad really hit the spot.

3 tablespoons peanut butter, such as
  Smart Balance

3 tablespoons freshly squeezed orange
  juice

1 tablespoon water

¼ teaspoon grated fresh ginger (optional)

⅛ teaspoon salt

3 cups sugar snap peas

1 cup sprouts, any type (if sprouts aren't
  available, use 1 cup baby greens or
  chopped romaine)

1. Combine the peanut butter, orange juice, water, ginger, if desired, and salt in a food processor and puree until smooth, about 1 minute.

2. Put the peas and sprouts in a large bowl and dress with the peanut butter dressing. Serve.

Optional: Garnish with 2 teaspoons shredded orange peel.

PREP TIME: 5 minutes   **TOTAL TIME:** 5 minutes

PER SERVING, ABOUT: Calories: 104 Protein: 5 g Carbohydrate: 9 g Dietary Fiber: 3 g Sugars: 4 g Total Fat: 6 g Saturated Fat: 1 g Cholesterol: 0 mg Calcium: 30 mg Sodium: 78 mg

Marinated Mushrooms

SERVES 4

THIS SIMPLE SIDE IS full of minerals and antioxidants from the mushrooms.

4 cups sliced button mushrooms

Juice of 1 lemon

½ cup diced chives

1 tablespoon olive oil

⅛ teaspoon salt

Place the mushrooms in a medium bowl and toss with the other ingredients. Serve.

PREP TIME: 5 minutes   **TOTAL TIME:** 5 minutes

PER SERVING, ABOUT: Calories: 50 Protein: 2 g Carbohydrate: 4 g Dietary Fiber: 1 g
Sugars: 2 g Total Fat: 4 g Saturated Fat: 1 g Cholesterol: 0 mg Calcium: 9 mg Sodium: 77 mg

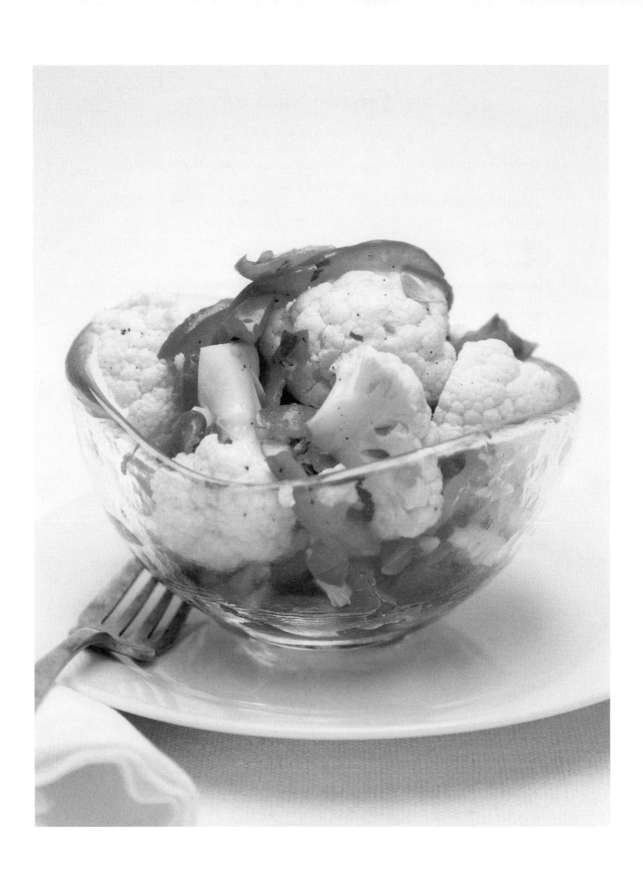

Pickled Cauliflower

SERVES 4

THIS QUICK PICKLING RECIPE makes a delicious side dish that is tasty over greens or as a complement to a variety of main dishes. Pickling is a great way to add variety to the preparation of standard vegetables.

1 cup red wine vinegar

2 cups water

1 tablespoon fresh oregano, or
   2 teaspoons dried

2 bay leaves

2 cloves garlic, minced

1 head cauliflower, cut into florets

1 red pepper, seeded and thinly sliced

1 tablespoon olive oil

⅛ teaspoon salt

Black pepper to taste

1. Bring the vinegar, water, oregano, bay leaves, and garlic to a boil in a large pot.

2. Add the cauliflower and red pepper and return to a full boil. Cover and cook for 1 minute.

3. Remove from the heat and let the vegetables cool in the hot liquid. Remove the vegetables from the cooking liquid and season with the oil, salt, and pepper. Serve.

PREP TIME: 5 minutes   **TOTAL TIME:** 20 minutes

PER SERVING, ABOUT: Calories: 91 Protein: 3 g Carbohydrate: 11 g Dietary Fiber: 5 g
Sugars: 5 g Total Fat: 4 g Saturated Fat: 1 g Cholesterol: 0 mg Calcium: 57 mg Sodium: 122 mg

Shredded Zucchini and Carrots

SERVES 4

ALTHOUGH THIS SALAD CAN be enjoyed year-round, try it in midsummer when zucchini is plentiful and tasty. The dressing acts as a marinade to bring out the delicious fresh taste of the raw vegetables.

2 zucchinis, shredded using a hand grater or with the grater attachment on a food processor

2 carrots, shredded using a hand grater or with the grater attachment on a food processor

2 tablespoons finely chopped red onion

1/4 teaspoon finely chopped fresh sage

2 tablespoons cider vinegar

1 tablespoon olive oil

1 tablespoon honey

1/8 teaspoon salt

1. Combine the zucchini, carrots, red onion, and sage in a large bowl.

2. Mix the vinegar, oil, honey, and salt in a small bowl until smooth.

3. Dress the zucchini mixture with the vinegar mixture and serve.

PREP TIME: 10 minutes   TOTAL TIME: 10 minutes

PER SERVING, ABOUT: Calories: 77 Protein: 2 g Carbohydrate: 11 g Dietary Fiber: 2 g Sugars: 8 g Total Fat: 4 g Saturated Fat: 1 g Cholesterol: 0 mg Calcium: 27 mg Sodium: 104 mg

Calcium-Rich Snacks

Spicy Wasa Melt

SERVES 1

AN UNEXPECTED TOUCH OF hot spice makes for an out-of-the-ordinary between-meal bite.

2 crispbreads, such as Wasa (any variety with the Best Life seal)

Red pepper flakes to taste

⅓ cup shredded part-skim mozzarella

1. Heat the oven or toaster oven to broil.

2. Top the crispbreads with cheese and sprinkle with red pepper flakes. Place in the oven until the cheese is melted, about 2 minutes. Serve.

PREP TIME: 3 minutes   TOTAL TIME: 5 minutes

PER SERVING, ABOUT: Calories: 154 Protein: 12 g Carbohydrate: 11 g Dietary Fiber: 2 g Sugars: 1 g Total Fat: 7 g Saturated Fat: 4 g Cholesterol: 27 mg Calcium: 333 mg Sodium: 343 mg

Apple Cheddar Melt

SERVES 1

THE APPLE AND CHEDDAR complement each other perfectly in this quick and delicious snack.

1 small apple, cored and thinly sliced

3 tablespoons reduced-fat grated Cheddar cheese

1. Heat the oven or toaster oven to broil.

2. Place the apple in a small ovenproof dish and top with the Cheddar. Cook until the cheese is melted and browned, about 3 minutes. Serve.

PREP TIME: 5 minutes   TOTAL TIME: 8 minutes

PER SERVING, ABOUT: Calories: 116 Protein: 8 g Carbohydrate: 10 g Dietary Fiber: 2 g Sugars: 7 g Total Fat: 5 g Saturated Fat: 3 g Cholesterol: 16 mg Calcium: 261 mg Sodium: 206 mg

Celery with Creamy Herb Dip

SERVES 1

THIS SNACK IS EASY to make ahead and take with you on the road or to the office.

6 tablespoons nonfat ricotta cheese

½ teaspoon finely chopped fresh thyme, or your favorite herb

½ teaspoon olive oil

5 stalks celery

1. Combine the ricotta, thyme, and oil in a small bowl.

2. Serve the dip with celery.

PREP TIME: 5 minutes   TOTAL TIME: 5 minutes

PER SERVING, ABOUT: Calories: 164 Protein: 13 g Carbohydrate: 8 g Dietary Fiber: 2 g
Sugars: 5 g Total Fat: 9 g Saturated Fat: 1 g Cholesterol: 8 mg Calcium: 348 mg Sodium: 216 mg

Cucumbers with Yogurt Dip

SERVES 1

THIS REFRESHING DIP PROVIDES plenty of calcium.

¾ cup low-fat plain yogurt

2 teaspoons chopped chives, mint, or parsley

½ teaspoon lemon juice

1 tablespoon chopped walnuts

Black pepper to taste

5 cucumber slices, about ½ inch thick

1. Combine the yogurt, chives, lemon juice, walnuts, and pepper in a small bowl.

2. Serve the dip with the cucumber slices.

PREP TIME: 5 minutes   TOTAL TIME: 5 minutes

PER SERVING, ABOUT: Calories: 172 Protein: 11 g Carbohydrate: 18 g Dietary Fiber: 1 g
Sugars: 2 g Total Fat: 7 g Saturated Fat: 2 g Cholesterol: 11 mg Calcium: 360 mg Sodium: 132 mg

Apple Tea Latte

SERVES 1

THIS DRINKABLE SNACK IS filling and provides 300 milligrams of calcium.

1 cup plain soymilk, such as Silk, or fat-free
    or 1 percent milk

1 teaspoon honey

½ apple, chopped, skin and seeds included

1 black tea bag, such as Lipton Black Pearl
    Pyramid Tea

1. Bring the soymilk, honey, and apple to a boil in a small saucepan. Reduce the heat and simmer for 3 minutes, stirring frequently.

2. Remove the mixture from the heat, add the tea bag, and stir. Remove the tea bag after 3 minutes. Strain the mixture and serve.

PREP TIME: 2 minutes   TOTAL TIME: 13 minutes

PER SERVING, ABOUT: Calories: 108 Protein: 6 g Carbohydrate: 9 g Dietary Fiber: 0 g
Sugars: 14 g Total Fat: 3 g Saturated Fat: 1 g Cholesterol: 0 mg Calcium: 301 mg Sodium: 166 mg

Chocolate Mint Latte

SERVES 1

THIS LUSCIOUS-TASTING DRINK BLENDS the flavors of chocolate and mint.

1 cup vanilla soymilk, such as Silk

1 mint herbal tea bag

1 tablespoon cocoa powder

1. Bring the soymilk and tea bag to a boil in a small pot over medium heat. Whisk in the cocoa powder until thoroughly incorporated.

2. Remove from the heat, stir, and let sit for 3 minutes. Remove the tea bag and serve.

PREP TIME: 5 minutes   TOTAL TIME: 8 minutes

PER SERVING, ABOUT: Calories: 114 Protein: 8 g Carbohydrate: 12 g Dietary Fiber: 3 g
Sugars: 6 g Total Fat: 5 g Saturated Fat: 1 g Cholesterol: 0 mg Calcium: 307 mg Sodium: 127 mg

Cherry Milk

SERVES 1

THIS COMFORTING SNACK, WHICH isn't too sweet, is a tasty way to satisfy your hunger between meals.

1 cup fat-free milk

¼ cup frozen cherries, pitted

¼ teaspoon sugar

Combine the ingredients in a blender until smooth, about 2 minutes. Serve.

PREP TIME: 5 minutes   **TOTAL TIME:** 5 minutes

PER SERVING, ABOUT: Calories: 105 Protein: 9 g Carbohydrate: 18 g Dietary Fiber: 1 g
Sugars: 17 g Total Fat: 0 g Saturated Fat: 0 g Cholesterol: 5 mg Calcium: 311 mg Sodium: 103 mg

Orange Cream Smoothie

SERVES 1

THIS RICH AND CREAMY smoothie delivers nearly a day's worth of vitamin C.

¾ cup calcium-enriched orange juice,
   frozen in an ice-cube tray (measure
   juice before freezing)

¼ cup fat-free milk or plain soymilk, such
   as Silk

Combine the ingredients in a blender until smooth, about 2 minutes. Serve.

PREP TIME: 2 minutes   **TOTAL TIME:** 3 hours (this includes freezing the orange juice)

PER SERVING, ABOUT: Calories: 99 Protein: 3 g Carbohydrate: 21 g Dietary Fiber: 0 g
Sugars: 19 g Total Fat: 0 g Saturated Fat: 0 g Cholesterol: 1 mg Calcium: 300 mg Sodium: 29 mg

Desserts

Frozen Banana Chocolate Chip "Ice Cream"

SERVES 4

THIS QUICK RECIPE IS so decadent tasting, you might have a hard time believing it's actually good for you. Dark chocolate contains powerful antioxidants that may help promote heart health. And it's a great way to use up a surplus of bananas; peeled bananas can be stored in the freezer for several weeks.

3 bananas, peeled and frozen in a resealable plastic bag

¼ cup dark chocolate, such as Hershey's Extra Dark, chopped coarsely

1. Slice the bananas and process in a food processor for 2 minutes. If the bananas are too hard to slice, let thaw at room temperature for 2 minutes before slicing.

2. Add the chocolate and process for 1 more minute. Spoon the mixture into chilled bowls and serve immediately.

PREP TIME: 5 minutes   TOTAL TIME: 3 hours 5 minutes (this includes freezing the bananas)

PER SERVING, ABOUT: Calories: 127 Protein: 1 g Carbohydrate: 26 g Dietary Fiber: 3 g Sugars: 16 g Total Fat: 4 g Saturated Fat: 2 g Cholesterol: 0 mg Calcium: 7 mg Sodium: 2 mg

SAVVY SPLURGING

If you're watching your weight—whether you're trying to lose or simply maintain—you need to keep a lid on sweets and other treats. But what would life be like without a little candy, a cookie, or some chips and salsa? It would be like a restrictive fad diet, one that you'd soon grow tired of! So, I encourage you to go ahead and indulge a little in these foods; they help you stay motivated to stick with an otherwise healthful diet.

On my Best Life Diet plan, I've even allotted a designated amount of treat calories called "Anything Goes Calories." The more daily calories you can afford (largely influenced by the amount of exercise you get), the more treat calories you get. The chart below breaks it down for you; remember, you can skip a splurge one day and save your calories for a higher-calorie indulgence the next. For examples, check out the meal plans in this book (under "Treats") or go to my Web site, www.thebestlife.com.

IF YOU EAT . . .	YOU GET THIS MANY DAILY ANYING GOES CALORIES
1,500 calories per day	0 That's because you can barely squeeze in all the nutritious staples you need on 1,500 calories!
1,600 calories per day	100
1,700 calories per day	150
1,800 calories per day	210
2,000 calories per day	280
2,500 calories per day	300 (men may be able to go up to 350)

Pomegranate with Grapefruit and Mint

SERVES 4

ENJOY THIS DESSERT IN the fall and winter, when pomegranates and grapefruit are in season. The fresh taste of mint enhances the citrusy grapefruit and the intense, deep flavor of pomegranate.

1 tablespoon sugar

2 tablespoons finely chopped fresh mint

2 cups pomegranate seeds (see page 349)

2 grapefruits, sectioned (see page 346)

2 tablespoons toasted pine nuts (see page 346)

1. Combine the sugar and mint in a large bowl. Add the pomegranate and grapefruit and let sit for at least 5 minutes, or up to 24 hours tightly covered and refrigerated.

2. Stir in the pine nuts right before serving.

   PREP TIME: 10 minutes   **TOTAL TIME:** 10 minutes

PER SERVING, ABOUT: Calories: 121 Protein: 2 g Carbohydrate: 24 g Dietary Fiber: 2 g Sugars: 22 g Total Fat: 3 g Saturated Fat: 0 g Cholesterol: 0 mg Calcium: 20 mg Sodium: 2 mg

---

LABEL LOOKOUT! BEST LIFE APPROVED TREAT

Even when you're watching your weight, a little chocolate, ice cream, or other favorite treat is in order. A little indulgence prevents feelings of deprivation—a killer to any healthy eating plan. The key, of course, is sticking to portions that won't tip the scale. That's where this seal comes in: 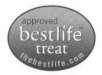 you'll find it on treats that offer a 150-calorie (or less) portion; often the products come individually wrapped. Skinny Cow ice cream sandwiches, Edy's and Dreyer's Fruit Bars, Nonni's Biscotti, and Hershey's Extra Dark chocolates are among the brands sporting this seal.

Peaches with Herbs and Almond Crunch

SERVES 4

THIS IS FANTASTIC IN the summertime with just-picked peaches, but it's also good with frozen peaches. Lavender or mint works in concert with the peaches to highlight their subtle flavors, while the nuts add a satisfying crunch. Make sure you're using lavender that has not been sprayed with pesticides.

2 cups sliced fresh peaches or frozen, defrosted at room temperature

1 tablespoon minced fresh lavender or mint

1 tablespoon sugar

¼ cup almonds

1 tablespoon honey

1. Toss the peaches, lavender, and sugar in a medium bowl. Let sit for at least 5 minutes or up to an hour at room temperature or several hours refrigerated.

2. Combine the almonds and honey in a food processor and pulse until the almonds are in small pieces but not pureed, about 1 minute.

3. Divide the peaches into individual serving bowls, top with the almond mixture and serve.

PREP TIME: 10 minutes   **TOTAL TIME:** 10 minutes

PER SERVING, ABOUT: Calories: 113 Protein: 3 g Carbohydrate: 17 g Dietary Fiber: 2 g Sugars: 15 g Total Fat: 5 g Saturated Fat: 0 g Cholesterol: 0 mg Calcium: 31 mg Sodium: 1 mg

Marinated Cherries with Chocolate Biscotti

SERVES 4

THIS INDULGENT DESSERT IS just as good served hot or cold.

2 cups fresh pitted or frozen cherries

½ cup dry red wine

4 chocolate biscotti (with 110 to 120 calories per biscotti, such as Nonni's Biscotti, or see page 342 to make your own)

1. Place the cherries and wine in a medium saucepan. Bring to a boil, reduce heat to low, and simmer for 5 minutes. If you'd like to serve cold, refrigerate.

2. Serve with the biscotti.

PREP TIME: 2 minutes   **TOTAL TIME:** 12 minutes

PER SERVING, ABOUT: Calories: 170 Protein: 3 g Carbohydrate: 26 g Dietary Fiber: 2 g Sugars: 15 g Total Fat: 5 g Saturated Fat: 1 g Cholesterol: 10 mg Calcium: 22 mg Sodium: 35 mg

Uncooked Stone Fruit Tart

SERVES 4

FOR JUST A LITTLE bit of work, you'll be rewarded with an unbelievably delicious dessert. It's best during the summer when stone fruit is in season, or you could make it with apples or pears during the winter.

2 cups sliced ripe peaches, plums, or apricots, or a mixture of these

1 tablespoon sugar

4 biscotti (with 110 to 120 calories per biscotti, such as Nonni's Biscotti, or see page 342 to make your own)

1 tablespoon peanut butter, such as Smart Balance

1. Place the peaches and sugar in a medium mixing bowl and set aside.

2. Grind the biscotti in a food processor for 1 minute. Add the peanut butter and process until combined, about 1 minute.

3. On individual serving plates, make a full circle of biscotti dough 3 to 4 inches in diameter and top with the sliced fruit. Serve.

PREP TIME: 5 minutes   **TOTAL TIME:** 5 minutes

PER SERVING, ABOUT: Calories: 216 Protein: 5 g Carbohydrate: 32 g Dietary Fiber: 3 g Sugars: 19 g Total Fat: 9 g Saturated Fat: 2 g Cholesterol: 14 mg Calcium: 25 mg Sodium: 59 mg

Lemon Oatmeal Cookies

SERVES 4

THESE TART AND SWEET cookies are great with a cup of herbal tea after a meal.

1 cup rolled oats	2 teaspoons lemon juice
2 tablespoons olive oil	1/2 teaspoon lemon zest
1/2 tablespoon plain soymilk or fat-free milk	1/2 teaspoon baking powder
2 tablespoons sugar	Pinch of salt
1 tablespoon honey	Vegetable oil cooking spray

1. Preheat the oven to 350°F.

2. Combine the oats, oil, milk, sugar, honey, lemon juice and zest, baking powder, and salt in a mixer for 2 minutes.

3. Coat a cookie sheet with cooking spray. Divide the dough evenly to make 4 individual cookies and place on the cookie sheet. Wet your palm with a little water and flatten the cookies with your palm. Bake until golden brown, about 7 minutes. Serve.

PREP TIME: 5 minutes   **TOTAL TIME:** 15 minutes

PER SERVING, ABOUT: Calories: 171 Protein: 4 g Carbohydrate: 22 g Dietary Fiber: 2 g
Sugars: 8 g Total Fat: 8 g Saturated Fat: 1 g Cholesterol: 0 mg Calcium: 55 mg Sodium: 104 mg

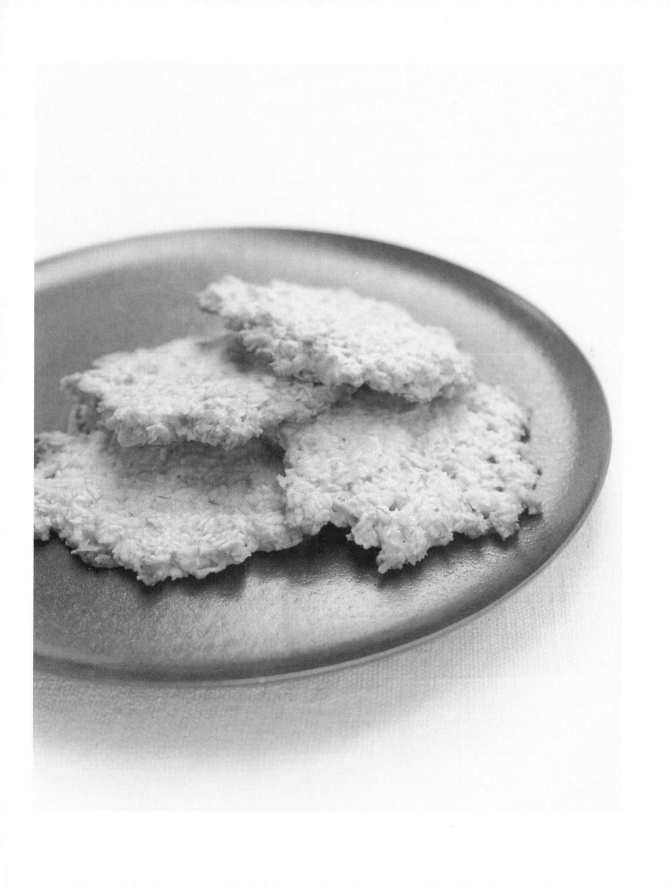

Sesame Seed Biscotti

MAKES 16 COOKIES

THE RICH UNIQUE TASTE of sesame is a pleasant surprise in this cookie. Many cultures around the world incorporate sesame into their desserts. These biscotti store very well; you can keep them in an airtight container for up to 10 days.

3 tablespoons silken tofu	½ cup unbleached all-purpose flour
¼ cup sugar plus 1 teaspoon for rolling	¼ cup whole wheat flour
1 teaspoon baking powder	2 tablespoons sesame seeds
2 tablespoons sesame oil	Vegetable oil cooking spray

1. Preheat the oven to 375°F.

2. Process the tofu in a food processor and puree until smooth, about 30 seconds. Add ¼ cup sugar, baking powder, oil, both flours, and sesame seeds and process for 1 more minute.

3. Remove the dough and roll first into a ball and then into a log with a 1-inch diameter. Place the remaining 1 teaspoon sugar on a plate and roll biscotti through the sugar until it is evenly coated.

4. Coat a baking sheet with cooking spray, place the log on sheet, and cook for 10 minutes.

5. Remove from the oven, let cool for 5 minutes, and slice into ½-inch-thick slices. You should have about 16 cookies.

6. Return the slices to the baking sheet and place in the oven. Turn the oven off and let the biscotti dry for 15 minutes in the oven or overnight in the oven before serving. The longer you dry biscotti, the harder the cookies will be. They are different, but delicious either soft in the middle or hard all the way through.

PREP TIME: 10 minutes   **TOTAL TIME:** 40 minutes

PER 2 COOKIES, ABOUT: Calories: 113 Protein: 2 g Carbohydrate: 16 g Dietary Fiber: 1 g
Sugars: 7 g Total Fat: 5 g Saturated Fat: 1 g Cholesterol: 0 mg Calcium: 78 mg Sodium: 63 mg

Pear and Banana Crisp

SERVES 4

THE UNEXPECTED COMBINATION OF pear and banana creates a rich and delicious dessert.

2 large pears, cored and sliced

1 banana, sliced

1 teaspoon sugar

½ cup oats

1 tablespoon honey

Pinch of salt

2 tablespoons ground walnuts (see note below)

5 tablespoons fat-free milk or plain soymilk, such as Silk Unsweetened (1 for oat mixture, 4 for topping)

1. Preheat the oven to 375°F.

2. Combine the pears, banana, and sugar in a medium bowl. Place the mixture into a 9-inch pie plate or 4 individual ramekins.

3. Combine the oats, honey, salt, walnuts, and 1 tablespoon soymilk in a food processor and puree for 1 minute, scraping the sides down into the bowl if necessary.

4. Top the pear mixture with the oatmeal mixture and bake for 20 minutes.

5. Remove from the oven and drizzle the remaining 4 tablespoons soymilk around the edges of the crisp. Serve immediately.

NOTE: To make 2 tablespoons of ground walnuts, start with 2 heaping tablespoons walnut halves or pieces and grind for 1 minute in a food processor.

PREP TIME: 5 minutes   TOTAL TIME: 25 minutes

PER SERVING, ABOUT: Calories: 175 Protein: 3 g Carbohydrate: 37 g Dietary Fiber: 6 g Sugars: 21 g Total Fat: 3 g Saturated Fat: 0 g Cholesterol: 0 mg Calcium: 43 mg Sodium: 51 mg

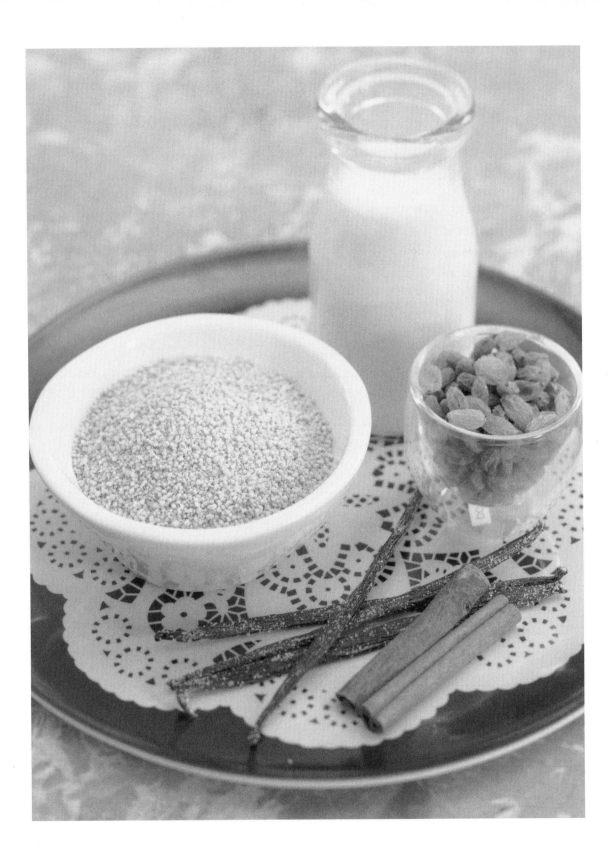

Whole Wheat Couscous Pudding

SERVES 4

SATISFY A SWEET TOOTH without adding too many extra calories to your diet with this creamy dessert. The combination of cinnamon, vanilla, and raisins are a real treat for your taste buds. You can substitute cardomom for the cinnamon for a more exotic taste.

2 cups plain soymilk or fat-free milk

$^1/_2$ cup whole wheat couscous

$^1/_2$ cup golden raisins

1 vanilla bean, cut in half, seeds removed and reserved, or 1 teaspoon vanilla extract

3 teaspoons sugar

$^1/_2$ teaspoon cinnamon or cardamom

$^1/_8$ teaspoon salt

1. Bring the milk to a boil in a medium pot.

2. Stir in the couscous, raisins, vanilla bean seeds, sugar, cinnamon, and salt. Cover and remove the pot from the heat.

3. Let the pot sit covered for 5 minutes. Open, stir, and serve, or cool and serve at room temperature.

PREP TIME: 5 minutes   TOTAL TIME: 10 minutes

PER SERVING, ABOUT: Calories: 237 Protein: 9 g Carbohydrate: 42 g Dietary Fiber: 5 g Sugars: 19 g Total Fat: 3 g Saturated Fat: 0 g Cholesterol: 0 mg Calcium: 252 mg Sodium: 127 mg

Grape Crumble with Frozen Grapes

SERVES 4

SERVE THIS ELEGANT DESSERT warm out of the oven with frozen grapes as a garnish. You can also crush the frozen grapes in a blender to make a mock sorbet. You'll get a taste of sweet plus the health benefit of antioxidants from the grapes.

³/₄ cup seedless green grapes, cut in half

³/₄ cup oatmeal

¹/₄ teaspoon baking powder

2 tablespoons soymilk or fat-free milk

2 tablespoons olive oil

1 tablespoon honey

3¹/₄ cups red, black, or a mixture seedless grapes

1. Place the green grapes on a sheet pan in the freezer for at least 3 hours.

2. Preheat the oven to 375°F.

3. Combine the oatmeal, baking powder, milk, oil, and honey in a food processor and blend for 1 minute.

4. Place the red grapes in a 9-inch pie plate. Cover with the oatmeal mixture and bake for 20 minutes.

5. Garnish with frozen green grapes and serve.

   PREP TIME: 10 minutes   TOTAL TIME: 3 hours 30 minutes

PER SERVING, ABOUT: Calories: 198 Protein: 3 g Carbohydrate: 31 g Dietary Fiber: 2 g Sugars: 20 g Total Fat: 8 g Saturated Fat: 1 g Cholesterol: 0 mg Calcium: 54 mg Sodium: 37 mg

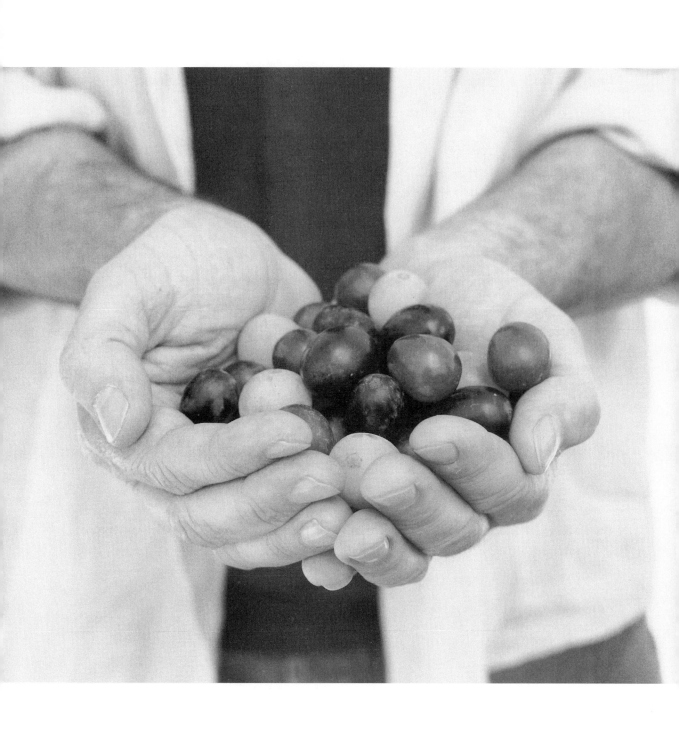

Blueberry Slump

SERVES 4

A MEMORABLE WAY TO end your meal, this dessert is full of antioxidants from the blueberries.

Vegetable oil cooking spray

2 cups fresh blueberries or frozen, such as Cascadian Farm, defrosted

1/4 cup cornmeal, preferably whole grain

1/4 cup silken tofu, pureed in a food processor for 1 minute

1 1/2 teaspoons melted healthy spread, such as Smart Balance Buttery Spread

1/2 teaspoon baking powder

1/8 teaspoon baking soda

1/4 cup soymilk, such as Silk, or fat-free milk

4 teaspoons reduced-fat sour cream

1 tablespoon brown sugar

1. Preheat the oven to 350°F.

2. Coat a 9-inch pie plate or 4 individual baking dishes with cooking spray and fill with the blueberries. Make sure the pie plate or baking dishes have at least an inch of room above the blueberries.

3. In a medium bowl, combine the cornmeal, tofu, spread, baking powder, baking soda, and milk.

4. Pour the cornmeal mixture over the berries and bake for 25 minutes.

5. Mix together the sour cream and brown sugar. Garnish the slump with the sour cream mixture. Serve.

PREP TIME: 5 minutes   **TOTAL TIME:** 30 minutes

PER SERVING, ABOUT: Calories: 134 Protein: 4 g Carbohydrate: 23 g Dietary Fiber: 3 g Sugars: 12 g Total Fat: 3 g Saturated Fat: 1 g Cholesterol: 2 mg Calcium: 77 mg Sodium: 208 mg

Apple Pie with Oatmeal Crust

SERVES 8

APPLE PIE CAN BE enjoyed year-round, but it's even better in the fall when you can use your favorite variety of locally grown apples.

2 cups oatmeal

4 tablespoons healthy spread, such as
    Smart Balance

2 tablespoons water

Vegetable oil cooking spray

5 apples, cored and sliced

¼ cup sugar

2 teaspoons cinnamon

2 tablespoons flour

1. Preheat the oven to 375°F.

2. Combine the oatmeal, spread, and water in a food processor for 1 minute.

3. Coat a 9-inch pie plate with cooking spray and press the oatmeal mixture into the bottom of the plate.

4. Bake the crust for 10 minutes.

5. Toss together the apples, sugar, cinnamon, and flour in a large bowl.

6. Place the apple mixture on top of the crust and bake, covered with aluminum foil, for 45 minutes. Remove the foil and bake for an additional 5 minutes. Serve.

PREP TIME: 15 minutes   **TOTAL TIME:** 1 hour 15 minutes

PER SERVING, ABOUT: Calories: 195 Protein: 4 g Carbohydrate: 34 g Dietary Fiber: 4 g Sugars: 16 g Total Fat: 6 g Saturated Fat: 2 g Cholesterol: 0 mg Calcium: 23 mg Sodium: 47 mg

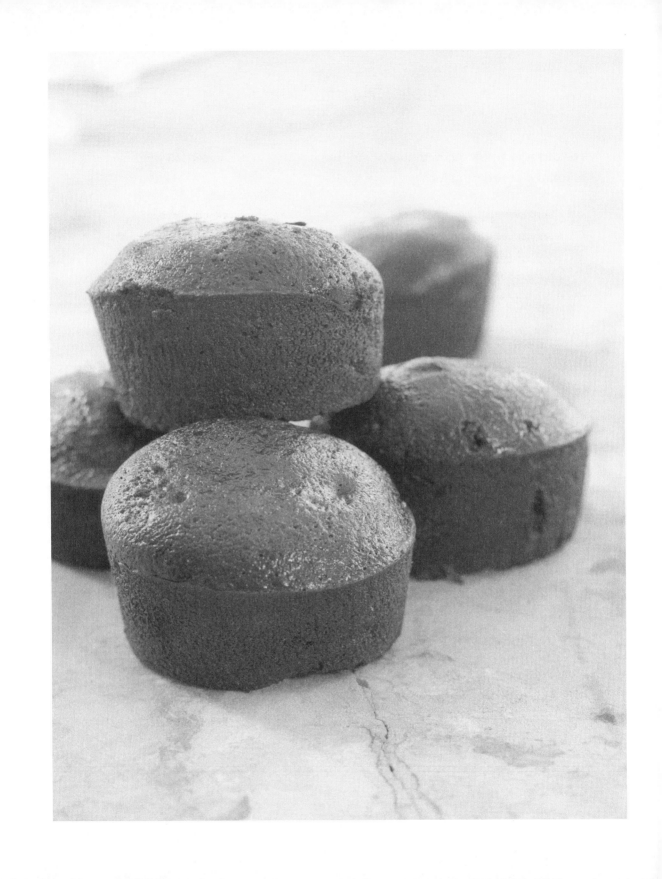

Chocolate Cake

SERVES 5

FORGET ABOUT DEATH BY chocolate—these individual chocolate cakes are a smart way to indulge.

$1/2$ cup unbleached all-purpose flour

$1/4$ cup sugar

Pinch of salt

$1/2$ teaspoon baking soda

2 tablespoons vegetable oil

2 tablespoons unsweetened cocoa, such as Hershey's Natural Cocoa

$1/2$ teaspoon vanilla extract

1 teaspoon vinegar

$1/2$ cup water

Vegetable oil cooking spray

1. Preheat the oven to 350°F.

2. Combine the flour, sugar, salt, baking soda, oil, cocoa, vanilla, vinegar, and water in a mixer and blend just until the lumps disappear, about 1 minute.

3. Coat a muffin tin with cooking spray. Pour the batter into the individual cups.

4. Bake until a toothpick inserted into the middle of a muffin comes out clean, about 20 minutes. Serve.

PREP TIME: 5 minutes   **TOTAL TIME:** 25 minutes

PER SERVING, ABOUT: Calories: 180 Protein: 2 g Carbohydrate: 26 g Dietary Fiber: 1 g Sugars: 13 g Total Fat: 7 g Saturated Fat: 1 g Cholesterol: 0 mg Calcium: 4 mg Sodium: 164 mg

SWEET NEWS ABOUT CHOCOLATE

Isn't it great when you discover that foods you love are actually *good* for you? If chocolate happens to be one of your favorite treats, then you're in luck! Chocolate lovers (I include myself in this group) have reason to celebrate, mainly because chocolate just happens to be the third highest source of antioxidants for Americans (behind coffee and tea), according to a study from the University of Scranton in Pennsylvania. These disease-fighting antioxidants (flavonols) keep your arteries healthy by offering a one-two punch that:

Reduces cholesterol. In a Finnish study, healthy people who ate 2.6 ounces of dark chocolate daily for three weeks had less damage to LDL, or bad cholesterol, than those who ate white chocolate. This is important because damaged cholesterol settles in your arteries, setting you up for a heart attack and stroke. Dark-chocolate eaters also had higher levels of HDL (good cholesterol), which transports cholesterol out of the body. (Although chocolate is high in saturated fat, which usually spikes your cholesterol and contributes to clogged arteries, most of it is stearic acid, the one type of saturated fat that does not raise cholesterol.)

Lowers blood pressure. Chocolate's polyphenols also relax and open up the arteries, which keeps blood flowing and reduces blood pressure. This also means a decreased risk for heart disease and stroke. A recent review of chocolate research in the *Archives of Internal Medicine* found that in most studies, consuming a chocolate-rich diet for just two weeks helped reduce blood pressure by 4 to 5 systolic points (top number) and 2 to 3 diastolic points (bottom number). This might seem modest, but the authors of the study note that it's enough to cut the stroke risk in the general population by 20 percent, heart disease risk by 10 percent, and death from all causes by 8 percent!

But before you hit the vending machine, you should know that these benefits aren't associated with all forms of chocolate. It has to be antioxidant-rich, and that usually means dark chocolate. While there's no definition for "dark," any bar that contains 50 percent cocoa, cacao, or cocoa solids (check the label) most likely has a decent amount of antioxidants, says Joe Vinson, PhD, professor of chemistry at Scranton University. Cocoa mixes, chocolate milk mixes, and syrups aren't all that antioxidant-rich, but pure cocoa powder that has not been "Dutch processed" or alkalized (which removes antioxidants) are good sources.

Although participants in some studies ate up to 500 calories per day of the sweet stuff, other research suggests that a lot less may be beneficial. For instance, a German study of people with mildly high blood pressure found that just 30 calories—about ¼ ounce—a day of dark chocolate helped reduce blood pressure, says Vinson. To figure out how many calories you can afford to spend on chocolate, check out Savvy Splurging, page 201.

Angel Food Cake

SERVES 4

THIS QUICK CAKE RECIPE is the ultimate light dessert. Fill the empty muffin tins halfway with water so they don't burn.

⅓ cup liquid egg whites, such as AllWhites, or 3 egg whites

½ teaspoon cream of tartar

Pinch of salt

¼ plus 1 tablespoon sugar

¼ cup flour

Vegetable oil cooking spray

1. Preheat the oven to 350°F.

2. Beat the egg whites in a mixer using the whisk attachment until frothy, about 2 minutes. Add the cream of tartar and salt.

3. Continue beating until stiff, about 3 minutes. Add the sugar and beat for another 2 minutes.

4. Sift the flour over the egg whites and fold in gently with a spatula.

5. Coat 4 muffin tins with cooking spray. Pour the mixture into the muffin tins and cook until browned on top, about 20 minutes. Cool before removing from the muffin tins. Serve.

VARIATIONS

You can also add 1 teaspoon vanilla extract, 1 teaspoon lemon zest, or 1 teaspoon orange zest when the egg whites are nearly stiff.

PREP TIME: 10 minutes   **TOTAL TIME:** 30 minutes

PER SERVING, ABOUT: Calories: 103 Protein: 4 g Carbohydrate: 22 g Dietary Fiber: 0 g Sugars: 16 g Total Fat: 0 g Saturated Fat: 0 g Cholesterol: 0 mg Calcium: 3 mg Sodium: 119 mg

Summer Pudding

SERVES 4

THIS IS A SIMPLER version of a traditional English dessert. It's not at all like a cooked pudding but it's equally delicious and satisfying. It's a good choice on a warm day when it's too hot to turn on the oven.

3 cups mixed fresh berries or frozen, such as Cascadian Farm (pitted cherries are also good to mix in)

1 tablespoon sugar

1 whole wheat 100-calorie wrap, tortilla, or flatbread, such as Multi-Grain Flatout Flatbread, cut into 8 pieces

4 teaspoons nonfat sour cream

1. Put the fruit and sugar in a medium pot and slowly bring to a simmer over low heat. Cook for 15 minutes, stirring every few minutes.

2. Place 1 tablespoon of the fruit mixture into four 1-cup ramekins. Place a piece of flatbread on top, followed by 2 tablespoons of fruit, another layer of flatbread, and the remaining fruit.

3. Wrap with plastic and place in the refrigerator for at least 1 hour or up to 24 hours.

4. Garnish with the sour cream before serving.

    PREP TIME: 5 minutes   **TOTAL TIME:** 1 hour 25 minutes (this includes chilling summer pudding)

PER SERVING, ABOUT: Calories: 116 Protein: 3 g Carbohydrate: 25 g Dietary Fiber: 6 g Sugars: 10 g Total Fat: 1 g Saturated Fat: 0 g Cholesterol: 0 mg Calcium: 38 mg Sodium: 76 mg

Best Life Recipes from World-Class Chefs

WHO SAID HAUTE CUISINE CAN'T be healthful? I asked a group of world-renowned chefs to share recipes that met the Best Life requirements and they all rose to the challenge. While some of these are definitely special-occasion dishes and require some time and effort, most are surprisingly easy, and will make any meal an event.

MOLLIE AHLSTRAND

Owner and executive chef of Trattoria Mollie
in Santa Barbara, California

FOR FIFTEEN YEARS MOLLIE AHLSTRAND has been serving simple, fresh Italian food at Trattoria Mollie. It might be a surprise to learn that the chef behind such dishes as homemade fresh pasta Bolognese and margherita pizza is Ethiopian, but the Italian culture was something Mollie had been interested in ever since she was a child. Exposed to the language by her father as a young girl, she eventually went on to train at some of the biggest restaurants in Rome. The cooking philosophy that she learned at these eateries—

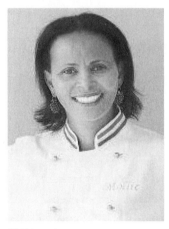

Ali Ahlstrand

use high-quality ingredients and you won't need to rely on adornments or fancy cooking techniques—works perfectly in her new home in Santa Barbara; after all, Californians had been buying locally grown, seasonal foods long before it became trendy to do so. There are several wonderful farmers' markets that take place each week in Santa Barbara, one of which is held right in front of the restaurant.

Not surprisingly, the restaurant has attracted some famous fans, including Oprah Winfrey, John Cleese, Michael Douglas and Catherine Zeta-Jones. Perhaps it's because Mollie has found the perfect balance between health and flavor. Her dishes contain a well-rounded mix of protein (often fish) served with fresh vegetables, preceded by a small serving of pasta and vegetable-based antipasto, and everything is eaten in relatively modest portions. When you add up all the courses, you end up with a satisfying, but not overindulgent meal.

Trattoria Mollie is listed as one of the ten best destinations and restaurants in the world in National Geographic's *The 10 Best of Everything: An Ultimate Guide for Travelers.* Her famous meatballs have been featured on *The Oprah Winfrey Show* and in *O, The Oprah Magazine.* Mollie has also served as a guest chef at the Grand Hyatt's Italian restaurant in Hong Kong twice, and at the Grand Hyatt in Dubai, United Arab Emirates. In May 2007, she was presented with the Star Diamond Award by the Academy of Hospitality of Sciences.

Mollie Ahlstrand's Tagliolini con Gamberi e Rucola

SERVES 4

THE FIRST TIME I had dinner at Trattoria Mollie, I knew that she was something special. The fresh, homemade pastas, the perfectly prepared fish dishes, the wonderful appetizers, and her insistence on inspecting every element that goes into each meal makes dining there such a special experience. Both Oprah and I became regulars after the first visit. Now *you* can enjoy a taste of Mollie's cooking with this tasty shrimp and pasta recipe.

1 tablespoon extra virgin olive oil	1 tablespoon brandy
1 clove garlic, chopped	¼ teaspoon salt
1 shallot, chopped	Ground white pepper to taste
½ pound fresh thin spinach pasta	1½ cups diced tomatoes, organic, if possible
1 tablespoon butter	
16 shrimp (31 to 40 shrimp per pound), peeled and deveined	4 cups baby arugula, well washed
	1 tablespoon chopped fresh Italian parsley

1. Heat a medium pan over medium heat. Add the oil and sauté the garlic and shallot until lightly browned, about 5 minutes.

2. At the same time, cook the fresh pasta in boiling water for 4 to 5 minutes. Drain the pasta, reserving 2 tablespoons of water, and toss with the butter.

3. Continue stirring the garlic and shallot and add the shrimp. Add the brandy and 2 tablespoons of water from the pasta, or more if necessary, to prevent dryness. Cook until the shrimp are pink, about 5 minutes.

4. Transfer the pasta to the pan with the shrimp sauce and toss to combine.

5. Add the salt and pepper. Add the diced tomatoes and arugula and toss.

6. Transfer to a serving plate, sprinkle with parsley, and serve.

PREP TIME: 10 minutes   **TOTAL TIME:** 30 minutes

PER SERVING, ABOUT: Calories: 278 Protein: 14 g Carbohydrate: 37 g Dietary Fiber: 2 g Sugars: 3 g Total Fat: 8 g Saturated Fat: 3 g Cholesterol: 86 mg Calcium: 139 mg Sodium: 216 mg

Mollie Ahlstrand's Zuppa di Pomodoro

SERVES 4

THERE ARE SO MANY days when tomato soup is the ideal food. Luckily, you can now add this recipe with its well-balanced flavor to your repertoire.

1 tablespoon extra virgin olive oil

1 clove garlic, chopped

1 shallot, chopped

24 ounces tomatoes, organic, if possible, cut in half, seeds removed and chopped, to make about 4 cups

1 sprig fresh rosemary

½ tablespoon brandy

½ cup water

⅛ teaspoon salt

Ground white pepper to taste

1½ tablespoons freshly squeezed orange juice

1 ounce thinly sliced Parmesan

1. Heat a medium pot over medium heat. Add the oil and sauté the garlic and shallot until lightly browned, about 5 minutes.

2. Add the tomatoes and rosemary, stirring, and cook for 5 minutes.

3. Continue to stir the tomatoes while adding the brandy and water (or more if the soup is too thick; the thickness will vary, depending on the water content of the tomatoes you use) for 10 minutes, until the tomatoes are soft.

4. Remove the rosemary and add the salt and pepper.

5. Carefully transfer the contents of the pot into a blender and blend until pureed, about 2 minutes.

6. Put the soup in a serving bowl and add the orange juice. Mix well.

7. Place the Parmesan on top and serve immediately.

PREP TIME: 10 minutes   TOTAL TIME: 35 minutes

PER SERVING, ABOUT: Calories: 101 Protein: 4 g Carbohydrate: 8 g Dietary Fiber: 2 g Sugars: 5 g Total Fat: 6 g Saturated Fat: 2 g Cholesterol: 6 mg Calcium: 99 mg Sodium: 190 mg

DAN BARBER

*Executive chef/co-owner, Blue Hill in Manhattan
and Blue Hill at Stone Barns in Pocantico Hills, New York*

DAN BARBER STARTED COOKING FOR family and friends at a young age at Blue Hill Farm, a 138-acre farm in the Berkshires that his grandmother bought in the sixties. It was also the place where he was first introduced to, and gained respect for, locally grown and seasonal produce. Dan learned that cooking with fresh foods that are in season not only benefits the environment but also leads to more flavorful dishes. This may be one of the reasons why Blue Hill, which he, his brother David, and sister-in-law Laureen opened in 2000, quickly went from a noted neighborhood eatery to a *New York Times* 3-star restaurant.

In May 2004, Dan and his family opened Blue Hill at Stone Barns located within the Stone Barns Center for Food and Agriculture in Pocantico Hills, New York. Locally grown produce, meats, seafood, and cheeses are the centerpieces of most dishes on the menus at both of his restaurants. Typical offerings include This morning's soft/ fried farm egg or Stone Barns shelling beans.

As the restaurants' chef/co-owner and a member of the Stone Barns Center's board of directors, Dan focuses on the issues of pleasure, taste, and regional bounty, and how these imperatives are threatened. Dan helped create the philosophical and practical framework for Stone Barns Center for Food and Agriculture and continues to help guide it in its mission to create a consciousness about the effects of everyday food choices.

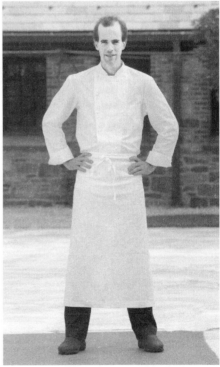

Nicholas Basilion

Dan was featured as one of the country's "Best New Chefs" in 2002 by *Food & Wine* magazine. He was also awarded Best Chef: New York City in 2006 by the James Beard Foundation and the "Chef of Merit" Award by *Bon Appétit* magazine in 2007. Both Blue Hill and Blue Hill at Stone Barns have received Best New Restaurant nominations from the James Beard Foundation.

Dan Barber's Four Bean Salad

SERVES 4

THIS SALAD CALLS FOR a variety of fresh beans that should be available at your local farmers' market in late spring and summer. The pine nut oil (available at gourmet or specialty food stores) is a bit pricier than other oils, but a little goes a long way, plus the flavor will transform a good salad to an extraordinary salad. This recipe calls for only one-quarter of the salad dressing that you make; put the rest aside and use to dress green salads or other vegetables.

½ teaspoon salt

½ cup shelled fava beans

½ cup haricot verts, stem end removed

½ cup yellow wax beans, stem end removed

½ cup romano beans, stem end removed

2 tablespoons pine nuts

1 tablespoon pine nut oil

DRESSING

¼ cup balsamic vinegar

1½ tablespoons diced shallots

½ tablespoon mustard

½ cup fine-quality extra virgin olive oil

1. Bring a medium pot of water with salt to a boil. Fill a large bowl with ice and water.

2. Pour the balsamic vinegar over the shallots in a medium bowl and let sit for 30 minutes. Stir in the mustard. While whisking, pour in the olive oil to emulsify. Set aside.

3. Cook each type of bean separately for about 1 minute. Remove from the pot with a slotted spoon or small strainer and immediately plunge into the bowl of ice water. Drain the beans and set aside. Peel and discard the skin from the fava beans.

4. Combine the beans and pine nuts and divide among 4 plates. Lightly dress with one-quarter of the balsamic vinaigrette and drizzle the pine nut oil on top. Serve.

PREP TIME: 30 minutes **TOTAL TIME:** 30 minutes

PER SERVING, ABOUT: Calories: 354 Protein: 3 g Carbohydrate: 12 g Dietary Fiber: 2 g Sugars: 3 g Total Fat: 34 g Saturated Fat: 4 g Cholesterol: 0 mg Calcium: 36 mg Sodium: 368 mg

SUZANNE GOIN

Co-owner and executive chef at Lucques
in West Hollywood and A.O.C. in Los Angeles

SUZANNE GOIN HAS WORKED IN some of the top restaurants all across the world, including Ma Maison in Los Angeles, Olives in Boston, Le Mazarin in London, Chez Panisse in Berkeley, California, and Arpege in Paris. After gaining years of valuable experience at these and other outstanding restaurants, she decided to venture out on her own. The result: Lucques, which she opened in 1998 with her business partner, Caroline Styne. The restaurant, which serves seasonal market-driven Mediterranean cuisine, received rave reviews from *Condé Nast Traveler, Gourmet, Bon Appétit, Saveur,* and the *Los Angeles*

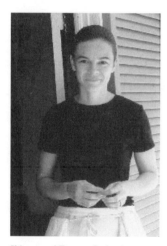

Shimon and Tammar Rothstein

Times, which gave it a prestigious 3 stars. In 2002, she opened her second restaurant, A.O.C., Suzanne's take on a wine bar with an extensive cheese and charcuterie selection, as well as a large menu of dishes served in small plate format to be shared family style. As if running two critically acclaimed establishments wasn't enough, she went on to open her third restaurant, The Hungry Cat, with her husband, fellow chef David Lentz in 2005. The casual seafood restaurant located in Hollywood was so popular that they decided to open a second location in Santa Barbara in 2007.

Suzanne's philosophy is to seek out the best locally grown organic ingredients and show them off as much as possible. She loves taking traditional dishes and remaking them in a modern way; for example, heavy sauces are replaced with fresh salsas and bright herb-based accompaniments. And with many of her offerings, the vegetables, rather than the protein, are the guiding inspiration for a dish.

If you can't make it to one of her four eateries, you can get a taste of her cooking by purchasing her cookbook *Sunday Suppers at Lucques* (Knopf, 2005). The book won the James Beard Foundation award for *Best Cookbook from a Professional Viewpoint* in May 2006. Suzanne also won the *Best Chef California* award from the James Beard Foundation in 2006 and was nominated for their Outstanding Chef Award in 2008. She was also named the "Best Creative Chef" by *Boston* magazine in August 1994 and was featured as one of the "Best New Chefs" by *Food & Wine* magazine in July 1999.

Suzanne lives in Los Angeles with her husband and two children.

Suzanne Goin's Succotash Salad with Sweet Corn, Summer Squash, and Cherry Tomatoes

SERVES 4

THIS UNFORGETTABLE SALAD FEATURES a mixture of delicious summer vegetables.

2 teaspoons finely diced shallot

2 tablespoons fresh lemon juice, or more to taste

³⁄₈ teaspoon kosher salt (¹⁄₈ for dressing, ¹⁄₈ for onion and squash, ¹⁄₈ for corn)

4 tablespoons extra virgin olive oil (3 for dressing, ¹⁄₂ for onion and squash, ¹⁄₂ for corn)

¹⁄₂ cup diced red onion

1¹⁄₂ teaspoons fresh thyme leaves

1¹⁄₃ cups diced summer squash

2 cups fresh corn kernels, from about 3 ears

Freshly ground black pepper to taste

²⁄₃ cup cherry tomatoes, cut in half

²⁄₃ cup cooked fresh lima beans, well drained (see page 345)

2 teaspoons chopped fresh parsley

3 tablespoons sliced fresh opal and green basil

2 teaspoons minced chives

1¹⁄₂ cups watercress and arugula, mixed

1. Combine the shallot, lemon juice, and ¹⁄₈ teaspoon salt in a small bowl and let sit for 5 minutes. Whisk in 3 tablespoons oil and taste the dressing for balance and seasoning.

2. Heat a large sauté pan over high heat for 2 minutes. Add ¹⁄₂ tablespoon oil, red onion, and thyme. Sauté for about 1 minute and add the squash. Season with ¹⁄₈ teaspoon salt and cook until the squash is tender and has a little color, about 4 minutes. Cool on a platter or baking sheet.

3. Wipe the sauté pan with paper towels, return it to the stove, and heat over high for 2 minutes. Add ¹⁄₂ tablespoon oil, corn, ¹⁄₈ teaspoon salt, and pepper. Sauté quickly, tossing often, for about 2 minutes, until the corn is just tender. Remove from the pan and cool.

(continued)

4. Place the tomatoes and beans in a large salad bowl. Add the squash, and more lemon juice, if desired. Gently toss the parsley, basil, and chives into the succotash.

5. Toss the watercress and arugula with the dressing and season with pepper. Place the greens on a large chilled platter and arrange the succotash on top. Serve.

PREP TIME: 10 minutes   **TOTAL TIME:** 25 minutes

PER SERVING, ABOUT: Calories: 237 Protein: 6 g Carbohydrate: 25 g Dietary Fiber: 6 g Sugars: 4 g Total Fat: 15 g Saturated Fat: 2 g Cholesterol: 0 mg Calcium: 78 mg Sodium: 142 mg

Suzanne Goin's Persimmon and Pomegranate Salad with Arugula and Hazelnuts

SERVES 4

IN THE WINTER MONTHS when there is noticeably less variety of seasonal produce available, the arrival of both pomegranates and persimmons are always welcome. This salad utilizes both of these outstanding fresh, flavorful, and often underused fruits.

½ cup blanched hazelnuts, toasted (see page 346), cooled, and chopped coarsely

2 teaspoons plus ½ teaspoon hazelnut oil

⅜ teaspoon kosher salt (⅛ for nuts, ⅛ for shallot, ⅛ for persimmons)

2 teaspoons finely diced shallot, plus 2 shallots, thinly sliced

2 tablespoons fresh pomegranate juice (see page 349), plus 3 tablespoons pomegranate seeds (see page 349)

2 teaspoons sherry vinegar

1½ teaspoons rice vinegar

2 tablespoons extra virgin olive oil

1½ small Fuyu persimmons, thinly sliced

Freshly ground black pepper to taste

Juice of ½ lemon

2½ cups arugula

1. Toss the nuts with ½ teaspoon hazelnut oil and ⅛ teaspoon salt. Set aside.

2. Place 2 teaspoons of the finely diced shallot, pomegranate juice, vinegars, and ⅛ teaspoon salt in a medium bowl and let sit for 5 minutes.

3. Whisk in the olive oil and the remaining 2 teaspoons hazelnut oil. Taste for balance and seasoning.

4. In a large salad bowl, toss the persimmons, 2 thinly sliced shallots, and pomegranate seeds with the dressing. Season with ⅛ teaspoon salt, pepper, and lemon juice. Gently toss in the arugula and taste for seasoning.

5. Arrange the salad on a platter and scatter the hazelnuts over the top. Serve.

PREP TIME: 25 minutes   **TOTAL TIME:** 25 minutes

PER SERVING, ABOUT: Calories: 262 Protein: 4 g Carbohydrate: 21 g Dietary Fiber: 4 g
Sugars: 12 g Total Fat: 20 g Saturated Fat: 2 g Cholesterol: 0 mg Calcium: 52 mg Sodium: 158 mg

THOMAS KELLER

*Chef/owner of eight restaurants, including
The French Laundry, Per Se, Bouchon,
Bouchon Bakery, and Ad Hoc*

A NATIVE OF CALIFORNIA, THOMAS began his culinary career at a young age, working in the Palm Beach restaurant managed by his mother. After serving apprenticeships in Rhode Island, Florida, and the Catskills, Thomas moved to France to work at several prestigious restaurants, including the Michelin-starred houses Guy Savoy and Taillevent. He eventually returned to New York, where he had successful runs at La Reserve and Restaurant Raphael, before he opened his first restaurant, Rakel, in 1986. The eatery gained extensive critical acclaim and a loyal clientele.

Five years later, Thomas moved to California to work as executive chef at Checkers Hotel in Los Angeles. In 1994, he opened The French Laundry in Yountville, which quickly became a destination restaurant known for its innovative, compelling cuisine. His bistro, Bouchon, opened in Yountville in 1998, with Bouchon Bakery following five years later. In February 2004, Thomas brought his distinct style back to New York City again with Per Se, which features Thomas's French-influenced contemporary American cuisine. *The Michelin Guide New York City* has given Per Se its most prestigious recognition, a three-star rating, for the past three consecutive years. In addition, the *Michelin Guide San Francisco* awarded The French Laundry a three-star rating (and a one-star rating for Bouchon) in 2007 and 2008, making Thomas the only American-born chef to hold multiple 3-star ratings since the guide's inception in 1900.

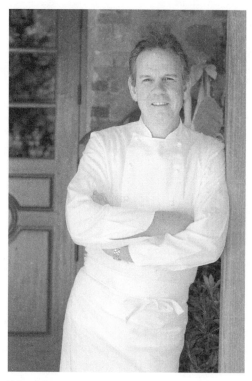

Deborah Jones

One of the most recognized American chefs today, Thomas is as renowned for his well-honed culinary skills as he is for his ability to establish a restaurant that's both relaxed yet exciting. Good food coupled with a memorable social and sensual experience has always been Thomas's focus. A man of exceptionally high personal standards, Thomas values genuine collaboration. He has successfully assembled an expert staff that shares his philosophy and vision, thus enabling him to concentrate on his many varied interests.

Thomas is the author of the award-winning *The French Laundry Cookbook* and *Bouchon.* In 2001, Thomas was named America's Best Chef by *Time* magazine. In 2003, Johnson & Wales University conferred upon him the honorary Degree of Doctor of Culinary Arts for his contributions to the industry. Thomas has collected many accolades within the last decade, including consecutive Best Chef awards from the James Beard Foundation, the first chef ever to achieve this honor. He most recently added their Outstanding Restaurateur award to the roster. The Culinary Institute of America also named him Chef of the Year in 2007. And the Monterey Bay Aquarium recently chose Thomas as the recipient of their 2009 Cooking for Solutions Conservation Leadership award for his leadership and advocacy for sustainable seafood.

Thomas now has eight restaurants in the United States. In addition to The French Laundry, Per Se, and Bouchon, branches of Bouchon and Bouchon Bakery opened in Las Vegas in 2004. In early 2006, Bouchon Bakery opened in the TimeWarner Center in New York City. Ad Hoc, a casual dining establishment inspired by the comfort food he enjoyed growing up, opened later that year in Yountville, California. Keller will open an outpost of Bouchon and Bouchon Bakery in Beverly Hills in the fall of 2009.

Thomas Keller's Watermelon Sorbet

SERVES 4

THESE FEW INGREDIENTS RESULT in an icy, refreshing dessert with intense watermelon flavor.

¼ small watermelon, about 1½ pounds	2 tablespoons water
¼ cup corn syrup	Cubed honeydew, cantaloupe, and
2 tablespoons sugar	watermelon, for garnish (optional)

1. Place the watermelon on a chopping board and cut into 1-inch-thick slices. Remove the skin of the melon from each slice with a small, sharp knife. Roughly dice the melon into 1- to 2-inch cubes. Remove as many of the black seeds as you can.

2. Place the watermelon in a blender and blend for about 30 seconds, until the melon is pureed.

3. Bring the corn syrup, sugar, and water to a rolling boil in a small pan. Pour over the pureed watermelon and stir well.

4. Pass the mixture through a fine sieve.

5. Refrigerate until cool. Turn in a sorbet machine until smooth and firm. If you don't have one you can create a refreshing watermelon ice by pouring the mix into a foil container (like the ones for cooking meat) or a clean metal dish that is no more than 4 inches high. Place the dish in the freezer and whisk with a hand whisk every 30 minutes to make flakes of ice. Keep whisking at 30-minute intervals until mixture has formed lots of small flakes of ice, about 2 hours.

6. Once frozen, scoop into cold sundae glasses. If desired, serve with cubes of honeydew, cantaloupe, and watermelon for color.

PREP TIME: 15 minutes   **TOTAL TIME:** 2 hours 15 minutes

PER SERVING, ABOUT: Calories: 159 Protein: 2 g Carbohydrate: 41 g Dietary Fiber: 1 g Total Sugars: 38 g Total Fat: 0 g Saturated Fat: 0 g Cholesterol: 0 mg Calcium: 22 mg Sodium: 35 mg

Thomas Keller's Salad of Riesling-Poached Tokyo Turnips with Brussels Sprouts, Pickled French Laundry Garden Onion, and Toasted Mustard Seed Emulsion

SERVES 4

THESE COOL WEATHER VEGETABLES have never been so brilliant as they are in this dish, which balances their earthy tones and the flavors of Riesling and mustard.

Tokyo turnips are small turnips with a mild flavor. Any tender young turnip may be used.

TURNIPS

1½ cups Riesling wine (preferably Gunderlooh Nackenheimer Rothenberg Auslese Rheingau, 2004)

12 small Tokyo turnips

1 tablespoon sugar

Pinch of kosher salt

1. Reduce the wine by half in a medium saucepan over medium heat for about 15 minutes.

2. Add the turnips, sugar, and salt.

3. Reduce until dry, about 15 minutes. The turnips should be tender. If not, add a touch more water to finish cooking, making sure to cook until dry. Set aside in a medium bowl.

BRUSSELS SPROUTS AND ONIONS

¼ teaspoon salt

12 small Brussels sprouts

4 Vidalia onion shoots (if onion shoots are not available use 1 tablespoon very finely chopped Vidalia onion)

4 small cipollini onions (a small and flat variety of onion)

1 tablespoon sugar

1. Bring a large pot of water with the salt to a boil. Fill a large bowl with ice and water.

2. Cook the Brussels sprouts in boiling water until tender, about 4 minutes.

(continued)

3. Submerge in ice water for 5 minutes. Drain and set aside in a small bowl.

4. Repeat with the onion shoots.

5. Place the cipollini onions in a small pot with sugar and fill with enough water to cover.

6. Cook over medium heat until the water has evaporated. The onions should be completely tender. If not, add a touch more water and continue cooking until dry. Don't drain because they will be dry. Set aside.

MUSTARD SEED EMULSION

1½ large Spanish onions, thinly sliced

1 tablespoon sugar

1½ teaspoons champagne vinegar

2½ tablespoons Dijon mustard

⅓ cup vegetable oil

1½ teaspoons mustard seeds, toasted (see page 346) and cooked in boiling water until tender, about 5 minutes

1. Preheat the oven to 350°F. Toss the Spanish onions with the sugar and wrap in aluminum foil. Bake in the oven until completely tender, 1 to 1½ hours.

2. Unwrap the onions and place into a fine sieve. Press with a spoon to extract as much liquid as possible.

3. Add the vinegar and mustard to the liquid. Slowly whisk in the oil.

4. Whisk in the mustard seeds.

5. Combine the Brussels sprouts, onions, and turnips in a large salad bowl and dress lightly with one-quarter of the mustard seed emulsion.

6. Arrange on a plate and garnish with a little bit of additional sauce. Serve.

PREP TIME: 35 minutes   **TOTAL TIME:** 2 hours

PER SERVING, ABOUT: Calories: 334 Protein: 4 g Carbohydrate: 33 g Dietary Fiber: 6 g Sugars: 21 g Total Fat: 19 g Saturated Fat: 1 g Cholesterol: 0 mg Calcium: 98 mg Sodium: 441 mg

ANITA LO

Co-owner and executive chef at Annisa, Bar Q,
and Rickshaw Dumpling Bar in New York City

ANITA LO, A SECOND GENERATION Chinese American, has had a lifelong love for eating and cooking. In fact, she took her first step into the restaurant industry at an early age, while studying for a degree in French at Columbia University. To satisfy both her hunger for fine food and her desire to learn the language, Lo traveled to Paris to study the art of cooking during her junior year.

After graduating, she went to work at Bouley restaurant in New York City, but decided to return to France a year later to get her degree in cooking at the prestigious École Ritz-Escoffier in Paris. She graduated first in her class with honors, which set her up for internships at several 2-star Michelin-rated restaurants in Paris. She went on to work at a number of New York City restaurants, including Chanterelle, Can, Maxim's, and finally, Mirezi. As chef of this pan-Asian hot spot, she won rave reviews from the local press, including a glowing 2-star write-up from the *New York Times*.

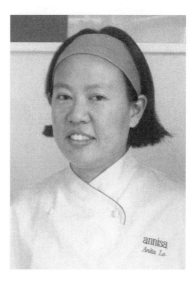

Despite her growing popularity—she made several TV appearances on CNN, the Food Network, and *Martha Stewart Living*, and her recipes were published in the *New York Times, Time Out New York*, and *Food & Wine*—Anita was still looking for more. After two years, she left her position at Mirezi to travel with her partner Jennifer Scism, whom she'd met while working at Can. They spent a year searching for the ultimate meal throughout Southeast Asia and Mediterranean Europe, all the while planning for a place they could eventually call their home. Annisa, which opened in 2000, would be that place; it gave Anita complete freedom to create her contemporary American style of cooking. The eatery, which is consistently top rated in Zagat, also earned 1 star in Michelin's guide.

In 2005, Anita consulted as chef/partner on a new project, Rickshaw Dumpling Bar, also in New York; Rickshaw will expand to more locations locally. Anita most recently opened a third restaurant, Bar Q, in New York City in April 2008.

Anita Lo's Barbecued Breast of Chicken

SERVES 4

CHICKEN CAN SOMETIMES BE dry and bland; marinating, then quickly grilling the boneless breasts helps lock in the flavor.

4 boneless skinless chicken breasts, about 4 ounces each

2 tablespoons canola oil

MARINADE

2 cloves garlic, finely chopped

2 tablespoons fish sauce plus a few drops for salad

4 tablespoons brown sugar

2 teaspoons lemongrass, finely chopped, or substitute a little less dried powdered (optional)

Freshly ground black pepper to taste

SALAD

½ avocado, skin and pit removed, flesh diced

2 thin slices red onion, rinsed

½ cup grape tomatoes, cut in half

2 small Kirby or Persian cucumbers, cut in half and sliced, or 1 cup peeled and sliced regular cucumber

8 large mint leaves, roughly chopped

2 tablespoons roughly chopped fresh cilantro (optional)

1 small clove garlic, finely chopped and pasted (see note)

3 tablespoons fresh lime juice

1 teaspoon sugar

½ teaspoon fish sauce

Freshly chopped red chile pepper to taste

⅛ teaspoon salt

1. Place the individual chicken breasts between two damp pieces of plastic wrap and pound with a mallet or a small sauté pan until flattened to ½-inch thickness. Place the chicken breasts in a container in a single layer but without much space between them. Set aside.

2. Combine the marinade ingredients in a medium bowl. Pour over the chicken breasts, making sure to coat all sides evenly. Marinate, covered in the refrigerator, for at least 4 hours or overnight.

3. Heat a large grill to medium heat. Or substitute a grill pan, if a grill isn't available, over high heat.

4. In a large bowl, mix the avocado, red onion, tomatoes, cucumbers, mint, cilantro, if desired, and garlic together. Add the lime juice, sugar, fish sauce, chile pepper, and salt and mix thoroughly.

5. Wipe the excess marinade from the chicken breasts and coat with oil. Place chicken breasts on grill or in grill pan. Cook until caramelized, about 3 minutes on each side. Serve immediately with the salad on top.

NOTE: To paste, crush finely chopped garlic a tiny bit at a time with the side of a chef's knife; lean firmly on the knife with the heel of your hand.

PREP TIME: 15 minutes   **TOTAL TIME:** 4 hours 25 minutes

PER SERVING, ABOUT: Calories: 252 Protein: 28 g Carbohydrate: 9 g Dietary Fiber: 2 g Sugars: 5 g Total Fat: 11 g Saturated Fat: 1 g Cholesterol: 68 mg Calcium: 46 mg Sodium: 407 mg

Anita Lo's Seasonal Fruit Soup with Jicama and Mint

SERVES 4

FRESH, IN-SEASON FRUIT IS always a good way to end a meal. The addition of crunchy jicama, sweet white wine, and fresh mint make this a standout fruit dessert.

2 cups mixed seasonal fresh fruit, diced

¼ cup jicama, diced

1 cup freshly squeezed seasonal fruit juice

½ teaspoon finely grated ginger

¼ cup sweet white wine or champagne

1 teaspoon sugar, or less, depending on the sweetness of the fruit

4 large mint leaves, thinly sliced

Mix the diced fruit, jicama, fruit juice, ginger, and wine together in a large bowl. Add the sugar, if desired. Divide into 4 bowls, garnish with mint, and serve.

PREP TIME: 10 minutes   **TOTAL TIME:** 10 minutes

PER SERVING, ABOUT: Calories: 74 Protein: 1 g Carbohydrate: 16 g Dietary Fiber: 1 g Sugars: 14 g Total Fat: 0 g Saturated Fat: 0 g Cholesterol: 0 mg Calcium: 18 mg Sodium: 9 mg

NOBU MATSUHISA

Chef/owner of twenty-one restaurants in seventeen cities around the world

NOBUYUKI MATSUHISA, KNOWN AS "NOBU," was born in Saitama, Japan. He traces the beginnings of his professional ambition to the day his older brother took him to a sushi restaurant for the first time. Fascinated by the environment, he knew then that he was destined for a career in the kitchen.

Nobu took his first job right out of high school, working at a sushi restaurant called Matsuei in Tokyo. When he was twenty-four, he accepted an offer from one of his customers that took him to Lima, Peru, to open a restaurant. There he began weaving Peru-

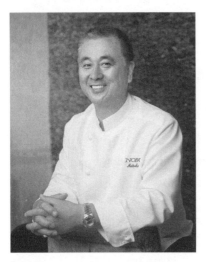

Steven Freeman

vian influences into his dishes, the beginnings of his signature style. After three years, he left Lima to do a brief stint in Buenos Aires, Argentina, before returning to Japan. Soon after, he was given an opportunity to open a restaurant in Alaska, but it burned to the ground during one of his rare nights away from the restaurant.

With debts to pay, Nobu went to Los Angeles on the advice of a friend. He took a job at a sushi bar, and no less than nine years later, after earning his way back to solvency, he opened his own restaurant Matsuhisa in Beverly Hills in 1987. Matsuhisa was an instant success and became a magnet for food lovers and celebrities alike. It was here that his longtime friendship and business relationship with Robert De Niro began. At De Niro's urging, they opened Nobu in New York City in 1994 with restaurateur Drew Nieporent. Like Matsuhisa, Nobu was a hit.

The awards and citations that Nobu's restaurants have racked up are almost too numerous to name. Some of the highlights: Matsuhisa was named one of the Top Ten Restaurant Destinations in the world by the *New York Times* in 1993; Nobu was awarded Best New Restaurant by the James Beard Foundation in 1995; Nobu London was awarded 1 Michelin star in 1997; Nobu Berkeley St. was awarded 1 Michelin star in 2005; and Matsuhisa Beverly Hills and Nobu Las Vegas were awarded 1 Michelin star in 2007.

His personal honors are just as impressive. He was named one of America's 10 Best New Chefs by *Food & Wine* magazine in 1989 and Southern California's Rising Stars by the *Los Angeles Times* magazine in 1998. He was inducted into Who's Who of Food and Beverage in America by the James Beard Foundation in 2002, and was nominated for Outstanding Chef by the James Beard Foundation nine times.

Nobu is also the author of five cookbooks: *Nobu* the cookbook, *Nobu Now, Japanese Finger Food—Nobu Style* (in Japanese only), *Nobu West,* and *Nobu Miami: The Party Cookbook.*

Nobu resides in Beverly Hills with his wife. His two grown daughters now live in Tokyo.

Nobu Matsuhisa's Steamed Clams with Ginger and Garlic

SERVES 4

THE GINGER AND GARLIC infuse the broth and clams in this outstanding yet easy-to-prepare dish.

2¼ pounds fresh cherrystone clams, or other variety if not available

2 cloves garlic, sliced

1-inch piece ginger, peeled and cut into thin strips

1 tablespoon grapeseed oil

1½ teaspoons toasted sesame oil

1 leek, white part only, well washed and cut lengthwise into long strips

1 cup sodium-free chicken broth

2 teaspoons soy sauce

Freshly ground black pepper to taste

1. Wash the clams thoroughly with your hands and running water and place in a saucepan with the garlic, ginger, oils, leek, and chicken broth. Cover with a lid and cook over high heat for 10 minutes, or until the clams have opened.

2. Transfer the clams to a large serving dish, discarding any that have stayed closed. Add the soy sauce and pepper to the cooking liquid and pour over the top of the clams. Serve.

PREP TIME: 10 minutes   **TOTAL TIME:** 20 minutes

PER SERVING, ABOUT: Calories: 108 Protein: 7 g Carbohydrate: 7 g Dietary Fiber: 1 g
Sugars: 1 g Total Fat: 6 g Saturated Fat: 1 g Cholesterol: 13 mg Calcium: 38 mg Sodium: 135 mg

Nobu Matsuhisa's Parmesan Baked Small Scallops

SERVES 4

THE RICH FLAVOR OF scallops is heightened by the addition of Parmesan and soy sauce in this fuss-free dish.

16 ounces bay scallops

½ ounce butter

2 teaspoons soy sauce

1 teaspoon grated garlic

1 tablespoon chopped fresh parsley

3 tablespoons grated Parmesan

1 lemon, sliced into thin round slices

1. Preheat the oven to 400°F. Divide the scallops evenly between 4 small baking dishes, placing the scallops in a single layer.

2. On each scallop, place a tiny bit of butter, a drop of soy sauce, a little grated garlic, chopped parsley, and a little Parmesan.

3. Bake in the oven for 5 minutes. Serve hot with lemon slices.

PREP TIME: 5 minutes   **TOTAL TIME:** 10 minutes

PER SERVING, ABOUT: Calories: 151 Protein: 21 g Carbohydrate: 3 g Dietary Fiber: 0 g Sugars: 0 g Total Fat: 5 g Saturated Fat: 3 g Cholesterol: 50 mg Calcium: 89 mg Sodium: 353 mg

SARMA MELNGAILIS

*Proprietor and executive chef of Pure Food and Wine
in New York City*

SARMA MELNGAILIS HAS DEDICATED HERSELF to achieving one very important dream: presenting raw food as accessible, uplifting, and appealing, thereby exposing more and more people to the health value of the raw lifestyle. One huge step toward making this a reality is the restaurant she co-founded, Pure Food and Wine, where she surprises diners with raw food such as White Corn Tamales with Raw Cocoa Mole and Zucchini and Tomato Lasagna, which many prefer to their favorite conventionally prepared meals.

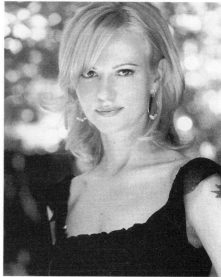

Erika Michelsen

Another step toward realizing her dream is One Lucky Duck Holdings, LLC. As founder and president of the company, which operates www.oneluckyduck.com, an online boutique that offers products for the ultimate raw and organic lifestyle, Sarma is bringing the raw lifestyle to people who otherwise may not have had a chance to learn about it. The company also labels and distributes a line of snack products made and packaged by hand at Pure Food and Wine, and sold exclusively at her e-commerce boutique as well as at her café and retail store, One Lucky Duck Juice and Takeaway, also in New York's historic Gramercy Park neighborhood.

Sarma is coauthor of *Raw Food Real World* (HarperCollins, 2005), a beautifully illustrated book of recipes and practical advice related to raw foods, and she has another cookbook, *Living Raw Food,* in the works. Sarma is a graduate of the French Culinary Institute. She also holds a B.S. in Economics and a B.A. in Economics from the Wharton School at the University of Pennsylvania.

Sarma Melngailis's Avocado, Tomato, and Fennel Salad with Walnut–Mint Dressing

SERVES 4

THIS SALAD IS COMFORTING, satisfying, *and* raw, and the dressing might just become your new favorite.

¼ cup walnuts

¼ cup capers, drained

Zest of 1 lemon

1 tablespoon chopped shallot

2 tablespoons raw walnut oil

½ cup olive oil

1 tablespoon fresh lemon juice

¼ cup chopped fresh mint, plus extra leaves for garnish

¼ teaspoon salt

Freshly ground black pepper to taste

2 tablespoons water

1 fennel bulb, thinly sliced

1½ large tomatoes, preferably organic heirloom tomatoes, sliced

1 avocado, peel and pit removed, flesh sliced

1. Grind the walnuts, capers, lemon zest, and shallot into a paste in a food processor, about 1 minute.

2. Transfer to a medium bowl and whisk in the oils, lemon juice, mint, salt, pepper, and water.

3. Divide the fennel, tomatoes, and avocado slices evenly between 4 bowls and drizzle the walnut-mint dressing over the top. Garnish with more pepper and mint leaves and serve.

PREP TIME: 15 minutes　**TOTAL TIME:** 15 minutes

PER SERVING, ABOUT: Calories: 435　Protein: 3 g　Carbohydrate: 13 g　Dietary Fiber: 6 g
Sugars: 2 g　Total Fat: 44 g　Saturated Fat: 6 g　Cholesterol: 0 mg　Calcium: 64 mg　Sodium: 440 mg

Sarma Melngailis's Avocado Soup with Blood Orange and Mango Salsa

SERVES 4

THIS CREAMY SOUP HAS a base of rich avocado highlighted by tart citrus and the flowery flavor of mango.

SOUP

½ cup chopped cucumber, skin and seeds included if organic

1 small avocado, skin and pit removed

1½ teaspoons roughly chopped shallot

1 small stalk celery, roughly chopped

1 tablespoon fresh lemon juice

¼ teaspoon coriander

¼ teaspoon cumin

⅛ teaspoon orange zest

1 cup water

¼ teaspoon salt

¼ cup fresh cilantro, leaves only

SALSA

½ cup small diced red bell pepper (make cubes same size)

2 blood oranges or other type of orange, sectioned (see page 346) and chopped into big chunks, juice squeezed into salsa

½ cup small diced mango (make cubes same size)

½ cup chopped fresh cilantro leaves, plus extra leaves for garnish

⅛ teaspoon salt

1. Blend all the soup ingredients in a high speed blender until very smooth, about 2 minutes. If the soup is too thick, add a little water, 1 tablespoon at a time.

2. Toss all the salsa ingredients in a medium bowl until well combined.

3. Evenly distribute the soup into medium bowls and garnish with the salsa and cilantro leaves. Serve.

PREP TIME: 15 minutes   **TOTAL TIME:** 15 minutes

PER SERVING, ABOUT: Calories: 112 Protein: 2 g Carbohydrate: 17 g Dietary Fiber: 5 g Sugars: 11 g Total Fat: 6 g Saturated Fat: 1 g Cholesterol: 0 mg Calcium: 44 mg Sodium: 227 mg

VITALY PALEY

Chef/owner of Paley's Place and creator of The Paley Bar

LURED TO PORTLAND, OREGON, FROM New York in 1995 by the bounty of the Pacific Northwest, Vitaly Paley has become one of the region's leading chefs. His cooking is based on local, sustainably grown ingredients, and he prides himself on being instrumental in the movement to define regional Northwest cuisine. As he explains, his goal is to bring the farmer closer to the restaurant guest. Indeed, the relationship he has with local growers dictates everything about the menu and preparations.

Vitaly, who was born near Kiev in the former Soviet Union and immigrated to the United States in 1976, brings an artist's sensitivity to his cooking. A childhood concert pianist who studied at Juilliard, he eventually shifted his creative energies to cooking, and in 1989 he earned a Grand Diploma from the French Culinary Institute in New York. He refined his skills at the Union Square Café, Remi, and Chanterelle in New York, and then went on to apprentice at the Michelin-starred restaurant, Moulin de la Gorce in France.

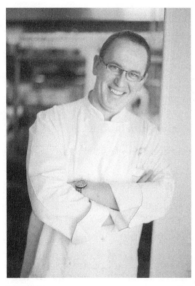

John Valls

Paley's Place, which Vitaly opened in 1995, and his inspired cuisine, consistently draws praise, both locally and nationally. He received the Best Chef Northwest Award from the James Beard Foundation in 2005. He was recently featured in a Food Network award segment honoring Portland as "Delicious Destination of the year." The restaurant has been featured in *Gourmet* magazine several times: as one of America's Top 50 Restaurants in October 2006, as one of the Best Farm-to-Table restaurants in October 2007, and in their restaurant issues in 2006 and 2007. *O, The Oprah Magazine* called Paley's Place "the place for foodies" in November 2006. Paley's Place recipes have also been featured in the *Food & Wine* 2007 Cookbook, *Bon Appétit*, and *Food Arts*. Vitaly is also coauthor (along with his wife, Kimberly, and Robert Reynolds) of *The Paley's Place Cookbook: Recipes and Stories from the Pacific Northwest* (Ten Speed Press, October 2008).

Vitaly took his culinary talents one step further in 2004 when he designed an alternative energy bar for his own personal use. An avid cyclist, he wanted to reenergize the typical sports bar with new flavors and wholesome organic ingredients—from apricots and raisins to strawberries, figs, and dry roasted hazelnuts.

Vitaly lives in Portland with his wife Kimberly, who is the co-owner/general manager of Paley's Place.

Vitaly Paley's Spice Grilled Chicken Breasts with Couscous Salad and Sesame Sauce

SERVES 4

THIS SPICE MIX IS used with both the chicken and couscous.

COUSCOUS

½ tablespoon turmeric powder	Freshly ground black pepper to taste
½ tablespoon cumin powder	½ cup whole grain couscous
¼ teaspoon ground cayenne	¼ cup coarsely chopped roasted unsalted almonds
¼ teaspoon cinnamon	
¼ teaspoon ground star anise	4 teaspoons dried cranberries
½ cup water	2 tablespoons chopped fresh mint leaves
Pinch of saffron	Juice of 1 lemon
⅛ teaspoon salt	1½ tablespoons olive oil

1. Place the turmeric, cumin, cayenne, cinnamon, and star anise in a small mixing bowl and stir until incorporated. Separate about half of the spice mix and reserve for the chicken breasts. Place the rest in a small pot, add water, saffron, salt, and pepper. Bring the mixture to a boil over high heat.

2. Place the couscous in a medium mixing bowl and pour the boiling spice water over the couscous. Cover the bowl tightly with plastic wrap and let the couscous steam for 7 to 10 minutes (any longer and the couscous will overcook). Remove the plastic wrap and fluff up the couscous with a fork.

3. Add the almonds, cranberries, mint, lemon juice, and oil. Season with pepper. Set aside and keep at room temperature while assembling the other components of the dish.

(continued)

SAUCE

¼ cup tahini

2 cloves garlic, peeled and finely minced

Juice of ½ lemon

¼ cup water

⅛ teaspoon salt

Freshly ground black pepper to taste

Place the tahini, garlic, and lemon juice in the bowl of a food processor and puree until well incorporated, about 1 minute. Add the water. If the sauce is still too thick, add enough water to loosen it up so it is thin enough to pour. Season with the salt and pepper and set aside.

CHICKEN

2 skinless chicken breasts, bone in, about
   8 ounces each

⅛ teaspoon salt

Freshly ground black pepper to taste

2 teaspoons canola oil

1. Heat an outdoor grill, or a large heavy-bottomed ovenproof skillet over high heat, and preheat the oven to 375°F. Sprinkle the chicken breasts on both sides with the reserved spice mix and salt and pepper. Drizzle with the oil.

2. To grill, place the chicken breasts bone side down on the coldest portion of the grill. Cover and cook until the chicken has lost its translucency and is a bit springy to the touch, about 10 minutes. Flip and place over a hot part of the grill to finish, another 5 minutes or so. Check with a probe thermometer to make sure the core temperature is at least 160°F. Cook longer if necessary. To cook on the stove, place the chicken in a hot skillet breastbone side down. Cook until browned, about 5 minutes. Flip and place the skillet in the oven for an additional 10 minutes. Check with a probe thermometer to make sure the core temperature is at least 160°F. Cook longer if necessary.

3. Once the chicken is cooked, remove the breastbone, slice thinly, and serve with the couscous salad and sesame sauce drizzled over the whole dish.

PREP TIME: 30 minutes   **TOTAL TIME:** 45 minutes

PER SERVING, ABOUT: Calories: 452 Protein: 35 g Carbohydrate: 33 g Dietary Fiber: 6 g Sugars: 2 g Total Fat: 22 g Saturated Fat: 3 g Cholesterol: 66 mg Calcium: 85 mg Sodium: 300 mg

Vitaly Paley's Grilled Lamb Paillard with Summer Vegetable Salad and Herbed Yogurt

SERVES 4

THIS ELEGANT SALAD IS equally at home as a picnic or a formal dinner. To retain moistness and flavor, take care not to overcook the lamb.

SPICES

1 teaspoon cumin seeds

1 teaspoon fennel seeds

1 teaspoon coriander seeds

2 bay leaves

1 tablespoon paprika

Place the cumin seeds, fennel seeds, coriander seeds, and bay leaves in a small skillet. Over medium heat, toast the spices until you begin to smell a rich, spicy aroma, about 3 minutes. Remove from the heat and let cool slightly. Transfer to a spice mill or food processor and finely grind them. Transfer to a small mixing bowl, stir in the paprika, and set aside.

LAMB

1 pound boneless leg of lamb, trimmed of fat and sinew, cut into 4 pieces, about 4 ounces each

⅛ teaspoon salt

Freshly ground black pepper to taste

2 tablespoons extra virgin olive oil

1. Lay out a 12-inch square piece of plastic wrap on a cutting board. Place one piece of lamb on it. Loosely place another piece of plastic wrap over the top of it. Using the smooth side of a meat mallet, pound out the piece of lamb until it is about ⅛ inch thick all the way around. It may be irregularly shaped with jagged edges; this will only add to the rustic look of the finished dish.

2. Lift off the top layer of the plastic. Sprinkle the lamb with a little spice mixture and season with salt and pepper. Drizzle ¼ teaspoon oil over the lamb. Turn the lamb over and repeat the process. Refrigerate. Repeat the process with the rest of the lamb pieces.

(continued)

SALAD

3 tablespoons fresh mint, finely chopped except for a few leaves

3 tablespoons fresh parsley, finely chopped except for a few leaves

1½ tablespoons fresh cilantro, finely chopped except for a few leaves

2 tablespoons fresh basil, finely chopped except for a few leaves

2 cloves garlic, peeled and finely chopped

1 cup reduced-fat plain yogurt

Zest and juice of 1 lemon

⅛ teaspoon salt

Freshly ground black pepper to taste

1 large sweet onion, peeled, halved, and cut into 8 wedges

2 teaspoons olive oil (1½ for onion, ½ for tomato mixture)

1 large ripe tomato, cored and cut into 8 wedges

1 medium seedless cucumber, peeled and cut into ¼-inch-thick disks

¼ cup black olives with pits

1. Put the chopped mint, parsley, cilantro, and basil into a medium mixing bowl. Add the garlic, yogurt, and half the lemon juice. Stir together until well combined. Season with the salt and pepper.

2. Heat an outdoor grill to hot or, if you don't have a grill available, heat the broiler in your oven to high.

3. Season the onion wedges with pepper. Drizzle with 1½ teaspoons oil.

4. To grill, place the onion over the hot part of the grill until it develops well-defined grill marks, about 3 minutes per side. To broil, place the onion on a sheet pan and cook for 3 minutes on each side.

5. Transfer the onion to a large mixing bowl. Add the tomato, cucumber, olives, the reserved herb leaves, lemon zest, and the remaining half of the lemon juice. Drizzle with ½ teaspoon oil. Season the salad with pepper and mix well to incorporate. Set aside while cooking the lamb.

6. To grill, place the lamb over the hottest part of the grill and cook for 30 seconds. Carefully turn it over and cook for 30 seconds more. To broil, place the lamb on a sheet pan under the broiler at its highest setting. Cook for 30 seconds. Carefully turn it over and cook for 30 seconds more.

7. Transfer the lamb onto a dinner plate, top with the salad, and drizzle the yogurt sauce over the whole dish. Serve.

PREP TIME: 30 minutes   **TOTAL TIME:** 30 minutes

PER SERVING, ABOUT: Calories: 328 Protein: 29 g Carbohydrate: 18 g Dietary Fiber: 4 g Sugars: 7 g Total Fat: 16 g Saturated Fat: 4 g Cholesterol: 79 mg Calcium: 197 mg Sodium: 431 mg

TAL RONNEN

Executive chef and founder of Veg Advantage

TAL RONNEN, A GRADUATE OF New York City's Natural Gourmet Institute, has worked at the top vegan restaurants in the country, including Sublime in Fort Lauderdale, Florida, and Candle 79 in New York City. In 2007, Tal teamed up with Rock and Roll Hall of Famer Chrissie Hynde to open her new vegetarian restaurant, VegiTerranean, in Akron, Ohio. Most recently, he has provided recipes for *New York Times* bestselling author Kathy Freston's latest book, *Quantum Wellness,* as well as preparing meals for Oprah Winfrey during her twenty-one-day cleanse.

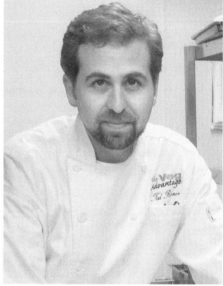

Tal's approach to vegan cuisine is based on classic French techniques, but he's not afraid to give his creations a contemporary twist. His signature dishes include a Key lime and avocado-cream dessert parfait, Old Bay tofu cakes with vegan horseradish crème, and artichoke tortellini with saffron "cream" sauce.

Tal's passion for vegan food goes beyond cooking. In 2004, Tal started the Veg Advantage program, which is designed to help food-service operators integrate vegan options into their menus. He has worked with many of the top vegetarian food manufacturers, such as Turtle Island Foods, Garen Protein International, Follow Your Heart, and Gardenburger. He has also performed cooking demonstrations on numerous television shows and often assists hotels, schools, including New York University, and corporate dining halls, including America Online's headquarters, with vegan menu options. And he conducts master vegetarian workshops for students and staff at several Le Cordon Bleu–affiliate culinary schools nationwide.

Tal Ronnen's Shaved Fennel, Orange, and Quinoa Salad

SERVES 4

THIS DISH OFFERS AN elegant presentation with exceptionally fresh and bright flavors. Tangy orange and nutty quinoa complement the unique sweetness of fennel.

FENNEL SLAW

1½ pounds fresh fennel, shaved very thinly

1 cup julienned carrots

2 tablespoons fresh lemon juice

1 tablespoon extra virgin olive oil

1 tablespoon chopped fresh dill

½ teaspoon finely grated fresh lemon zest

⅛ teaspoon salt

Mix all ingredients together in a large bowl. Set aside.

QUINOA LAYER

1 cup quinoa, rinsed

2 cups vegetable stock (with no more than 350 mg sodium per cup)

1 tablespoon extra virgin olive oil

1 tablespoon diced red onion

2 oranges, peeled and sectioned (see page 346)

1 cup microgreens

2 teaspoons champagne vinegar

1 teaspoon olive oil

1 tablespoon finely chopped fresh chives

1. Cook the quinoa in the stock in a medium pot over medium heat until the quinoa is translucent and the stock is absorbed, about 10 minutes.

2. Place the cooked quinoa in a large bowl and let cool. Add the extra virgin oil and onion to the quinoa. Set aside.

3. Using a ring mold, layer the fennel slaw, oranges, and quinoa. Press down firmly and smooth the top. Carefully turn over onto a plate.

4. Toss the microgreens in vinegar and olive oil. Place on top of the fennel layer.

5. Garnish with fresh chives and serve.

PREP TIME: 20 minutes   **TOTAL TIME:** 30 minutes

PER SERVING, ABOUT: Calories: 341 Protein: 9 g Carbohydrate: 54 g Dietary Fiber: 10 g Sugars: 8 g Total Fat: 12 g Saturated Fat: 2 g Cholesterol: 0 mg Calcium: 1,401 mg Sodium: 345 mg

Tal Ronnen's Black Bean Cakes with Lime–Peppered "Mayo"

SERVES 4

THESE CAKES ARE CRISPY on the outside, moist on the inside and full of flavor.

3 cups canned black beans, drained and rinsed, or cooked (page 345)

2 tablespoons vegan margarine, such as Earth Balance, softened

2 tablespoons chopped fresh cilantro

2 tablespoons chopped shallots

2 teaspoons minced garlic

2 teaspoons Creole seasoning (or make your own by combining ⅛ teaspoon sea salt, ½ teaspoon chili powder, ½ teaspoon smoked paprika, pinch of onion powder, pinch of black pepper, pinch of dried thyme, pinch of dried

basil, pinch of dried oregano, pinch of ground coriander, small pinch of cayenne, very small pinch of cumin)

1 slice multi-grain bread, toasted and processed in a food processor for 1 minute to make bread crumbs

Black pepper to taste

¼ cup vegan mayonnaise

1½ teaspoons fresh lime juice

1 jalapeño pepper, minced

¼ cup canola oil

1. Preheat the oven to 300°F.

2. Place the beans on paper towels to soak up the excess moisture. Bake the beans on a sheet pan for 20 minutes. Let cool.

3. Combine the beans, margarine, cilantro, shallots, garlic, Creole seasoning, bread crumbs, and pepper in a food processor and blend for 1 minute. Place in a bowl and refrigerate, covered, for 1 to 2 hours.

4. Mix the vegan mayonnaise, lime juice, and jalapeño in a medium bowl. Season with pepper and refrigerate, covered, until ready to serve.

5. Heat the oil in a large skillet over medium heat. Form the bean mixture into patties and fry the cakes for 4 minutes, until browned and crispy, then flip and cook on the other side until crispy, about 3 minutes. Drain on paper towels.

6. Serve patties garnished with the lime mayo.

PREP TIME: 15 minutes   TOTAL TIME: 1 hour 50 minutes (this includes refrigerating bean mixture)

PER SERVING, ABOUT: Calories: 448 Protein: 12 g Carbohydrate: 34 g Dietary Fiber: 12 g Sugars: 0 g Total Fat: 29 g Saturated Fat: 3 g Cholesterol: 0 mg Calcium: 49 mg Sodium: 226 mg

CHARLIE TROTTER

Owner and executive chef at Charlie Trotter's in Chicago

CHARLIE TROTTER IS AN ALUMNI of the University of Wisconsin Madison, where he studied literature and political science before he followed his passion to cook. He opened Charlie Trotter's restaurant in 1987, and since then it has become known as one of the finest restaurants in the world. He has been instrumental in establishing new standards for fine dining.

All of Charlie's dishes are designed to highlight the finest, freshest food obtainable. A network of more than ninety purveyors provides the healthful ingredients that inspire him to create flavorful masterpieces. From the naturally raised meat and game to the line-caught seafood to the organic produce, every component of each dish is the purest available. Indiana bobwhite quail, petite greens from Farmer Jones, heirloom tomatoes from Illinois, North Dakota buffalo, and Hawaiian gindai are just a few of the products that arrive each day at Charlie Trotter's.

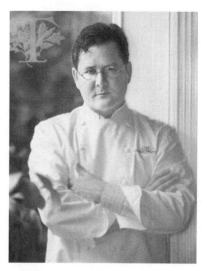

Kipling Swehla

The restaurant has been recognized by a variety of prestigious national and international institutions. In 1995, Charlie Trotter's was inducted into the esteemed Relais & Chateaux, and in 1998 was accepted as a member by Traditions & Qualité. The restaurant has also received 5 stars from the Mobil Travel Guide and 5 diamonds from the AAA. Charlie and his restaurant have also racked up 10 James Beard Foundation awards, including Outstanding Restaurant (2000) and Outstanding Chef (1999). *Wine Spectator* named the eatery The Best Restaurant in the World for Wine & Food (1998) and America's Best Restaurant (2000).

Building on his success, Charlie opened Trotter's To Go, a gourmet take out retail shop in the Lincoln Park neighborhood in 2000. He also produces a line of private label organic products. In February 2008, Charlie expanded his culinary offerings with the addition of a new restaurant, Restaurant Charlie, located in the Palazzo Hotel Resort and Casino in

Las Vegas, Nevada. Future restaurant plans include two new restaurants in The Elysian, a luxury hotel project currently being built in the Gold Coast neighborhood of Chicago.

Charlie is the author of fourteen cookbooks, three management books, and is the host of the award-winning PBS cooking series, *The Kitchen Sessions with Charlie Trotter.*

His culinary accolades are matched only by his philantrophic honors: he was recognized by President Bush and Colin Powell for his work with his nonprofit organization, Trotter Culinary Education Foundation, which benefits people seeking a career in the culinary arts. He was named one of only five "heroes" to be honored by Colin Powell's charity, America's Promise. In 2005, Charlie was awarded the Humanitarian of the Year award by the International Association of Culinary Professionals for his overall service to the community.

Charlie Trotter's Passion Fruit Pudding Cake

SERVES 16

THIS RECIPE CREATES A combination of creamy custard and silky cake. If you can't find fresh passion fruit, substitute a citrus juice, such as Meyer lemon, Key lime, or orange juice. And feel free to use any seasonal fruit for garnish.

4 tablespoons unsalted butter, softened

1 cup plus 2 tablespoons sugar

Pinch of salt

6 egg yolks

6 tablespoons unbleached all-purpose flour

2 cups fat-free milk

1/2 cup fresh passion fruit juice or citrus juice

8 egg whites

GARNISH

3/4 cup nonfat plain yogurt

1 tablespoon honey

2 passion fruits, cut in half, seeds and juice scooped into a medium bowl, or finely dice or mash a substitute seasonal fruit

4 teaspoons honeycomb (available in the honey section in many grocery stores)

1 cup wild strawberries, stems on, large berries cut in half lengthwise, or another seasonal fruit

(continued)

1. Preheat the oven to 325°F. Line a 8½ x 12-inch pan with plastic wrap.

2. Combine the butter, sugar, and salt in a large bowl and cream with an electric mixer until smooth and fluffy, 2 to 3 minutes. Add the egg yolks one at a time, mixing well after each addition. Add the flour and mix well. Add the milk and ½ cup juice and mix until combined.

3. In a separate mixer bowl, beat the egg whites until stiff peaks form, 3 to 4 minutes. Gently fold the egg whites into the batter just until combined. Immediately pour the batter onto the prepared pan. Place the pan in a large roasting pan and add hot water to the roasting pan until the water reaches halfway up the sides of the sheet pan.

4. Bake for about 45 minutes, or until golden brown and firm to the touch. Carefully remove the sheet pan from the water bath and let the cake cool to room temperature. Refrigerate, covered, until well chilled, 45 minutes.

5. To unmold, invert onto a cutting board. Lift off the pan and peel off the plastic wrap. Trim all 4 edges to even them, and then cut the cake into 16 pieces, each 4 by 1½ inches.

6. Add the yogurt and honey to the bowl with the juice and seeds of two passion fruits and stir until combined.

7. To assemble, place a piece of the chilled pudding cake on each plate. Drizzle 1 tablespoon of fruit-yogurt sauce over the cake and around the plate. Place ¼ teaspoon honeycomb in front of the cake, and sprinkle the strawberries around the plate. Serve.

PREP TIME: 35 minutes   **TOTAL TIME:** 2 hours

PER SERVING, ABOUT: Calories: 150 Protein: 5 g Carbohydrate: 22 g Dietary Fiber: 1 g
Sugars: 19 g Total Fat: 5 g Saturated Fat: 2 g Cholesterol: 87 mg Calcium: 74 mg Sodium: 61 mg

Charlie Trotter's Sea Scallops with Fresh Soybeans and Ginger-Soy-Hijiki Broth

SERVES 4

THE BROTH IN THIS dish explodes with complex flavors imparted by the seaweed, soy, mirin, and ginger. The buttery scallops take on just enough of the ginger and soy sauce to complement their meaty flesh. Hijiki, mirin, and rice wine vinegar can be found in Asian markets, online, or in the international section of well-stocked supermarkets.

PRESERVED GINGER

4 teaspoons very thinly sliced fresh ginger

½ cup sugar

2 cups water

BROTH

¼ cup dried hijiki or wakame seaweed

2 cups water

1 tablespoon finely diced jalapeño

1 tablespoon finely diced shallot

1 tablespoon minced fresh ginger

1 teaspoon minced garlic

2 tablespoons rice vinegar

1 tablespoon mirin

2 tablespoons reduced-sodium soy sauce

SCALLOPS

1 pound sea scallops

¼ teaspoon kosher salt

Freshly ground black pepper to taste

2 teaspoons grapeseed oil

2 tablespoons freshly squeezed lemon juice

2 tablespoons sesame seeds, toasted (see page 346)

1 tablespoon thinly sliced fresh cilantro

GARNISH

½ cup shelled soybeans (edamame), blanched (see page 350)

¾ cup diced firm silken tofu

4 water chestnuts, thinly sliced

4 teaspoons fresh flat-leaf parsley leaves

1. Place the ginger, 2 tablespoons sugar, and ½ cup water in a small saucepan over medium heat. Bring to a simmer and cook for 10 minutes. Drain the ginger, discarding the liquid, and return the ginger to the saucepan. Add 2 tablespoons sugar and ½ cup water and again simmer for 10 minutes. Repeat two more times, then remove from the heat, reserving the liquid the last time. Let cool, and refrigerate the ginger in the liquid for up to 2 weeks. Drain the liquid before using the ginger.

(continued)

2.   Soak the hijiki in cold water to cover completely for 30 minutes then drain. Place the seaweed and 2 cups water, jalapeño, shallot, ginger, garlic, vinegar, mirin, and soy sauce in a medium saucepan and simmer over medium heat for 15 minutes.

3.   Season the scallops with salt and pepper. Heat a large sauté pan over high heat and pour in the oil. Add the scallops and cook, turning once, for 1½ minutes on each side, or until slightly underdone. Scallops should fit comfortably in the pan in a single layer. Use 2 pans or cook in 2 batches if your pan can't accommodate the scallops.

4.   Add the lemon juice, sesame seeds, and cilantro. Cook, spooning the mixture over the scallops in the sauté pan, turning them once, for 1 minute longer, or until the scallops are coated with the mixture.

5.   To assemble, place one-quarter each of soybeans, tofu, water chestnuts, and parsley in each bowl. Place an equal amount of scallops in the center of each bowl and sprinkle with the preserved ginger. Ladle in ½ cup broth. Serve.

PREP TIME: 25 minutes   **TOTAL TIME:** 1 hour 15 minutes

PER SERVING, ABOUT: Calories: 268 Protein: 28 g Carbohydrate: 22 g Dietary Fiber: 2 g Sugars: 11 g Total Fat: 8 g Saturated Fat: 1 g Cholesterol: 37 mg Calcium: 76 mg Sodium: 697 mg

ROY YAMAGUCHI

Chef and founder of Roy's restaurants with thirty-five locations around the world

ROY YAMAGUCHI WAS BORN AND raised in Tokyo; his mother was from Okinawa and his father, a career military man, was born in Hawaii. Roy could not help but absorb much of Japan's culture, although he was also influenced by his Hawaiian heritage. It was during one of his visits to see his grandparents in Maui that he got his first taste of fresh seafood—lobster and octopus. He eventually left his home in Tokyo to come to America, where he attended the Culinary Institute of America, located in Hyde Park, New York. After graduating in 1976, his devotion to French cooking was nurtured in Southern California, where he signed on for an apprenticeship at L'Escoffier, followed by one at L'Ermitage.

After working at a number of other Los Angeles restaurants, including his own, 385 North, he decided to uproot his young family in 1988 and move to Hawaii, settling on the eastern side of Honolulu known as Hawaii Kai. Soon after, he opened Roy's, which has become well known throughout the world for its Hawaiian Fusion® Cuisine, featuring the freshest local ingredients, European sauces, and bold Asian spices with a focus on seafood.

He was honored with the James Beard Foundation's Best Pacific Northwest Chef award in 1993. The California Restaurant Writers Association also chose him as the California Chef of the Year in 1986 and 1987, and he was named among the Honolulu 100 who were recognized at the Centennial Gala Celebration of Honolulu in November 2005.

Aside from hosting *Hawaii Cooks with Roy Yamaguchi* on PBS, Roy was selected to be among the Iron Chef USA world-class contingent in 2001. The following year, he taped a segment with the Food Network for their series, *My Country, My Kitchen,* and in 2004 he was featured on the Home Shopping Network, where his signature line of cookware was sold. He has also appeared on *Good Morning America, Emeril,* the *Today* show, *CBS This Morning, The Early Show on CBS,* Bravo's *Top Chef, iVillage Live,* and *Live with Regis and Kelly.*

Roy has published four cookbooks: *Pacific Bounty* (Ten Speed Press, 1994), *Roy's Feasts from Hawaii* (Ten Speed Press, 1995), *Hawaii Cooks with Roy Yamaguchi* (Ten Speed Press, 2003), and *Roy's Fish & Seafood* (Ten Speed Press, 2005). He is currently working on his fifth book.

Roy Yamaguchi's Slow-Baked Pepper-Crusted Salmon with Roasted Beets and Crispy Garlic Lemon Vinaigrette

SERVES 4

THE METHOD OF CURING the salmon and then cooking it at a very low temperature results in a very tender, moist, and flaky piece of fish.

BEETS

2 medium beets, unpeeled

1/8 teaspoon salt

1/8 teaspoon freshly cracked black pepper

1 teaspoon extra virgin olive oil

1. Preheat the oven to 325°F.

2. Season the beets with salt and pepper. Coat the beets with oil and place on a baking sheet pan. Roast the beets for 1 hour.

3. Let the beets cool, then remove the skin by cutting off the tops, then pressing the blade of your knife against the meat of the beets to peel the skin off from top to bottom. Cut the beets into thin strips.

NOTE: Working with beets can be messy, so you might consider wearing disposable gloves and placing a sheet of wax paper on your cutting board for easy clean up.

SALMON

Rinds of 2 lemons

2 tablespoons salt

4 tablespoons sugar

4 salmon steaks, about 5 ounces each, 1 inch thick, 2 inches wide, and 5 1/2 to 6 inches long

1. Reduce the heat of the oven to 200°F.

2. Combine the lemon rinds, salt, and sugar in a small bowl and mix thoroughly. Sprinkle the mixture evenly on both sides of the salmon. Let the salmon cure for about 15 minutes.

SEASONING

1 teaspoon freshly cracked black pepper

2 teaspoons extra virgin olive oil

1/8 teaspoon salt

1. Rinse the salmon lightly under cold water and place on a sheet pan. Sprinkle the salmon with pepper and salt.

2. Rub the salmon with oil. Cover the sheet pan with aluminum foil and bake for 6 minutes. Turn the salmon over and cook for another 6 minutes, until the fish is opaque or to your desired doneness.

CRISPY GARLIC VINAIGRETTE

2 tablespoons extra virgin olive oil

1 teaspoon Dijon mustard

1 tablespoon minced garlic

Zest of 1/2 lemon

Juice of 1/2 lemon

1/8 teaspoon freshly cracked black pepper

2 tablespoons finely minced shallot

1 teaspoon honey

2 teaspoons tarragon

1/8 teaspoon salt

2 teaspoons fresh basil

1/8 teaspoon soy sauce

2 tablespoons water

1. Pour the oil in a medium sauté pan and heat over medium heat. Add the garlic, spreading it throughout the oil. Continue to move the garlic around in the pan until the garlic turns golden brown. Remove from the pan and place in a blender.

2. Add the remaining vinaigrette ingredients to the blender and blend to a coarse consistency, about 1 minute.

3. Mix the beets with 2 tablespoons of the vinaigrette.

4. To serve, place the salmon on one side of the plate and the beets on the other side.

PREP TIME: 25 minutes   **TOTAL TIME:** 1 hour 40 minutes

PER SERVING, ABOUT: Calories: 259 Protein: 29 g Carbohydrate: 5 g Dietary Fiber: 1 g Sugars: 3 g Total Fat: 13 g Saturated Fat: 2 g Cholesterol: 78 mg Calcium: 30 mg Sodium: 249 mg

Roy Yamaguchi's Grilled Teriyaki Tuna with Shrimp and Orange

SERVES 4

THIS DISH COMBINES A bright tasting shrimp salsa with flavorful seared tuna.

SALSA

1 teaspoon olive oil

5 large shrimp (about 3 ounces) peeled, deveined, and each cut into 5 pieces

9 sections from 1 orange, each cut into 4 pieces (see page 346)

1/2 teaspoon Tabasco sauce

1/8 cup finely minced sweet onion

2 tablespoons finely minced green onions (scallions)

2 ounces (4 tablespoons) orange juice concentrate

1/2 large ripe tomato, heirloom if possible, cut into 1/2-inch squares, skin intact

2 1/2 teaspoons roughly chopped fresh cilantro

1 1/2 teaspoons roughly chopped fresh mint

1/8 teaspoon salt

1. Heat a large sauté pan over low heat. Add the oil and then the shrimp. Cook for about 2 minutes, until the shrimp is opaque.

2. Combine the orange, Tabasco, sweet and green onions, concentrate, tomato, cilantro, mint, and salt together in a medium bowl with the shrimp and chill for 2 hours before using.

TERIYAKI

4 teaspoons soy sauce

4 teaspoons sugar

4 teaspoons minced fresh ginger

2 teaspoons minced green onion (scallion)

1 teaspoon minced garlic

1 teaspoon toasted white sesame seeds (see page 346)

1 teaspoon dark sesame oil

TUNA

4 pieces ahi tuna, about 2 1/2 ounces each, cut into about 1-inch-thick pieces, 1 1/2 inches wide by 2 3/4 inches long

1 teaspoon olive oil

GARNISH

1 teaspoon toasted white sesame seeds (see page 346)

4 fresh cilantro sprigs

1. Combine all the teriyaki ingredients in a medium bowl.

2. Marinate the tuna in the teriyaki for as little as 10 minutes or up to 5 hours, refrigerated.

3. Heat a sauté pan over high heat. Add the olive oil and sear the tuna for 15 seconds on all 4 sides. Or, you may also cook the tuna in this style on the grill. Remove from the pan or the grill.

4. To serve, slice each piece of tuna into 6 or 7 slices. Arrange the tuna on one side of the plate in layers. Sprinkle the toasted sesame seeds over the tuna and place the cilantro sprig on top. On the other side of the plate, in line with the tuna, place one-quarter of the shrimp.

PREP TIME: 30 minutes   **TOTAL TIME:** 2 hours 35 minutes (this includes chilling shrimp)

PER SERVING, ABOUT: Calories: 302 Protein: 25 g Carbohydrate: 44 g Dietary Fiber: 8 g
Sugars: 35 g Total Fat: 5 g Saturated Fat: 1 g Cholesterol: 64 mg Calcium: 156 mg Sodium: 213 mg

ERIC ZIEBOLD

ERIC ZIEBOLD'S AFFINITY FOR COOKING started in his mom's kitchen as a young child growing up in Iowa. He started working in restaurants when he was sixteen years old and hasn't looked back since.

Eric went on to attend the Culinary Institute of America, and graduated with honors in 1994. From there, he has held positions at some of the best restaurants in the country, including Vidalia restaurant in Washington, D.C., Spago Restaurant in Los Angeles, and Thomas Keller's The French Laundry in Yountville, California. He's currently the executive chef at City Zen in Washington. His style is rooted in tradition but infused with new flavors and interpretations. Eric's vision is presented in two menus: a six-course chef's tasting menu, drawing inspiration from his traditional background and presented with a modern flair, and a three-course prix fixe menu prepared with a creative French twist.

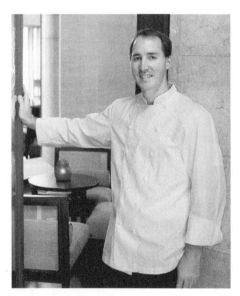

Courtesy of Mandarin Oriental

Eric was named one of America's Best New Chefs by *Food & Wine* magazine in 2005. He recently won the James Beard Foundation's Best Chef: Mid-Atlantic award and the Restaurant Association of Metropolitan Washington's Best Chef award. In March 2007, Eric was named one of Forbes.com's Ten Tastemaking Chefs, ten of the most influential working chefs in America. In addition, City Zen has received numerous awards, including: AAA's Five Diamond Award (2007 and 2008); named one of *Gourmet*'s best 100 restaurants (October 2007); listed as one of the "hottest restaurants in the world" by *Food & Wine* magazine (May 2006 and 2007); Fine Dining Restaurant of the Year 2007 by the Restaurant Association of Metropolitan Washington; and one of America's Best New Restaurants by *Esquire* (November 2005).

Eric Ziebold's Falafel Sandwich with Marinated Red Onion and English Cucumber

SERVES 4

THIS DISH IS DEFINITELY time-consuming, but it will be the best falafel you have ever tasted.

FALAFEL

¹/₃ cup canned no-salt-added garbanzo beans, drained and rinsed, or cooked (see page 345)

²/₃ cup dried garbanzo beans

1 tablespoon bulgur wheat

¹/₂ onion, minced

3 cloves garlic, minced

1 teaspoon fresh mint

1 teaspoon cumin

¹/₃ cup fresh cilantro

¹/₃ cup fresh parsley

1 teaspoon baking soda

¹/₈ teaspoon salt

1 teaspoon olive oil

1. Soak the cooked and dried garbanzo beans and bulgur wheat in water overnight in the refrigerator. Make sure the water covers the beans and bulgur.

2. Drain any leftover water. Grind the beans, wheat, onion, garlic, mint, cumin, cilantro, parsley, baking soda, and salt through a small grinder, or pulse in a food processor to a fine mince, about 1 minute.

3. Mix in a bowl to make sure the falafel holds together and all the ingredients are fully incorporated.

4. Form into 12 patties, about 2 ounces each, and refrigerate for 4 hours on a plate covered with plastic wrap.

5. Heat a large heavy-bottomed and skillet over medium heat. Add the oil and sauté the patties for about 4 minutes on each side or until heated through.

NAAN

2 packages yeast

¹/₃ cup water

¹/₂ teaspoon sugar

¹/₈ teaspoon salt

¹/₂ cup unbleached all-purpose flour

¹/₂ cup whole wheat flour

5 teaspoons clarified butter (see page 350)

2 tablespoons plain low-fat yogurt

¹/₂ teaspoon olive oil

(continued)

1. Preheat the oven to 425°F.

2. Dissolve the yeast in the water in a large bowl.

3. Mix in the sugar, salt, flours, butter, and yogurt. Knead for 2 minutes and allow to sit at room temperature until double in size, about 30 minutes.

4. Portion the dough into 4 pieces and roll out by hand to approximately ⅛ inch thick.

5. Brush with oil and bake in a large ovenproof skillet for about 2 minutes per side.

MARINATED RED ONION AND CUCUMBER

1 tablespoon very thinly sliced red onion

1 teaspoon rice vinegar

⅛ teaspoon salt

1 teaspoon sugar

1 tablespoon very thinly sliced English cucumber

1 teaspoon olive oil

1. Mix the onion with ½ teaspoon vinegar, pinch of salt, and ½ teaspoon sugar. Marinate for 15 minutes, then drain well.

2. Mix the cucumber with the remaining ½ teaspoon vinegar, salt, and ½ teaspoon sugar. Marinate for 1 minute, then rinse with cool water and drain.

3. Toss the onion and cucumber together with the oil.

GARNISH

½ teaspoon low-fat yogurt

1. To serve, place 3 pieces of falafel on 1 piece of naan and top with the yogurt and onion mixture.

2. Fold in half and serve.

PREP TIME: 45 minutes

TOTAL TIME: 13 hours (this includes prep, cooking, and refrigeration time)

PER SERVING, ABOUT: Calories: 412 Protein: 17 g Carbohydrate: 62 g Dietary Fiber: 13 g Sugars: 8 g Total Fat: 12 g Saturated Fat: 4 g Cholesterol: 14 mg Calcium: 104 mg Sodium: 562 mg

Eric Ziebold's Grilled Shrimp with Romaine Lettuce and Sweet Pepper Coulis

SERVES 4

THE SWEET AND TANGY pepper sauce pairs perfectly with the shrimp. The simplicity and speed of preparation make this a dish that you can enjoy often.

2 tablespoons plus 1 teaspoon olive oil
(1 teaspoon for shallot and garlic,
1 tablespoon for red pepper sauce,
1 teaspoon for shrimp, 1 teaspoon for
romaine, 1 teaspoon for bread)

1 shallot, sliced

1 clove garlic, sliced

1 sweet pepper, seeds removed and sliced

1 tablespoon red wine vinegar

1 tablespoon white wine

1 teaspoon sugar

1/4 teaspoon salt

20 fresh gulf shrimp (**16/20** count), shelled and deveined

2 heads romaine, split in half lengthwise

3 slices whole wheat bread, cut into cubes

3 tablespoons minced red onion

3 tablespoons diced fresh basil

1. Heat a heavy-bottomed skillet over medium heat. Add 1 teaspoon oil and cook the shallot and garlic until tender, about 3 minutes. Add the sweet pepper, vinegar, and wine. Simmer for 15 minutes. Puree in a food processor with the sugar, salt, and 1 tablespoon oil.

2. Toss the shrimp with 1 teaspoon oil. Toss the romaine lightly with 1 teaspoon oil. Grill the lettuce on a grill or in a grill pan over medium heat or cook in a heavy-bottomed skillet heated over medium heat for about 1 minute on each side.

3. Once the lettuce is lightly cooked, grill the shrimp on a grill or in the grill pan or cook it in a heated heavy-bottomed skillet until pink on each side, about 2 minutes per side.

4. Sauté the bread cubes in a medium pan with 1 teaspoon oil. Cook until they are lightly crisp, about 5 minutes.

5. Spoon the pepper sauce onto individual plates and place a piece of grilled lettuce next to the sauce. Toss the hot shrimp in a bowl with the red onion, basil, and sautéed whole wheat bread cubes, and arrange on top of the lettuce.

PREP TIME: 10 minutes   **TOTAL TIME:** 50 minutes

PER SERVING, ABOUT: Calories: 275 Protein: 16 g Carbohydrate: 34 g Dietary Fiber: 15 g
Sugars: 10 g Total Fat: 11 g Saturated Fat: 2 g Cholesterol: 46 mg Calcium: 250 mg Sodium: 346 mg

Meal Plans

NO MATTER WHAT YOUR LEVEL of skill in the kitchen or your time constraints, one of these plans will work for you. Go for the Quick and Easy Meal Plan when you're most pressed for time. The Family-Friendly Plan also has plenty of quick meals, but some dishes require a little more time and are meant to satisfy the whole gang. The Kitchen Connoisseur Plan will be lots of fun for those of you who have more time to spend preparing food or are simply looking for more of a challenge in the kitchen.

If you are trying to drop some pounds, or want to maintain your weight, these plans do all the calorie-calculating for you. For each plan, the basic menu offers about 1,700 calories. With some additions (or subtractions), it will cover a wide range of calorie levels: 1,500, 1,600, 1,800, 2,000, and 2,500, so you're sure to find one that works for you.

Here's how to use the meal plans:

- Pick a calorie level. Some of you know how many calories are right for you, but there's always some trial and error.

- Check the note under each meal to see if you need more or less food according to your calorie level. If you're on the 1,500-calorie plan, you'll notice you have no daily treat. Add a little more activity to your day and you can move up to 1,600 calories or more—all those levels include a treat.

- Follow the plans as written, or mix them up to create your own. The daily meals are just a suggestion; actually you can choose any breakfast, any lunch, any dinner, any high-calcium snack, and any of the treats and end the day at the calorie level of your choice. For instance, you can have Monday's breakfast with Tuesday's lunch, Thursday's dinner, Saturday's snack, and Sunday's treat and still come out at the daily calorie level of your choice. You can even mix and match from three different plans.

- Start on any day you'd like. Generally, there's more cooking involved on the weekends in these plans because you're likely to have more time to spend in the kitchen.

- Make substitutions if you like, but substitute similar foods. For instance, instead of 3 ounces of lean roast beef, eat 3 ounces of chicken. Drink 1 cup of calcium-enriched soymilk (with no more than 100 calories) in place of 1 cup of fat-free milk or have 2 cups of cauliflower instead of 2 cups of broccoli. When substituting cereals, bars, and tortillas, make sure you pick products with the same amount of fiber (or more). This plan is designed to provide at least 25 g of fiber—many meal combos will offer more. If you want to bolster your fiber intake, add a supplement, such as Benefiber.

- Look for low sodium (LS) meals. No matter which LS meals you choose, you won't exceed the recommended 2,300 mg sodium per day. Specifically, it means that no breakfast is more than 450 mg sodium; no lunch tops 600 mg; no dinner exceeds 750 mg; no snack has more than 300 mg, and the treats max out at 200 mg sodium. This applies to meals in the 1,500, 1,600, and 1,700 daily calorie levels; meals in higher daily caloric levels may have higher sodium levels.

- Look for the V if you want a vegetarian meal. These meals contain no fish, red meat, or poultry. They may include dairy and eggs.

- Stay Hydrated. You'll notice that the meal plans include only a few beverages, such as fat-free milk or soymilk, both of which are high in calcium; tea, which is virtually calorie-free and loaded with antioxidants; and smoothies, which are easy breakfasts that often contain a serving of fruit. You'll need to drink more than these each day to stay hydrated, though, and zero-calorie water is your best bet. If you're on the go or at your desk, a bottle of water is especially convenient. Look for the Best Life Seal of Approval on Nestlé Pure Life Purified Water, a nationally available brand that is committed to using less plastic, which means it's good for you and kinder to the planet. If you want to add flavor, squirt a little lemon or lime juice into plain water. And if you're looking for a change of pace, try sparkling water; Perrier and San Pellegrino are two of my favorites.

A NOTE ON COMMON INGREDIENTS: "Healthy spread" means a spread that contains no partially hydrogenated oil, and is about 80 calories per tablespoon, such as Smart Balance Buttery Spread. Soymilk on this plan should be no more than 110 calories and have at least 30 percent of the Daily Value for calcium per cup, like many of the Silk soymilks. A slice of whole wheat bread should be about 80 calories.

A NOTE ON SODIUM: In order to keep sodium in a healthy range, recipes in this book call for moderate amounts of salt. Salads and other mini-recipes in the meal plan call for no salt. If you'd like a little more salt, add a few crystals to the food on your plate (instead of adding it during preparation or cooking). The crystals hitting your tongue will give you a strong salt sensation.

Kitchen Connoisseur Plan

IF YOU'RE COMFORTABLE IN THE kitchen and ready to dive into some adventurous dishes, then this is your plan. You'll find lots of quick, easy-to-prepare meals, but you'll also come across more challenging dishes. This plan includes extraordinary recipes from such famous chefs as Charlie Trotter and Thomas Keller; those are saved for the weekends. *Bon appétit!*

WEEK 1

MONDAY, DAY 1

BREAKFAST LS V

- Peanut Butter and Banana "Sushi" (page 25)

- 1 cup fat-free milk

    2,500 CAL/DAY: Add ½ tablespoon peanut butter

SNACK LS V

    2,500 CAL/DAY ONLY: 1 cup vanilla soymilk with 45 calories of any whole grain cracker such as 1 Wasa crispbread, spread with 1 teaspoon peanut butter

LUNCH

- 1 cup minestrone soup (with no more than 500 mg sodium per cup)

- Salad: 1½ cups mixed greens, 5 cherry tomatoes, ½ cup cooked skinless chicken pieces (use leftover chicken or pull from a rotisserie chicken), tossed with 100 calories of dressing. Optional: 1 tablespoon fresh chopped basil, dill, or parsley, and a chopped scallion.

- 45 calories of any (100 percent) whole grain cracker, such as 1 piece Wasa crispbread

    2,000 CAL/DAY: Add another ¼ cup chicken to the salad

    2,500 CAL/DAY: Add another ½ cup soup. To the salad add another 5 cherry tomatoes and another ¼ cup chicken. Have the crackers with 1 tablespoon healthy spread

HIGH-CALCIUM SNACK LS V

▪ Apple Tea Latte (page 196)

▪ ½ small apple, spread with 1 teaspoon peanut butter

1,800, 2,000, AND 2,500 CAL/DAY: Have 2 teaspoons peanut butter

DINNER LS

▪ Pecan-Crusted Trout with Peaches (page 140)

▪ Raw Garlicky Kale (page 181)

▪ 1 slice whole grain bread or a roll (around 75 calories) with 1 tablespoon healthy spread

1,500–1,600 CAL/DAY: Have 1 teaspoon healthy spread instead of 1 tablespoon

2,000 CAL/DAY: Have ½ cup grapes for dessert

2,500 CAL/DAY: Have another roll, and another teaspoon healthy spread, and ½ cup grapes for dessert

TREAT *(anytime during the day)* LS V

▪ 150 calories dark chocolate, such as 3 tasting squares from a bag of Hershey's Extra Dark Cranberries, Blueberries, and Almonds

1,500 CAL/DAY: Skip the treat

1,600 CAL/DAY: Have 100 calories chocolate, such as 2 tasting squares

1,800 CAL/DAY: Have 210 calories chocolate, such as 4 tasting squares

2,000 CAL/DAY: Have 280 calories chocolate, such as 6 tasting squares

2,500 CAL/DAY: Have 300 calories chocolate, such as 6½ tasting squares

---

TUESDAY, DAY 2

BREAKFAST LS V

▪ Irish Oatmeal with Pears and Vanilla (page 17)

▪ 1 cup fat-free milk

2,500 CAL/DAY: Add 1 tablespoon unsalted nuts of your choice

SNACK LS V

2,500 CAL/DAY ONLY: 1 cup plain low-fat yogurt mixed with 2 tablespoons (about 40 calories) dried fruit

LUNCH

- Crab Salad Roll (page 95)

- Quickie coleslaw: Combine 2 teaspoons lemon juice, pinch of salt, black pepper to taste, 1 teaspoon red wine vinegar, ⅛ teaspoon sugar, 1 tablespoon olive oil, 1 cup shredded cabbage, ½ cup shredded carrot, 1 tablespoon chopped red onion

- ½ cup grapes

  2,000 CAL/DAY: Add another ½ cup grapes

  2,500 CAL/DAY: Add another ½ cup grapes and 3 tablespoons of a fruit and nut trail mix

HIGH-CALCIUM SNACK LS V

- Chocolate milk (1 cup fat-free milk mixed with 2 teaspoons Hershey's Chocolate Syrup) and 6 unsalted almonds

  1,800, 2,000, AND 2,500 CAL/DAY: Have 12 unsalted almonds

DINNER LS

- Chicken Breasts with Pumpkin Seeds (page 126)

- Large sweet potato, cooked, topped with 2 teaspoons healthy spread

- 2 cups all vegetable salad: 1½ cups mixed greens and ½ cup chopped vegetables, such as tomatoes or cucumbers, tossed with 10 sprays Wish-Bone Salad Spritzers

  1,500–1,600 CAL/DAY: Have a medium sweet potato (4 to 5 inches long) instead of a large

  2,000 CAL/DAY: Add ¼ avocado, chopped, to the salad

  2,500 CAL/DAY: Add 1 more teaspoon healthy spread to the potato, and ½ avocado, chopped, into the salad

TREAT *(anytime during the day)* LS V

- 1 ounce (140 to 150 calories) vegetable or tortilla chips, such as 14 Terra original chips or 6 Tostito's Natural Yellow Corn or Blue Corn

  1,500 CAL/DAY: Skip the treat

1,600 CAL/DAY: Have ⅔ ounce chips (about 100 calories), 9 Terra chips or 4 Tostitos

1,800 CAL/DAY: Have 1⅔ ounces chips (about 210 calories), 19 Terra chips or 8 Tostitos

2,000 CAL/DAY: Have 1¾ ounces chips (about 280 calories), 25 Terra chips or 11 Tostitos

2,500 CAL/DAY: Have 2 ounces chips (about 300 calories), 28 Terra chips or 12 Tostitos

Note: If taking the Refried Bean Wrap to work tomorrow, assemble the ingredients tonight.

WEDNESDAY, DAY 3

BREAKFAST LS V

- 2 eggs, scrambled in 1 teaspoon olive oil or 1½ teaspoons healthy spread

- 1 slice whole grain bread

- 1½ cups sliced strawberries, fresh, or frozen and thawed

- 1 cup fat-free milk

    2,500 CAL/DAY: Add 1½ teaspoons healthy spread to the bread

SNACK LS V

   2,500 CAL/DAY ONLY: Slim-Fast Optima Milk Chocolate Shake with 1 graham cracker

LUNCH LS V

- Refried Bean Wrap (page 92). Note: If taking this to work, make the bean mixture the night before. Refrigerate. Take 1 serving, along with a separately wrapped whole wheat tortilla and avocado slices to the office. At the office, do not refrigerate the bean mixture or tortilla. If possible, microwave the bean mixture and roll into the tortilla with the avocado.

    2,000 CAL/DAY: Have 1½ cups watermelon or 1 cup of any other fruit for dessert

    2,500 CAL/DAY: Add a salad with 2 cups mixed greens, ½ cup each sliced carrots and tomatoes, tossed with 1 tablespoon olive oil and a splash of red wine vinegar. Have 1½ cups watermelon or 1 cup of any other fruit for dessert

HIGH CALCIUM SNACK LS V

- Cucumbers with Yogurt Dip (page 195)

    1,800, 2,000, AND 2,500 CAL/DAY: Add another tablespoon of unsalted walnuts to dip

DINNER LS

▪ Scallops with Jicama and Oranges (page 72)

▪ Parmesan crisps: Spread 2 medium slices (2 ounces total) of crusty, whole grain bread with a total of 4 teaspoons olive oil and 2 tablespoons grated Parmesan. Toast in a toaster oven for about 3 minutes.

▪ 1 cup steamed vegetables of your choice seasoned with a spritz of lemon juice and 1 to 2 teaspoons chopped fresh parsley, basil, or other herb

   1,500–1,600 CAL/DAY: Use just 3 teaspoons olive oil in the Parmesan crisps

   2,000 CAL/DAY: Add another cup vegetables and toss with 1 teaspoon olive oil

   2,500 CAL/DAY: Add another cup vegetables and toss with 1 teaspoon olive oil, and have 1 cup grapes for dessert

TREAT *(anytime during the day)* LS V

▪ 1 Skinny Cow Ice Cream Sandwich

   1,500 CAL/DAY: Skip the treat

   1,600 CAL/DAY: Have 1 Skinny Cow Fudge Bar instead of the ice cream sandwich

   1,800 CAL/DAY: Have 1 Skinny Cow Ice Cream Sandwich along with 1 tablespoon chopped pecans

   2,000 CAL/DAY: Have 1 Skinny Cow Ice Cream Sandwich along with 3 tablespoons chopped pecans

   2,500 CAL/DAY: Have 1 Skinny Cow Ice Cream Sandwich along with 3½ tablespoons chopped pecans

---

THURSDAY, DAY 4

BREAKFAST LS V

▪ ¾ cup Kashi GoLean mixed with 3 tablespoons (60 calories) granola

▪ 1 cup fat-free milk

▪ 2 tablespoons unsalted walnuts

▪ 1 orange

   2,500 CAL/DAY: Have another ½ tablespoon walnuts

SNACK v

2,500 CAL/DAY ONLY: 1 sliced medium apple with 1 ounce reduced-fat cheese

LUNCH LS v

- Corn and Lima Bean Chowder (page 48)

- 1 slice whole grain bread or a roll (around 75 calories) spread with 2 teaspoons healthy spread

- 1 orange

    2,000 CAL/DAY: Have 1½ servings of chowder

    2,500 CAL/DAY: Have 2 servings of chowder and another teaspoon healthy spread on the bread

HIGH-CALCIUM SNACK LS v

- 12-ounce fat-free milk latte with 1 tablespoon trail mix

    1,800, 2,000, AND 2,500 CAL/DAY: Have 2 tablespoons trail mix

DINNER

- Frozen meal (with about 300 calories, at least 5 g fiber and no more than 4 g saturated fat and 700 mg sodium) such as Lean Cuisine Spa Cuisine Sesame Stir-Fry with Chicken

- 2 servings of Grape and Avocado Salad (page 70)

- Microwave 1½ cups broccoli to add to frozen dinner or have it on the side. Toss with 1 teaspoon olive oil and a spritz of lemon

    1,500–1,600 CAL/DAY: Have just ¾ cup broccoli with just ½ teaspoon olive oil

    2,000 CAL/DAY: Add 2 teaspoons slivered almonds to broccoli

    2,500 CAL/DAY: Add 1½ tablespoons slivered almonds to broccoli, and have 1 plum or other small fruit

Tip: If you're having Friday's breakfast, make the muffins tonight.

TREAT (*anytime during the day*) LS v

- 150 cookie calories, such as 2 Back to Nature Chocolate Chunk, with 1 cup of tea

    1,500 CAL/DAY: Skip the treat

1,600 CAL/DAY: Have 100 calories of cookies, such as 1½ Back to Nature cookies with 1 cup of tea

1,800 CAL/DAY: Have 210 calories of cookies with 1 cup of tea

2,000 CAL/DAY: Have 170 calories of cookies, along with ½ cup light vanilla ice cream and 1 cup of tea

2,500 CAL/DAY: Have 170 calories of cookies, along with ⅔ cup light vanilla ice cream and 1 cup of tea

---

FRIDAY, DAY 5

BREAKFAST LS V

- 1 Carrot Muffin (page 18) spread with 2 tablespoons almond butter

- Café au lait: Heat 1 cup fat-free milk and mix with 1 cup hot coffee (regular or decaf)

- ½ banana

  2,500 CAL/DAY: Have rest of banana

SNACK LS V

  2,500 CAL/DAY ONLY: ⅔ cup plain low-fat yogurt mixed with 2 teaspoons maple syrup drizzled over ¼ cup blueberries and ¼ cup strawberries

LUNCH

- ⅓ (instead of ¼) of the entire Tomato, Cucumber, and Mint Salad recipe (page 64)

- Piece of rotisserie chicken, skin removed; half breast or whole leg (drumstick and thigh)

- 1 medium whole wheat pita bread (around 120 calories)

  2,000 CAL/DAY: Add 3 tablespoons hummus to the pita

  2,500 CAL/DAY: Add 1 extra chicken leg or ½ breast, and have ¼ cup hummus

HIGH-CALCIUM SNACK V

- Spicy Wasa Melt (page 194)

  1,800, 2,000, AND 2,500 CAL/DAY: Add 1 cup cherry tomatoes tossed with ½ teaspoon olive oil and a dash of balsamic vinegar

DINNER LS

- Buffalo with Chilled Roasted Greens (page 84)

- Barley and Mushrooms (page 166)

- Dessert: ½ cup low-fat vanilla yogurt

    1,500–1,600 CAL/DAY: Skip the yogurt

    2,000 CAL/DAY: Add ⅓ cup sliced mango or other fruit to the low-fat vanilla yogurt

    2,500 CAL/DAY: Add another ½ cup low-fat vanilla yogurt with ¾ cup sliced mango or other fruit

TREAT *(anytime during the day)* LS V

- 140- to 160-calorie granola bar, such as Quaker Simple Harvest, any flavor

    1,500 CAL/DAY: Skip the treat

    1,600 CAL/DAY: Have 1 Kashi TLC cereal bar

    1,800 CAL/DAY: Have 1 Kashi Roll! bar

    2,000 CAL/DAY: Have 1 Kashi Roll! bar and 1 cup fat-free milk

    2,500 CAL/DAY: Have 1 Kashi Roll! bar and 12-ounce fat-free latte

---

SATURDAY, DAY 6

BREAKFAST LS, V

- Ginger Waffles (page 23) and 1 cup of tea. Try an interesting tea, such as Lipton Tuscan Lemon (a black tea) or Lipton Herbal Ginger Twist.

    2,500 CAL/DAY: Have 1 peach

SNACK LS

    2,500 CAL/DAY ONLY: 1 cup chocolate soymilk with 1 tablespoon unsalted peanuts

LUNCH LS V

- Portobello Sandwiches with White Beans and Roasted Garlic (page 93)

- Watercress, almond, and orange salad: combine 1 cup watercress, arugula, or other sharp green with 2 teaspoons slivered almonds and ½ orange, sectioned (for instructions, see page 346). Toss with 1 serving Mustard Vinaigrette (page 341)

2,000 CAL/DAY: Have a total of 2 tablespoons almonds

2,500 CAL/DAY: Have a total of 3 tablespoons almonds, another serving Mustard Vinaigrette, and the remaining ½ orange

HIGH-CALCIUM SNACK LS V

- Cherry Milk (page 197) with 1 tablespoon cashews

  1,800, 2,000, AND 2,500 CAL/DAY: Have another tablespoon of cashews

DINNER *(Invite guests, this meal is too good not to share!)* LS

- Steel-Cut Oats "Polenta" (page 167)
- Lamb Chops with Balsamic Roasted Garlic Puree (page 113)
- Roasted Root Vegetables (page 174)
- 1 small tangerine (dessert)

  1,500–1,600 CAL/DAY: Skip the tangerine

  2,000 CAL/DAY: Have 2 tangerines

  2,500 CAL/DAY: Have 1 thick slice crusty, whole grain bread and 2 tangerines

Note: If you're making the Barbecued Breast of Chicken for Sunday night dinner you should start marinating it tonight.

TREAT *(anytime during the day)* LS V

- Frozen Banana Chocolate Chip "Ice Cream" (page 200) with 1 teaspoon Hershey's Chocolate Syrup

  1,500 CAL/DAY: Skip the treat

  1,600 CAL/DAY: Have a little less than ¼ of the recipe

  1,800 CAL/DAY: Have ⅓ of the recipe with 2 teaspoons Hershey's Chocolate Syrup

  2,000 CAL/DAY: Have 2 servings of the recipe with 1 teaspoon Hershey's Chocolate Syrup

  2,500 CAL/DAY: Have 2 servings of the recipe with 2 teaspoons Hershey's Chocolate Syrup

SUNDAY, DAY 7

BREAKFAST LS V

- Spinach and Roasted Garlic Tart (page 28)

- ¾ cup nonfat plain yogurt mixed with 2 teaspoons honey and 1 cup fresh raspberries, or frozen, thawed

  2,500 CAL/DAY: Add ¼ cup low-fat plain yogurt and ⅛ cup raspberries

SNACK LS V

  2,500 CAL/DAY ONLY: Heaping ½ cup pistachios in shell, or 175 calories of any nut

LUNCH LS V

- Peanut butter and apple sandwich: 2 slices whole wheat bread, 2 tablespoons peanut butter (such as Smart Balance), and thin slices of 1 medium apple

- The rest of the apple, sliced

- ½ cup fat-free milk or soymilk

  2,000 CAL/DAY: Have another 2 teaspoons peanut butter

  2,500 CAL/DAY: Have a total of 4 tablespoons peanut butter, 2 teaspoons jam, and 1 cup fat-free milk or soymilk

HIGH-CALCIUM SNACK LS V

- 6 ounces flavored light yogurt mixed with ⅓ cup low-fat plain yogurt and topped with ½ cup sliced strawberries

  1,800, 2,000, AND 2,500 CAL/DAY: Have ½ cup low-fat plain yogurt and add ¾ cup sliced strawberries

DINNER LS

- Anita Lo's Barbecued Breast of Chicken (page 238)

- Sugar Snap Peas with Peanut Dressing (page 188)

- Cracked Wheat with Golden Raisins and Pumpkin Seeds (page 164)

  1,500–1,600 CAL/DAY: Have a little less than ¼ of the recipe of the Sugar Snap Peas with Peanut Dressing and the Cracked Wheat with Golden Raisins and Pumpkin Seeds

2,000 CAL/DAY: Have an extra ½ serving of Sugar Snap Peas with Peanut Dressing

2,500 CAL/DAY: Have an extra ½ serving of Sugar Snap Peas with Peanut Dressing and ⅓ of the recipe of Cracked Wheat with Golden Raisins and Pumpkin Seeds

TREAT *(anytime during the day)* LS V

■ Blueberry Slump (page 214) with 2 tablespoons frozen vanilla yogurt

1,500 CAL/DAY: Skip the treat

1,600 CAL/DAY: Have ⅓ cup frozen yogurt with the slump

1,800 CAL/DAY: Have ½ cup frozen yogurt with the slump

2,000 CAL/DAY: Have ⅔ cup frozen yogurt with the slump

2,500 CAL/DAY: Have ¾ cup frozen yogurt with the slump

WEEK 2

MONDAY, DAY 8

BREAKFAST LS V

■ Crunchy Yogurt with Fruit and Nuts (page 11)

2,500 CAL/DAY: Add 1 tablespoon unsalted nuts

SNACK LS V

2,500 CAL/DAY ONLY: 1 part-skim mozzarella string cheese with 80 calories of any whole grain cracker

LUNCH

■ Frozen meal (with about 300 calories, at least 4 g fiber, no more than 4 g saturated fat and 700 mg sodium), such as Lean Cuisine Spa Cuisine Ginger Chicken

■ 1¼ cups baby carrots

■ 3 tablespoons hummus (as dip for carrots)

2,000 CAL/DAY: Add 3 more tablespoons hummus

2,500 CAL/DAY: Add 3 more tablespoons hummus and have 3 tablespoons peanuts or other nuts

DINNER LS V

■ Cauliflower Curry with Red Lentils (page 155)

■ Brown Rice with Dates (page 163). You can make more brown rice and use it in the breakfast tomorrow.

    1,500–1,600 CAL/DAY: Have a small serving of the rice

    2,000 CAL/DAY: Add 1½ tablespoons slivered almonds to the rice

    2,500 CAL/DAY: Add 2 tablespoons slivered almonds

HIGH-CALCIUM SNACK LS V

■ 1 Slim-Fast Chocolate Mint bar with ¾ cup fat-free milk

    1,800, 2,000, AND 2,500 CAL/DAY: Have a total of 1 cup fat-free milk with 2 teaspoons Hershey's Chocolate Syrup

TREAT *(anytime during the day)* LS V

■ 1 ounce (140 to 150 calories) vegetable or tortilla chips, such as 14 Terra original chips or 6 Tostitos Natural Yellow Corn or Blue Corn

    1,500 CAL/DAY: Skip the treat

    1,600 CAL/DAY: Have ⅔ ounce chips (about 100 calories), such as 9 Terra chips or 4 Tostitos

    1,800 CAL/DAY: Have 1⅓ ounces chips (about 210 calories), such as 19 Terra chips or 8 Tostitos

    2,000 CAL/DAY: Have 1¾ ounces chips (about 280 calories), such as 25 Terra chips or 11 Tostitos

    2,500 CAL/DAY: Have 2 ounces chips (about 300 calories), such as 28 Terra chips or 12 Tostitos

---

TUESDAY, DAY 9

BREAKFAST LS V

■ Brown Rice Pudding (page 20)

- Café au lait: ½ cup hot fat-free milk mixed with ½ cup hot coffee (decaf or regular)

  2,500 CAL/DAY: Add ½ cup blackberries or blueberries

SNACK LS V

2,500 CAL/DAY ONLY: ½ cup low-fat vanilla yogurt mixed with ½ small peach or 2 tablespoons diced peaches and 2 tablespoons granola cereal

LUNCH V

- Pickled Cauliflower (page 191)

- Cheese sandwich: Spread 1 tablespoon of Hellmann's Canola Cholesterol Free Mayonnaise and 1 teaspoon spicy mustard on 2 slices whole grain bread. Stuff with 1½ ounces reduced-fat Cheddar cheese, 3 tomato slices, and ¼ cup alfalfa sprouts.

  2,000 CAL/DAY: Add 1 medium pear

  2,500 CAL/DAY: Add 1 medium pear and 2 cups mixed greens with ⅓ cup each sliced red bell pepper and carrots, with 1 tablespoon olive oil and 2 teaspoons balsamic vinegar

DINNER

- Baked Pork Tenderloin (page 106)

- Corn Pudding (page 169)

- Roasted broccoli: Spray 2 cups broccoli florets with vegetable oil cooking spray; broil on low, 4 inches from heat source, for 10 minutes. Toss with 2 tablespoons Mustard Vinaigrette (page 341).

- After dinner: ⅔ cup grapes

  1,500–1,600 CAL/DAY: Skip the grapes

  2,000 CAL/DAY: Add another 1 ounce pork

  2,500 CAL/DAY: Add 1½ ounces pork, 1 serving of corn pudding, and ½ cup grapes

HIGH-CALCIUM SNACK LS V

- 1 Slim-Fast Optima Creamy Milk Chocolate Shake

  1,800, 2,000, AND 2,500 CAL/DAY: Have 1 fresh apricot or plum or ½ cup fresh or frozen unsweetened raspberries

TREAT *(anytime during the day)* LS V

- Mini sundae: Top ½ cup light vanilla ice cream with 1 teaspoon chocolate syrup, such as Hershey's and 1 teaspoon chopped peanuts

  1,500 CAL/DAY: Skip the treat

  1,600 CAL/DAY: Skip the chocolate syrup and peanuts

  1,800 CAL/DAY: Have ¾ cup ice cream with 2 teaspoons chocolate syrup and 1 teaspoon chopped peanuts

  2,000 CAL/DAY: Have 1 cup ice cream with 2 teaspoons chocolate syrup and 2 teaspoons chopped peanuts

  2,500 CAL/DAY: Have 1 cup ice cream with 2 teaspoons chocolate syrup and 1 tablespoon chopped peanuts

  Note: If having the Muesli for breakfast tomorrow, you might want to assemble it tonight. Also, if taking the shrimp salad to work, save time in the a.m. by combining the sesame seeds, sesame oil, and vinegar in a bowl tonight. In the morning, toss with the remaining ingredients.

WEDNESDAY, DAY 10

BREAKFAST LS V

- Muesli (page 16)

- 1 cup fat-free milk

- ¾ cup fresh strawberries, or frozen, thawed

  2,500 CAL/DAY: Add 1 tablespoon unsalted walnuts

SNACK LS V

  2,500 CAL/DAY ONLY: Spread 2 teaspoons light mayonnaise on 1 slice whole wheat bread and top with 2 ounces turkey breast

LUNCH LS

- Shrimp, Avocado, and Sesame Seed Salad (page 74)

- 1 slice whole grain bread or roll (around 75 calories) spread with 1 teaspoon healthy spread

- 1 Orange or apple

  2,000 CAL/DAY: Use 1 tablespoon healthy spread

  2,500 CAL/DAY: Use 1 tablespoon plus 1 teaspoon healthy spread and have 1 more whole wheat roll

DINNER LS V

- Baked Beans on Grits (page 158)

- After dinner: 1 medium pear or other fruit of your choice, with a smear of goat cheese, (a little under 1 ounce) about 1 inch cubed

  1,500–1,600 CAL/DAY: Have ½ the pear with the cheese

  2,000 CAL/DAY: Add another ½ ounce cheese

  2,500 CAL/DAY: Add 1 slice whole grain bread or roll (around 75 calories) with 1 teaspoon healthy spread and another ½ ounce cheese

HIGH-CALCIUM SNACK: LS V

- Dip 1 to 2 celery stalks in ¾ cup 0 percent Greek yogurt mixed with 2 tablespoons feta and 1 scallion, chopped

  1,800, 2,000, AND 2,500 CAL/DAY: Add another 2 tablespoons feta

TREAT *(anytime during the day)* LS V

- 1 Edy's or Dreyer's fruit bar (80 calories) and 70 calories of a sweetened nut mixture, such as 3 pieces of True North Almond Clusters

  1,500 CAL/DAY: Skip the treat

  1,600 CAL/DAY: 1 Edy's or Dreyer's fruit bar and 20 to 25 calories of a sweetened nut mixture, such as 1 piece of True North Almond Clusters

  1,800 CAL/DAY: 1 Edy's or Dreyer's fruit bar and 130 calories of a sweetened nut mixture, such as 5 pieces of True North Almond Clusters

  2,000 CAL/DAY: 1 Edy's or Dreyer's fruit bar and 200 calories of a sweetened nut mixture, such as 8 pieces of True North Almond Clusters

  2,500 CAL/DAY: 1 Edy's or Dreyer's fruit bar and 210 calories of a sweetened nut mixture, such as 8½ pieces of True North Almond Clusters

THURSDAY, DAY 11

BREAKFAST LS V

- 2 eggs, any style. If scrambled or fried, use 1½ teaspoons healthy spread.

- 1 Whole wheat 100-calorie wrap or tortilla, such as Flatout Flatbread Multi-Grain, heated (If you don't use healthy spread to prepare eggs, use on flatbread.) Roll the eggs in the flatbread, if desired.

- 1 cup cherry tomatoes

- 1 cup fat-free milk

  2,500 CAL/DAY: Have a total of 12 ounces fat-free milk

SNACK LS V

  2,500 CAL/DAY ONLY: 3 tablespoons trail mix

LUNCH LS

- Quinoa and Grapefruit (page 160)

- 4-ounce piece of broiled salmon. Set the oven to "broil," rub the fish with 1 to 2 teaspoons olive oil, and place on a hot broiler pan about 6 inches from the heat source. Broil for 3 to 4 minutes on each side. Sprinkle with pepper, a dash of salt, and 1 tablespoon of chopped fresh herbs, if desired.

- ¾ cup fresh raspberries or frozen, unsweetened raspberries, thawed

  2,500 CAL/DAY: Have 45 calories of a whole grain cracker with 1 teaspoon healthy spread

  2,500 CAL/DAY: Have 90 calories of a whole grain cracker with 1 tablespoon healthy spread

DINNER LS V

- Vegetable Cottage Pie (page 150)

- 2 cups mixed greens with 70 calories of dressing of your choice or 1 serving Mustard Vinaigrette (page 341) topped with 2 tablespoons walnuts

  1,500-1,600 CAL/DAY: Have just 1 tablespoon nuts

  2,000 CAL/DAY: Add 1 whole wheat roll (75 calories)

  2,500 CAL/DAY: Add 1 whole wheat roll (75 calories) and 1 tablespoon healthy spread

HIGH-CALCIUM SNACK LS V

- Hot chocolate: In a mug, mix together 1 tablespoon sugar and 1½ tablespoons cocoa, such as Hershey's Natural Cocoa. Heat 1 cup fat-free milk in a microwave and gradually add hot milk to the cocoa mixture, stirring until blended. Stir in ¼ teaspoon vanilla extract. Alternately, mix all the ingredients in a small pot over medium heat.

   1,800, 2,000, AND 2,500 CAL/DAY: Add 2 squares graham crackers

TREAT *(anytime during the day)* LS V

- ½ cup sorbet, about 150 calories

   1,500 CAL/DAY: Skip the treat

   1,600 CAL/DAY: Have a heaping ⅓ cup sorbet, about 100 calories

   1,800 CAL/DAY: Have about ¾ cup sorbet, about 210 calories

   2,000 CAL/DAY: Have a heaping ¾ cup sorbet, about 230 calories, with 1 sliced kiwi

   2,500 CAL/DAY: Have about 1 cup sorbet, about 260 calories, with 1 sliced kiwi

---

FRIDAY, DAY 12

BREAKFAST LS V

- ¾ cup Kashi GoLean mixed with 3 tablespoons (60 calories) granola

- 1 cup fat-free milk

- ¾ cup strawberries

- 2 tablespoons almonds

   2,500 CAL/DAY: Add 2 tablespoons granola

SNACK LS V

2,500 CAL/DAY ONLY: 1 cinnamon or honey graham cracker spread with ¼ cup nonfat ricotta topped with ¼ teaspoon cinnamon, 2 teaspoons honey, and 1 tablespoon slivered almonds.

LUNCH LS V

- Vegetable Chili (page 57) or 1 cup of Amy's Reduced in Sodium Canned Chili, either "Medium" or "Spicy"

■ 1 ounce (140 to 150 calories) regular tortilla chips, such as 6 Tostitos Natural Yellow Corn

2,000 CAL/DAY: Add a salad: 2 cups mixed greens with ⅓ cup sliced carrots, ¼ cup chopped tomato, and ¼ cup sliced cucumber with 1 teaspoon olive oil and 1 splash red wine vinegar

2,500 CAL/DAY: Have the same salad as above, another ½ ounce (75 calories) tortilla chips, and top chili with ¼ cup shredded reduced-fat Cheddar

DINNER

■ Broiled Mahimahi with Grapes and Leeks (page 143)

■ Cracked Wheat with Golden Raisins and Pumpkin Seeds (page 164)

■ 4 cups spinach drizzled with 1 serving Mustard Vinaigrette (page 341) topped with 1 tablespoon slivered almonds

1,500–1,600 CAL/DAY: Omit the almonds and use just 1½ teaspoons olive oil in dressing

2,000 CAL/DAY: Add another tablespoon almonds

Add 2,500 CAL/DAY: Have 1½ servings Mustard Vinaigrette and add another tablespoon almonds

HIGH-CALCIUM SNACK: LS V

■ 1 cup vanilla soymilk with 1 small banana

1,800, 2,000, AND 2,500 CAL/DAY: Spread banana with 1½ teaspoons peanut butter

TREAT *(anytime during the day)* LS V

■ 1 tablespoon bittersweet chocolate chips with 1½ tablespoons unsalted peanuts

1,500 CAL/DAY: Skip the treat

1,600 CAL/DAY: Have 1 tablespoon chocolate chips with 2 teaspoons unsalted peanuts

1,800 CAL/DAY: Have 1 tablespoon chocolate chips with 2 tablespoons unsalted peanuts

2,000 CAL/DAY: Have 2½ tablespoons chocolate chips with 2 tablespoons unsalted peanuts

2,500 CAL/DAY: Have 3 tablespoons chocolate chips with 2 tablespoons unsalted peanuts

SATURDAY, DAY 13

BREAKFAST V

- Tofu Mushroom Scramble with Whole Wheat Tortilla (page 27)

- Café au lait: 1 cup hot fat-free milk mixed with 1 cup hot coffee (decaf or regular)

    2,500 CAL/DAY: Add 1 tangerine

SNACK LS V

    2,500 CAL/DAY ONLY: 3 tablespoons mixed unsalted nuts

LUNCH

- Crispbread Open-Faced Sandwich with Sardines and Sweet Pepper (page 94)

- Mozzarella salad: Mix together 1 ounce fresh mozzarella, diced, with 1 diced large tomato. Drizzle with 1 tablespoon olive oil and sprinkle with 1 tablespoon chopped basil.

    2,000 CAL/DAY: Add 1 orange

    2,500 CAL/DAY: Have the entire Crispbread recipe, which is 4 crispbreads topped with sardines. Add 1 orange.

HIGH-CALCIUM SNACK LS V

- 1 Luna Bar (with 180 calories, 35% DV for calcium)

    1,800, 2,000, AND 2,500 CAL/DAY: Add 1 tablespoon nuts, or spread bar with 2 teaspoons peanut butter

DINNER LS

- Vitaly Paley's Grilled Lamb Paillard with Summer Vegetable Salad and Herbed Yogurt (page 249)

- 2 slices (about 1¾ ounces, or 135 calories) crusty, bakery, whole grain bread

- ¾ cup grapes

    1,500–1,600 CAL/DAY: Have just 1 slice of bread

    2,000 CAL/DAY: Dip bread in 1 teaspoon olive oil

    2,500 CAL/DAY: Dip bread in 4 teaspoons olive oil

TREAT *(have this for dessert after dinner)* LS V

Thomas Keller's Watermelon Sorbet (page 234) for all calorie levels except 1,500 and 1,600 calories: Have a little less than ¼ of the recipe

Because the Watermelon Sorbet is just 159 calories, those of you at higher calorie levels also get an additional treat!

1,800 CAL/DAY: 1 Edy's or Dreyers fruit bar

2,000 CAL/DAY: 1 Skinny Cow Ice Cream Sandwich

2,500 CAL/DAY: 1 Skinny Cow Ice Cream Sandwich and 1 tablespoon chocolate chips

---

SUNDAY, DAY 14

BREAKFAST LS V

- Breakfast Pizza (page 33)

- 1 cup of tea, such as any of the Lipton Pyramid teas

    2,500 CAL/DAY: Add another tablespoon almonds to the pizza

SNACK LS V

    2,500 CAL/DAY ONLY: 1 small pear, sliced, spread with 1 tablespoon almond butter

LUNCH V

- 1½ cups lentil soup (with no more than 500 mg sodium per cup), simmered with 1½ cups arugula, spinach, or other green

- One 6-inch whole wheat pita dipped in 1½ teaspoons olive oil

    2,000 CAL/DAY: Have 1 apple

    2,500 CAL/DAY: Have an extra ½ cup soup, and another ½ teaspoon oil, and have 1 apple

HIGH-CALCIUM SNACK LS V

- Cucumbers with Yogurt Dip (page 195)

    1,800, 2,000, AND 2,500 CAL/DAY: Add another tablespoon of unsalted walnuts to dip

DINNER LS

- Roy Yamaguchi's Slow-Baked Pepper-Crusted Salmon with Roasted Beets and Crispy Garlic Lemon Vinaigrette (page 260)

- Suzanne Goin's Persimmon and Pomegranate Salad with Arugula and Hazelnuts (page 230)

- ½ cup fresh blackberries (for dessert)

  2,000 CAL/DAY: Add 1 small slice whole wheat crusty bread

  2,500 CAL/DAY: Add 1 small slice whole wheat crusty bread and brush with 2 teaspoons olive oil and grill

TREAT *(have this for dessert after dinner)* LS V

Charlie Trotter's Passion Fruit Pudding Cake (page 255) for all calorie levels except 1,500

1,600 CAL/DAY: Have a small piece

Because the Passion Fruit Pudding Cake is just 150 calories, those of you at higher calorie levels also get an additional treat:

1,800 CAL/DAY: 60 calories of any treat of your choice, such as ½ Nonni's biscotti

2,000 CAL/DAY: 130 to 140 calories of any treat of your choice, such as 1 Skinny Cow Ice Cream Sandwich

2,500 CAL/DAY: 150 calories of any treat of your choice, such as 3 Hershey's Extra Dark Tasting Squares, any flavor

Quick and Easy Meal Plan

ON THIS PLAN, YOU GET the benefits of home-cooked meals without having to spend hours in the kitchen. You'll see a combination of quick from-scratch dishes paired with convenience foods (case in point: Day 1 dinner has both canned soup and Rotisserie Chicken Salad with Oranges and Pistachios). There are even some fast-food meals thrown in the mix. It's a plan that fits into—and fuels—your busy lifestyle.

WEEK 1

MONDAY, DAY 1

BREAKFAST LS V

- 190 calories of whole grain cereal (with at least 3 g fiber per 100 calories), such as 1 cup Cascadian Farm Great Measure Cereal, topped with 2 tablespoons unsalted walnuts, pecans, or other nuts of your choice, and 1 cup fat-free milk

- ¾ cup strawberries or other berries

  2,500 CAL/DAY ONLY: Add another 40 calories of cereal, such as ¼ cup Cascadian Farm Great Measure Cereal

SNACK LS V

  2,500 CAL/DAY ONLY: 1 Kashi GoLean Crunchy! Bar, or another 150- to 180-calorie bar with at least 4 g fiber

LUNCH V

- Cheese and tomato sandwich: Spread 2 slices whole wheat bread with 1 tablespoon Hellmann's Canola Cholesterol Free Mayonnaise. Fill with 2 ounces (2 slices) reduced-fat Cheddar, such as Cabot 50%, or reduced-fat Swiss or Jack, and 2 tomato slices. Add chopped fresh basil or other herb, if desired.

- Have the rest of the tomato (use 1 medium or large tomato) sliced, sprinkled with a dash of salt, and a drizzle of balsamic vinegar

- 1 apple

  2,000 CAL/DAY: Have a 6-ounce container of light fruit yogurt

  2,500 CAL/DAY: Have a 6-ounce container of light fruit yogurt mixed with ¼ cup berries, and have 2 tablespoons unsalted walnuts, pecans, or other nuts of your choice

DINNER

- 1 cup lentil or black bean soup (with 500 mg sodium per cup or less)
- 90 calories of any whole grain cracker
- 1 serving Rotisserie Chicken Salad with Oranges and Pistachios (page 77)

  1,500–1,600 CAL/DAY: Have just 45 calories of any whole grain cracker

  2,000 CAL/DAY: Have another ⅓ cup soup

  2,500 CAL/DAY: Have another cup soup

HIGH-CALCIUM SNACK LS V

- 12-ounce fat-free milk latte, or 8-ounce glass of fat-free milk. Add 2 tablespoons unsalted nuts of your choice.

  1,800, 2,000, AND 2,500 CAL/DAY: Have one 16-ounce fat-free milk latte, or another ½ cup fat-free milk

TREAT *(anytime during the day)* LS V

- 150 calories of a sweetened nut mixture or bar, such as ¼ cup True North Peanut Crunches Honey Wheat

  1,500 CAL/DAY: Skip the treat

  1,600 CAL/DAY: 100 calories of a sweetened nut mixture or bar, such as 2½ tablespoons True North Peanut Crunches

  1,800 CAL/DAY: 210 calories of a sweetened nut mixture or bar, such as ⅓ cup True North Peanut Crunches

  2,000 CAL/DAY: 280 calories of a sweetened nut mixture or bar, such as a scant ½ cup True North Peanut Crunches

  2,500 CAL/DAY: 300 calories of a sweetened nut mixture or bar, such as ½ cup True North Peanut Crunches

---

TUESDAY, DAY 2

BREAKFAST LS V

- Peanut Butter Banana Smoothie (page 10)

   2,500 CAL/DAY ONLY: Have 1 tangerine

SNACK LS V

   2,500 CAL/DAY ONLY: 1 medium apple sliced and spread with 1 tablespoon nut butter, such as Smart Balance Peanut Butter

LUNCH V

- 90 calories of any whole grain cracker, such as 2 pieces Wasa Multi Grain crispbreads, topped with ½ cup nonfat ricotta, 5 chopped olives, and 6 slices tomato, drizzled with 2 teaspoons olive oil

- 2 cups mixed greens and 1 chopped red pepper tossed with 10 sprays Wish-Bone Salad Spritzer, any flavor, and topped with 1 tablespoon toasted pine nuts or other nuts of your choice

   2,000 CAL/DAY: Add another 45 calories of any whole grain cracker, such as 1 piece Wasa crispbread topped with another ¼ cup nonfat ricotta

   2,500 CAL/DAY: Add another 45 calories of any whole grain cracker, such as 1 piece Wasa crispbread topped with another ¼ cup nonfat ricotta and another 5 olives, and have ¾ cup grapes

DINNER LS

- Broil a 5-ounce piece of fish (trout, salmon, mackerel, or other fish of your choice). See page 287, Thursday, Day 11, of the Kitchen Connoisseur Meal Plan for instructions.

- 1 serving Raw Garlicky Kale (page 181)

- Garlic bread: 2 slices whole wheat bread with 2 teaspoons healthy spread, a smear of crushed garlic or a sprinkle of garlic salt, and a dash of black pepper. Heat in a toaster oven or oven until golden.

- ½ cup berries

   1,500–1,600 CAL/DAY: Have just 4 ounces fish and skip the berries

   2,000 CAL/DAY: Have another ½ cup berries

   2,500 CAL/DAY: Have another ½ cup berries and a second serving of Raw Garlicky Kale

HIGH-CALCIUM SNACK LS V

■ 1 Slim-Fast Optima Shake, any flavor

1,800, 2,000, AND 2,500 CAL/DAY: Have 1 tablespoon unsalted nuts

TREAT *(anytime during the day)* LS V

■ 150 calories of vegetable chips, such as Terra Sweet Potato or Sweets and Beets Chips (1 ounce, about 17 chips)

1,500 CAL/DAY: Skip the treat

1,600 CAL/DAY: Have 100 calories (about ⅔ ounce or 12 chips)

1,800 CAL/DAY: Have 210 calories (about 1⅓ ounces or 22 chips)

2,000 CAL/DAY: Have 280 calories (about 1¾ ounces or 31 chips)

2,500 CAL/DAY: Have 300 calories (about 2 ounces or 34 chips)

WEDNESDAY, DAY 3

BREAKFAST LS V

■ Crunchy Yogurt with Fruit and Nuts (page 11)

2,500 CAL/DAY ONLY: Add another tablespoon nuts

SNACK LS V

2,500 CAL/DAY ONLY: 1 part-skim mozzarella string cheese stick and ¾ cup grapes

LUNCH

Note: This, like other fast-food meals, is high in sodium, so have it only occasionally.

■ Fast-food lunch: Wendy's Small Chili, Side Salad with 1 packet Reduced-Fat Creamy Ranch Dressing, and a side of Mandarin oranges

2,000 CAL/DAY: Have a large chili

2,500 CAL/DAY: Have a large chili, skip the salad and the Mandarin oranges, and have a Sour Cream and Chives potato

DINNER LS

■ 1 serving Buffalo with Blackberries (page 102)

■ 1 cup raw sweet potato sticks spritzed with olive or canola oil cooking spray, seasoned with a dash of salt and any herbs of your choice, and baked at 400°F for 25 to 30 minutes. Or use frozen sweet potato sticks, such as Alexia brand.

■ 2 cups mixed greens, 1 cup chopped vegetable of your choice tossed with 1 tablespoon olive oil and 1 teaspoon balsamic vinegar. Top with 1 tablespoon walnuts.

   1,500–1,600 CAL/DAY: Skip the nuts on the salad

   2,000 CAL/DAY: Have another tablespoon nuts

   2,500 CAL/DAY: Have another tablespoon nuts and another ½ cup sweet potatoes

HIGH-CALCIUM SNACK V

■ 60 calories' worth of whole grain crackers, such as 2 slices Wasa Fiber Rye Crispbread, spread with ½ cup nonfat ricotta cheese and topped with 6 olives

   1,800, 2,000, AND 2,500 CAL/DAY: Add 45 calories of whole grain crackers

TREAT *(anytime during the day)* LS V

■ 3 tablespoons chocolate-covered peanuts

   1,500 CAL/DAY: Skip the treat

   1,600 CAL/DAY: Have 2 tablespoons chocolate-covered peanuts

   1,800 CAL/DAY: Have ¼ cup chocolate-covered peanuts

   2,000 CAL/DAY: Have ⅓ cup chocolate-covered peanuts

   2,500 CAL/DAY: Have ⅓ cup chocolate-covered peanuts plus ⅓ cup fat-free milk

THURSDAY, DAY 4

BREAKFAST LS V

- Oatmeal, ½ cup dry regular or ¼ cup steel-cut (Quaker, Arrowhead Mills, and McCann's make quick-cooking steel-cut). Top with 1 small apple, chopped; 1 tablespoon unsalted nuts of your choice; and 2 teaspoons brown sugar.

- 1 cup fat-free milk

  2,500 CAL/DAY ONLY: Add another tablespoon unsalted nuts of your choice

SNACK V

2,500 CAL/DAY ONLY: 1 small pita (around 70 calories) with ¼ cup hummus

LUNCH LS

- Chicken wrap. In a 90- or 100-calorie whole grain wrap or tortilla, such as Flatout Flatbread, place the following mix: ½ cup precooked chicken strips (or pulled from a rotisserie chicken) mixed with 1 tablespoon Hellmann's Canola Cholesterol Free Mayonnaise, 2 teaspoons mustard, and 3 tablespoons finely chopped shredded carrots (or mushrooms or celery or a combo of all; whatever you can find prechopped at the grocery store or have time to chop yourself)

- 1 cup grapes and 1 tablespoon unsalted nuts of your choice

  2,000 CAL/DAY: Add another ¼ cup chicken and 1 teaspoon mayonnaise

  2,500 CAL/DAY: Add another ¼ cup chicken, 1 teaspoon mayonnaise, 2 more tablespoons nuts, and another ½ cup grapes

DINNER

- Lean Cuisine Spa Cuisine Gourmet Mushroom Pizza, 1 package

- 1 serving Roasted Broccoli with Balsamic Vinegar (page 180)

- 1 cup fresh blueberries, or frozen, thawed, with 2 tablespoons slivered almonds

  1,500–1,600 CAL/DAY: Have just 1 tablespoon almonds

  2,000 CAL/DAY: Have a second serving of Roasted Broccoli with Balsamic Vinegar

  2,500 CAL/DAY: Have a second serving of Roasted Broccoli with Balsamic Vinegar and top berries and almonds with 100 calories of vanilla yogurt

HIGH-CALCIUM SNACK LS V

- Celery with Creamy Herb Dip (page 195)

  1,800, 2,000, AND 2,500 CAL/DAY: Add ¼ cup more ricotta and an extra ½ teaspoon olive oil to the dip

TREAT *(anytime during the day)* LS V

- One 100- to 110-calorie biscotti, such as Nonni's, with 1 café au lait: ½ cup hot fat-free milk mixed with ½ cup hot coffee (decaf or regular)

  1,500 CAL/DAY: Skip the treat

  1,600 CAL/DAY: Have just the biscotti

  1,800 CAL/DAY: Have another ½ biscotti

  2,000 CAL/DAY: Have another biscotti

  2,500 CAL/DAY: Have another biscotti and add another ½ cup each of hot fat-free milk and coffee to your café au lait.

FRIDAY, DAY 5

BREAKFAST LS V

- 1 slice whole wheat bread spread with 1 tablespoon nut butter, such as Smart Balance Peanut Butter, and topped with ½ banana, sliced. Drizzle with 1 teaspoon honey.

- 1 cup strawberries and ½ cup blueberries or other berries

- 1 cup fat-free milk (plain, or as part of a latte or heated and mixed with regular coffee)

  2,500 CAL/DAY ONLY: Add another ½ tablespoon nut butter

SNACK LS V

  2,500 CAL/DAY ONLY: ¾ cup Silk Vanilla Light soymilk or fat-free milk with 2 graham crackers

LUNCH V

- 1 cup minestrone soup (with no more than 500 mg sodium per cup), simmered with 1½ cups spinach

- 90 calories of any whole grain crackers, such as 2 pieces Wasa Multi Grain crispbreads, topped with 6 tablespoons nonfat ricotta, 1 tablespoon olive oil, and sprinkled with chopped fresh basil, parsley, or dill

- ½ cup sliced strawberries

   2,000 CAL/DAY: Add another ¼ cup soup and another ½ cup strawberries

   2,500 CAL/DAY: Have another ½ cup soup, and another 45 calories of any whole grain cracker, such as 1 piece Wasa crispbread, 3 more tablespoons ricotta, another 1½ teaspoons olive oil, and another ½ cup strawberries

DINNER LS

- ¼ cup dry whole wheat couscous (use regular if you can't find whole wheat), cooked according to package directions, mixed with 1 teaspoon olive oil and topped with ½ tablespoon toasted pine nuts or slivered almonds

- 1 serving Poached Wild Salmon with Zucchini and Mustard (page 131)

   1,500–1,600 CAL/DAY: Skip the oil in the couscous

   2,000 CAL/DAY: Add another tablespoon dry couscous

   2,500 CAL/DAY: Add another tablespoon dry couscous. When the couscous is ready, mix in ⅓ cup canned, drained chickpeas (garbanzo beans), preferably no-salt-added. Also add another ½ tablespoon pine nuts and have 1 cup grapes for dessert

HIGH-CALCIUM SNACK LS V

- ¾ cup nonfat plain yogurt mixed with 3 tablespoons dried fruit

   1,800, 2,000, AND 2,500 CAL/DAY: Add another 2 tablespoons dried fruit

TREAT *(anytime during the day)* LS V

- 2 Edy's or Dreyer's fruit bars (160 calories)

   1,500 CAL/DAY: Skip the treat

   1,600 CAL/DAY: Have 1 fruit bar

   1,800 CAL/DAY: Have 2 fruit bars with 1 tablespoon trail mix

   2,000 CAL/DAY: Have 2 fruit bars with 2 tablespoons trail mix

   2,500 CAL/DAY: Have 2 fruit bars with 2 tablespoons plus 2 teaspoons trail mix

---

SATURDAY, DAY 6

BREAKFAST v

■ ½ cup liquid eggs, such as Better'n Eggs, scrambled in 2 teaspoons healthy spread, rolled in 1 whole wheat wrap or tortilla, such as Flatout Flatbread Multi-Grain, with 2 tablespoons salsa

■ 1 cup fat-free milk

■ 1 grapefruit

2,500 CAL/DAY ONLY: Have a total of 1 tablespoon healthy spread and add 2 tablespoons shredded reduced-fat cheese to your wrap

SNACK v (LS *if your products meet the sodium limits listed below*)

2,500 CAL/DAY ONLY: 110 calories of baked or regular tortilla chips. For baked, have 1 ounce, about 18 chips. For regular, have ¾ ounce, preferably with no more than 90 mg sodium, such as some Tostitos and many of the Garden of Eatin' varieties like Blue Chips, about 11 chips. Dip chips in 2 tablespoons salsa, preferably with no more than 150 mg sodium, and 3 tablespoons guacamole, preferably with no more than 60 mg sodium.

LUNCH

■ Frozen meal (with around 400 calories, at least 3 grams of fiber, and no more than 4 grams of saturated fat), such as Lean Cuisine Chicken Fettuccine

■ 2 cups mixed greens topped with 10 sprays Wish-Bone Salad Spritzers

2,000 CAL/DAY: Add 1 teaspoon olive oil to the salad

2,500 CAL/DAY: Add 1 teaspoon olive oil to the salad and have 140 to 150 calories of fruit-flavored yogurt for dessert

DINNER v LS

■ 1 serving Angel Hair Pasta with Walnuts and Peas (page 148)

■ Salad: 2 cups mixed greens tossed with 100 calories of regular dressing

1,500–1,600 CAL/DAY: Have just 50 calories of dressing

2,000 CAL/DAY: Have 1 cup berries

2,500 CAL/DAY: Have ⅓ of the entire Angel Hair Pasta recipe instead of ¼, as the recipe specifies

HIGH-CALCIUM SNACK LS V

- 1 cup Silk Vanilla Soymilk or fat-free milk and 1 cup peach slices

  1,800, 2,000, AND 2,500 CAL/DAY: Have 1 tablespoon walnuts

TREAT *(anytime during the day)* LS V

- Banana cream pudding: Slice ½ banana and layer with 1 fat-free vanilla pudding cup

  1,500 CAL/DAY: Skip the treat

  1,600 CAL/DAY: Have just the pudding

  1,800 CAL/DAY: Have a full banana with the pudding

  2,000 CAL/DAY: Have a full banana with the pudding and top with 4 teaspoons unsalted chopped pecans or other nuts

  2,500 CAL/DAY: Have a full banana with the pudding and top with 2 tablespoons chopped unsalted pecans or other nuts

---

SUNDAY, DAY 7

BREAKFAST LS V

- 2 whole grain toaster waffles (about 170 calories for the 2, such as Kashi), topped with 1 teaspoon healthy spread, 1 cup berries, and 1 tablespoon maple syrup

- 1 cup fat-free milk

  2,500 CAL/DAY ONLY: Add 1 tablespoon unsalted almonds to the waffles

SNACK LS V

  2,500 CAL/DAY ONLY: 100 calories of yogurt with 1½ tablespoons unsalted nuts, such as pistachios

LUNCH V

- 1 cup reduced-sodium canned tomato soup

- 1 whole wheat pita stuffed with ½ cup chickpeas, 1 tablespoon chopped parsley, and 100 calories of vinaigrette dressing

  2,000 CAL/DAY: Add another ¾ cup soup

  2,500 CAL/DAY: Add another cup of soup and 1½ cups grapes

DINNER LS

▪ 1 serving Pan-Roasted Shrimp with Lemon, Garlic, and Spinach (page 135)

▪ Salad: 3 cups mixed greens, 1 cup chopped vegetables, such as tomatoes or red peppers, and 1 tablespoon toasted pine nuts or other nuts of your choice tossed with 1 tablespoon olive oil and 1 teaspoon balsamic vinegar

▪ 1 slice whole grain bread or roll (around 75 calories) with 2 teaspoons healthy spread

   1,500–1,600 CAL/DAY: Have only ½ roll

   2,000 CAL/DAY: Have another teaspoon nuts on your salad and another teaspoon healthy spread on your roll

   2,500 CAL/DAY: Have another roll, and a total of 4 teaspoons healthy spread for both rolls

HIGH-CALCIUM SNACK LS V

▪ 1 Luna Bar (with 180 calories, 35% DV for calcium)

   1,800, 2,000, AND 2,500 CAL/DAY: Add 1 tablespoon unsalted nuts

TREAT *(anytime during the day)* LS V

▪ 150 calories of light ice cream, about ¾ cup

   1,500 CAL/DAY: Skip the treat

   1,600 CAL/DAY: 100 calories light ice cream, about ½ cup

   1,800 CAL/DAY: 210 calories light ice cream, about 1 cup

   2,000 CAL/DAY: 280 calories light ice cream, about 1¼ cups

   2,500 CAL/DAY: 300 calories light ice cream, about 1½ cups

WEEK 2

MONDAY, DAY 8

BREAKFAST LS V

- Breakfast Pizza (page 33)

  2,500 CAL/DAY ONLY: Add 1 tangerine

SNACK LS V

  2,500 CAL/DAY ONLY: 1 Kashi GoLean Crunchy! Bar, or other 150- to 180-calorie bar with at least 4 g fiber

LUNCH

- Salad: 2 cups romaine, 10 cherry tomatoes, ½ cup cooked skinless chicken pieces (use leftover chicken or pull from a rotisserie chicken), tossed in 100 calories of Caesar dressing

- Parmesan crispbread: 90 calories of crispbreads, such as 2 pieces Wasa Hearty or Multi Grain crispbreads, each spread with 1 teaspoon healthy spread, topped with 1½ teaspoons grated Parmesan. Place in a toaster oven and broil for 2 minutes.

  2,000 CAL/DAY: Add another ½ cup chicken

  2,500 CAL/DAY: Add another ½ cup chicken and have 1¼ cups grapes

DINNER LS

- 1 serving Pork Chops with Apples and Onion (page 108)

- ¾ cup frozen baby lima beans, cooked according to package instructions, tossed with 1 teaspoon olive oil, ½ teaspoon lemon juice, and 1 to 2 teaspoons chopped dill or other herb

- 1 slice whole grain bread or roll (around 75 calories) with 2 teaspoons healthy spread

  1,500–1,600 CAL/DAY: Have just ½ teaspoon olive oil and a total of 1½ teaspoons healthy spread

  2,000 CAL/DAY: Add another ¼ cup lima beans

  2,500 CAL/DAY: Add another ¼ cup lima beans, another roll, and another 2 teaspoons healthy spread

HIGH-CALCIUM SNACK LS V

▪ Chocolate milk: 1 cup fat-free or 1% milk with 1 tablespoon Hershey's Chocolate Syrup with ½ cup sliced strawberries

   1,800, 2,000, AND 2,500 CAL/DAY: Have another ¾ cup sliced strawberries

TREAT *(anytime during the day)* LS V

▪ Peach Melba ice cream sundae: ½ cup light vanilla ice cream topped with ½ cup sliced peaches and ¼ cup raspberries

   1,500 CAL/DAY: Skip the treat

   1,600 CAL/DAY: Have just the ice cream

   1,800 CAL/DAY: Top with 1 tablespoon slivered almonds

   2,000 CAL/DAY: Add another ¼ cup ice cream and top with 1 tablespoon slivered almonds and 3 tablespoons whipped cream

   2,500 CAL/DAY: Add another ¼ cup ice cream and top with 1½ tablespoons slivered almonds and 3 tablespoons whipped cream

---

TUESDAY, DAY 9

BREAKFAST LS V

▪ 180 to 190 calories of whole grain cereal (with at least 3 g fiber per 100 calories), such as 1 cup Optimum Slim, topped with 2 tablespoons unsalted walnuts, pecans, or other nuts of your choice, and 1 cup fat-free milk

▪ ¾ cup strawberries or other berries

   2,500 CAL/DAY ONLY: Add another ¼ cup cereal

SNACK V

   2,500 CAL/DAY ONLY: ¾ cup 1% cottage cheese with ½ cup mandarin oranges canned in juice

LUNCH LS V

▪ Bean and corn salad: Combine ¾ cup black beans (either canned low sodium or no-salt-added, rinsed, and drained, or from scratch) with 1 cup canned, no-salt-added corn (such as Green Giant No Salt Added Niblets), drained, and ½ cup cherry tomatoes, halved. Toss with 100 calories of Italian dressing or vinaigrette (with no more than 250 mg sodium), such as Wish-Bone Olive Oil Vinaigrette. Optional: 1 tablespoon chopped fresh herbs such as dill, basil, or parsley.

2,000 CAL/DAY: Serve with ¾ ounce tortilla chips, about 12 chips

2,500 CAL/DAY: Add ½ chopped avocado to the salad and serve with 1 ounce baked tortilla chips, about 18 chips

DINNER LS

- Broil a 5-ounce piece of fish (trout, salmon, mackerel, or other fish of your choice). See page 287, Thursday, Day 11, for instructions.

- 1 serving Greens with Grapes (page 65)

- ¼ cup dry whole wheat couscous, cooked according to package directions, with 1 teaspoon olive oil

  1,500–1,600 CAL/DAY: Cook just 3 tablespoons couscous

  2,000 CAL/DAY: Have a second serving of Greens with Grapes

  2,500 CAL/DAY: Have a second serving of Greens with Grapes and have 1 cup blueberries for dessert

HIGH-CALCIUM SNACK LS V

- 1 medium apple with 1½ ounces reduced-fat Cheddar (such as Cabot 50%)

  1,800, 2,000, AND 2,500 CAL/DAY: Have 1 large apple

TREAT *(anytime during the day)* LS V

- 150 calories dark chocolate, such as 3 tasting squares Hershey's Extra Dark Cranberries, Blueberries, and Almonds

  1,500 CAL/DAY: Skip the treat

  1,600 CAL/DAY: 100 calories chocolate, such as 2 tasting squares

  1,800 CAL/DAY: 210 calories chocolate, such as 4 tasting squares

  2,000 CAL/DAY: 280 calories chocolate, such as 6 tasting squares

  2,500 CAL/DAY: 300 calories chocolate, such as 6½ tasting squares

---

WEDNESDAY, DAY 10

BREAKFAST LS V

■ Blueberry Smoothie (page 10)

■ 1 slice 100% whole wheat bread spread with 1 tablespoon almond butter

 2,500 CAL/DAY ONLY: Add ½ slice of bread

SNACK LS V

 2,500 CAL/DAY ONLY: 3 tablespoons trail mix

LUNCH LS V

■ Salad: 4 cups mixed greens, 1 tablespoon crumbled goat cheese, and 2 tablespoons each unsalted walnuts and dried cherries (or Craisins) tossed with 10 sprays Wish-Bone Salad Spritzers

■ 1 small whole wheat pita (about 75 calories) stuffed with 4 tablespoons hummus

 2,000 CAL/DAY: Have 1 medium whole wheat pita (120 calories) instead of a small one, and add another tablespoon of hummus

 2,500 CAL/DAY: Add another tablespoon goat cheese and 1 teaspoon olive oil to your salad. Have 1 medium whole wheat pita (120 calories) instead of a small one, and add another 2 tablespoons hummus. Have ½ cup grapes for dessert.

DINNER

■ 1 frozen entrée (with 290 to 300 calories, at least 3 grams of fiber, and no more than 4 grams of saturated fat and 700 mg sodium), such as Lean Cuisine Cheese Lasagna with Chicken Breast Scallopini.

■ Microwave along with (or steam): 2 cups mixed vegetables, tossed with 1 tablespoon healthy spread or 1½ teaspoons olive oil, 1 tablespoon Parmesan, and 1 tablespoon fresh chopped parsley or other herb

■ 1 slice whole grain bread or roll (around 75 calories) with 2 teaspoons healthy spread or 1 teaspoon olive oil

 1,500–1,600 CAL/DAY: Have just 2 teaspoons healthy spread or 1 teaspoon olive oil and 2 teaspoons Parmesan on the vegetables

 2,000 CAL/DAY: Have 1 orange for dessert

 2,500 CAL/DAY: Add 2 tablespoons slivered almonds to the vegetables, and have 1 orange for dessert

HIGH-CALCIUM SNACK LS V

- 1 Slim-Fast Optima Mint Crisp Snack Bar with ½ cup fat-free milk

  1,800, 2,000, AND 2,500 CAL/DAY: Have another ¾ cup fat-free milk

TREAT *(anytime during the day)* LS V

- 1 Skinny Cow Ice Cream Cone, any flavor

  1,500 CAL/DAY: Skip the treat

  1,600 CAL/DAY: Have 1 Skinny Cow Fudge Bar instead of the cone

  1,800 CAL/DAY: Have the cone and 1 Skinny Cow mini fudge bar, 50 calories

  2,000 CAL/DAY: Have the cone and 1 Skinny Cow mini fudge bar, 50 calories, sprinkled with 1½ tablespoons chopped nuts

  2,500 CAL/DAY: Have the cone and 1 Skinny Cow mini fudge bar, 50 calories, sprinkled with 2½ tablespoons chopped nuts

---

THURSDAY, DAY 11

BREAKFAST V

- Scramble together: ¼ cup liquid eggs (such as Better'n Eggs), ¼ cup sliced mushrooms (you can buy them presliced), and 2 tablespoons grated reduced-fat cheese in 2 teaspoons olive oil or 4 teaspoons healthy spread

- Serve with a warm, whole grain 100-calorie tortilla or wrap, such as Flatout Flatbread Multi-Grain

- 1 orange

- 1 cup fat-free milk

  2,500 CAL/DAY ONLY: Add another ¼ cup liquid eggs and another tablespoon cheese

SNACK LS V

  2,500 CAL/DAY ONLY: 1 medium apple sliced and spread with 1 tablespoon nut butter, such as Smart Balance Peanut Butter

LUNCH

Like most fast-food meals, these are high in sodium, so make them just an occasional lunch.

■ Subway sandwich: 6-inch Subway Club sandwich on Honey Oat or wheat bread with lettuce, tomatoes, pickles, onions, green peppers or olives, with a Veggie Delight salad with fat-free Italian dressing

2,000 CAL/DAY: Have a serving of Subway's minestrone soup

2,500 CAL/DAY: Have a serving of Subway's minestrone soup and the 100 calorie yogurt available at Subway

■ McDonald's sandwich: Grilled Honey Mustard Snack Wrap with a Southwest Salad (without chicken) with Newman's Own Balsamic Low Fat Balsamic Vinaigrette

2,000 CAL/DAY: Add apple dippers

2,500 CAL/DAY: Add a snack size Fruit and Walnut Salad

DINNER

■ 1 serving Tilapia with Carrot Ginger Puree (page 134)

■ Mixed greens with 100 calories of dressing and 2 tablespoons each crumbled feta and toasted pine nuts

■ 1 slice whole grain bread or roll (around 75 calories)

1,500–1,600 CAL/DAY: Have just ½ roll

2,000 CAL/DAY: Have 2 teaspoons healthy spread on the roll

2,500 CAL/DAY: Have 2 teaspoons healthy spread on the roll and have 1 cup grapes

HIGH-CALCIUM SNACK LS V

■ 12-ounce fat-free milk latte (or an 8-ounce glass of fat-free milk) plus 1 tablespoon unsalted nuts of your choice

1,800, 2,000, AND 2,500 CAL/DAY: Have another tablespoon of unsalted nuts

TREAT *(anytime during the day)* LS V

■ 110 calorie biscotti, such as Nonni's, with a café au lait: ½ cup hot fat-free milk mixed with ½ cup hot coffee

1,500 CAL/DAY: Skip the treat

1,600 CAL/DAY: Have just the biscotti

1,800 CAL/DAY: Have another ½ biscotti

2,000 CAL/DAY: Have another biscotti

2,500 CAL/DAY: Have another biscotti and a total of 1 cup hot milk and 1 cup coffee in your café au lait

---

FRIDAY, DAY 12

BREAKFAST LS V

- Oatmeal, ½ cup dry regular or ¼ cup steel cut (Quaker, Arrowhead Mills, and McCann's make quick-cooking steel cut), cooked according to package directions. Top with 1 small apple, chopped; 1 tablespoon unsalted nuts of your choice; 2 teaspoons brown sugar.

- 1 cup fat-free milk

  2,500 CAL/DAY ONLY: Add another tablespoon unsalted nuts

SNACK LS V

2,500 CAL/DAY ONLY: 1 small whole wheat pita (around 70 calories) with ¼ cup hummus

LUNCH

- Frozen meal (with around 250 calories, at least 3 grams of fiber, and no more than 4 grams of saturated fat and 700 mg sodium), such as Lean Cuisine Spa Cuisine Salmon with Basil

- 2 tablespoons unsalted almonds

- 1 orange

  2,000 CAL/DAY: Have 1 slice whole grain bread or roll around 75 calories

  2,500 CAL/DAY: Add another 2 tablespoons almonds; have 1 slice whole grain bread or roll around 75 calories spread with 2 teaspoons healthy spread

DINNER LS

- 1 serving Summer Steak Salad (page 82)

- 1 large ear of corn with 2 teaspoons healthy spread

- 1 small slice whole wheat garlic bread (spread 1 small piece of bread with 1 teaspoon olive oil, a smear of crushed garlic or a sprinkle of garlic salt, and a dash of pepper. Heat in toaster oven or oven until golden).

- ½ cup berries

  1,500–1,600 CAL/DAY: Skip the berries

  2,000 CAL/DAY: Add another teaspoon olive oil to your bread

  2,500 CAL/DAY: Have another ear of corn and a total of 1 tablespoon healthy spread

HIGH-CALCIUM SNACK LS V

- 2 part-skim mozzarella string cheese sticks

  1,800, 2,000, AND 2,500 CAL/DAY: Have 45 calories of any whole grain cracker, such as Wasa Hearty crispbread

TREAT *(anytime during the day)* LS V

- 150 calories dark chocolate

  1,500 CAL/DAY: Skip the treat

  1,600 CAL/DAY: 100 calories chocolate

  1,800 CAL/DAY: 210 calories chocolate

  2,000 CAL/DAY: 280 calories chocolate

  2,500 CAL/DAY: 300 calories chocolate

SATURDAY, DAY 13

BREAKFAST LS V

- Peanut Butter Banana Smoothie (page 10)

  2,500 CAL/DAY ONLY: Have 1 tangerine

SNACK LS V

  2,500 CAL/DAY ONLY: 45 calories any whole grain cracker, such as 1 Wasa crispbread, spread with 1 tablespoon peanut butter and 2 teaspoons jam

LUNCH v

- Fresh mozzarella, tomato, and basil salad: Layer 1 ounce fresh mozzarella slices, with slices from a medium tomato. Sprinkle with 1 tablespoon chopped fresh basil, and drizzle with 1 teaspoon olive oil

- 2 slices whole wheat bread

- 1 cup lentil soup (with no more than 500 mg sodium per cup)

  2,000 CAL/DAY: Have another ⅓ cup soup

  2,500 CAL/DAY: Have another ounce mozzarella and another cup soup

DINNER

- 1 serving Mussels with White Wine and Garlic (page 138)

- Spinach salad: 2 cups baby spinach with ¼ cup grated carrots, and 150 calories of dressing

- 2 slices crusty, whole grain bread, brushed with 2 teaspoons olive oil and grilled

  1,500–1,600 CAL/DAY: Have just 100 calories of dressing

  2,000 CAL/DAY: Add 1 tablespoon toasted pine nuts or other nuts to the salad

  2,500 CAL/DAY: Add 1 tablespoon toasted pine nuts or other nuts to the salad and have 2 cups diced cantaloupe or 1½ cups other fruit for dessert

HIGH-CALCIUM SNACK LS V

- 1 cup Silk Vanilla Soymilk with 1 large peach

  1,800, 2,000, AND 2,500 CAL/DAY: Add 9 almonds

TREAT (*anytime during the day*) LS V

- 1 Skinny Cow Ice Cream Sandwich

  1,500 CAL/DAY: Skip the treat

  1,600 CAL/DAY: Have 2 Skinny Cow mini fudge bars (100 calories total)

  1,800 CAL/DAY: Have 1 Skinny Cow Ice Cream Sandwich plus 2 tablespoons bittersweet chocolate chips

2,000 CAL/DAY: Have 1 Skinny Cow Ice Cream Sandwich plus 3 tablespoons bittersweet chocolate chips

2,500 CAL/DAY: Have 1 Skinny Cow Ice Cream Sandwich plus 1 banana and 1 tablespoon bittersweet chocolate chips

---

SUNDAY, DAY 14

BREAKFAST LS V

- 1 cup plain low-fat yogurt mixed with ½ banana, ½ cup raspberries or blackberries (frozen and thawed is fine), 1 teaspoon honey, 3 tablespoons granola, and 1 tablespoon ground flaxseeds

  2,500 CAL/DAY ONLY: Have another 2 tablespoons granola

SNACK LS V

  2,500 CAL/DAY ONLY: Kashi GoLean Crunchy! Bar, or another 150- to 180-calorie bar with at least 4 g of fiber

LUNCH V

- Lentil soup with spinach: Heat 1 cup lentil soup (with 500 mg sodium or less per cup). Simmer with 2 cups spinach or chopped arugula leaves for 2 minutes or until just wilted.
- 2 slices whole grain bread dipped in 2 teaspoons olive oil
- 1 apple

  2,000 CAL/DAY: Have another ⅓ cup soup

  2,500 CAL/DAY: Have 1 ounce reduced-fat Cheddar such as Cabot 50% with your bread, and another cup soup

DINNER

- 1 serving Cornmeal-Crusted Catfish with Spicy Slaw (page 145)
- 1 box (10 ounce) Kashi frozen Black Bean Mango, cooked according to package directions

  1,500–1,600 CAL/DAY: Leave 2 bites of the frozen dinner

  2,000 CAL/DAY: Have 1 tangerine

  2,500 CAL/DAY: Have 1 slice whole grain bread or roll around 75 calories with 1 teaspoon healthy spread

HIGH-CALCIUM SNACK LS V

- 1 Luna Bar (with 180 calories, 35% DV for calcium)

   1,800, 2,000, AND 2,500 CAL/DAY: Have 1 tablespoon unsalted nuts

TREAT *(anytime during the day)* LS V

- 150 calories popcorn (check package label for calorie counts) with no partially hydrogenated oil, such as Smart Balance Smart'N Healthy

   1,500 CAL/DAY: Skip the treat

   1,600 CAL/DAY: Have 100 calories popcorn

   1,800 CAL/DAY: Add 1 tablespoon mixed unsalted nuts

   2,000 CAL/DAY: Add 2 tablespoons mixed unsalted nuts

   2,500 CAL/DAY: Add 2½ tablespoons mixed unsalted nuts

Family–Friendly Plan

PEOPLE OFTEN COMPLAIN TO ME that their spouse is the reason they can't eat healthfully. If it's not the meat-and-potatoes husband, it's the vegetable-phobic children, or all the junk everyone in the family brings home. This plan can help bring some peace—and a lot of good nutrition—into the household. You'll find a mix of "safe" and familiar foods, such as Sloppy Joes, and slightly more adventurous, but delicious meals, such as Shrimp Curry. Serve yourself the portion that's in your calorie zone, and, depending on the age of your children, offer them a little more or less. And bring back the family meal!

MONDAY, DAY 1

BREAKFAST LS V

- Cereal. Adults: Mix ¾ cup Kashi GoLean with 3 tablespoons granola, ¼ cup Fiber One (or other 175- to 180-calorie serving of cereal that offers at least 6 g fiber). Children: Have 1 cup Kix, Cheerios, Barbara's Puffins, or other cereal children like that contains at least 3 g fiber per 100 calories.

- 1 banana, sliced

- 1 tablespoon walnuts or other unsalted nuts of your choice

- 1 cup fat-free milk (1% or fat-free for children)

    2,500 CAL/DAY: Add 1 tablespoon unsalted walnuts

SNACK LS V

   2,500 CAL/DAY ONLY: ¾ cup plain low-fat yogurt with 2 teaspoons honey and ¼ cup blueberries

LUNCH LS V

- Peanut butter and apple roll-up: 2 tablespoons peanut butter with thin apple slices rolled in a whole grain tortilla or wrap, such as Flatout Flatbread Multi-Grain

- Rest of the apple (small apple), sliced

- 1 cup fat-free milk

    2,000 CAL/DAY: Add 1 teaspoon peanut butter and ½ tablespoon raisins to the roll-up

2,500 CAL/DAY: Have 2 large apples instead of a small one, and add 1 tablespoon peanut butter and 1 tablespoon raisins to the roll-up

DINNER LS

- Sloppy Joes (page 109)

- Salad: 1½ cups mixed greens and ½ cup chopped vegetables of your choice tossed with 100 calories of dressing (with no more than 250 mg sodium per 2 tablespoons)

   1,500–1,600 CAL/DAY: Use just 50 calories of dressing

   2,000 CAL/DAY: Add ½ cup vegetables to the salad and have a total of 120 calories of dressing

   2,500 CAL/DAY: Add ¼ cup grated reduced-fat Cheddar to the Sloppy Joe; ½ cup more vegetables to the salad; and have a total of 120 calories of dressing

HIGH-CALCIUM SNACK LS V

- Orange Cream Smoothie (page 197) with 1½ tablespoons unsalted nuts of your choice

   1,800, 2,000, AND 2,500 CAL/DAY: Have another ½ tablespoon unsalted nuts

TREAT *(anytime during the day)* LS V

- 150 calories of cookies of your choice, made with no partially hydrogenated oil and, preferably, containing whole grain, such as Kashi or Back to Nature

   1,500 CAL/DAY: Skip the treat

   1,600 CAL/DAY: Have 100 calories of cookies, about 1 cookie

   1,800 CAL/DAY: Have 210 calories of cookies, about 3 cookies

   2,000 CAL/DAY: Have 280 calories of cookies, about 4 cookies

   2,500 CAL/DAY: Have 300 calories of cookies, about 4½ cookies

---

TUESDAY, DAY 2

BREAKFAST

- Peanut Butter Banana Smoothie (page 10) LS V

   2,500 CAL/DAY: Add ½ tablespoon peanut butter

SNACK LS V

2,500 CAL/DAY ONLY: 1 Slim-Fast Chocolate Mint Crisp snack bar with ½ cup fat-free milk

LUNCH LS V

■ Edamame and corn salad: Combine ¾ cup corn (canned no-salt-added, such as Green Giant Niblets, or frozen, thawed), with ½ cup shelled edamame (microwaved from frozen); ¼ cup each chopped red pepper and carrots. Toss with a mixture of 1½ teaspoons olive oil, ½ teaspoon Dijon mustard, 1 teaspoon balsamic vinegar, and 1 chopped scallion. Depending on your family's tastes, you can add 1 tablespoon chopped fresh basil, parsley, dill, or cilantro.

■ 1 cup orange and grapefruit sections

2,000 CAL/DAY: Have 1 small pita, around 75 calories

2,500 CAL/DAY: Have 1 small pita, around 75 calories, another ¾ cup orange and grapefruit sections, and 2 tablespoons unsalted nuts of your choice

DINNER LS

■ Chicken Noodle Soup (page 54)

■ 5 whole grain crackers (about 70 calories)

■ 1 cup broccoli florets sautéed with 1 clove of chopped garlic and ½ tablespoon olive oil, topped with 3 tablespoons (¾ ounce) reduced-fat Cheddar cheese

1,500–1,600 CAL/DAY: Use 1 teaspoon olive oil instead of ½ tablespoon and ½ ounce cheese instead of ¾ ounce

2,000 CAL/DAY: Use 1 tablespoon olive oil instead of ½ tablespoon

2,500 CAL/DAY: Use 1 tablespoon olive oil instead of ½ tablespoon, 1 ounce cheese instead of ¾ ounce, and have 5 more whole grain crackers

HIGH-CALCIUM SNACK LS V

■ Chocolate milk: 1 cup fat-free milk mixed with 2 teaspoons Hershey's Chocolate Syrup with 1 tablespoon trail mix

1,800, 2,000, AND 2,500 CAL/DAY: Have another tablespoon of trail mix

TREAT *(anytime during the day)* **LS V**

- 150 calories (1 ounce) of tortilla chips, about 6 chips, with 1 tablespoon salsa

  1,500 CAL/DAY: Skip the treat

  1,600 CAL/DAY: Have 100 calories (⅔ ounce), about 4 chips, with 1 tablespoon salsa

  1,800 CAL/DAY: Have 190 calories (1⅓ ounces), about 8 chips, with 2 tablespoons salsa

  2,000 CAL/DAY: Have 260 calories (1¾ ounces), about 10 chips, with 2 tablespoons salsa

  2,500 CAL/DAY: Have 280 calories (2 ounces), about 11 chips, with 2 tablespoons salsa

---

WEDNESDAY, DAY 3

BREAKFAST V

- 2 whole grain toaster waffles, 170 to 180 calories for 2 waffles, such as Kashi GoLean

- 1 teaspoon butter or healthy spread

- 1½ tablespoons pancake or maple syrup

- ¾ cup strawberries

- 1 cup fat-free milk

  2,500 CAL/DAY: Top the waffle with another 2 teaspoons butter or healthy spread

SNACK LS V

  2,500 CAL/DAY ONLY: 3 tablespoons trail mix

LUNCH V

- Cheese sandwich: 2 slices 100% whole wheat bread, spread with 1 tablespoon light mayonnaise; 2 ounces reduced-fat Cheddar, Swiss, or Jack; and 2 slices of a medium tomato and lettuce

- Rest of the tomato, sliced, tossed with a splash of balsamic vinegar

- 1 orange

  2,000 CAL/DAY: Toss 1 cup greens with the tomatoes, ½ teaspoon olive oil, a splash of vinegar, and 2 teaspoons sunflower seeds

2,500 CAL/DAY: Toss 2 cups greens with the tomatoes, 2½ teaspoons olive oil, a splash of vinegar, and 2 tablespoons sunflower seeds

DINNER LS

■ Pecan-Crusted Trout with Peaches (page 140)

■ Grape and Avocado Salad (page 70)

■ 1 slice whole grain bread or roll (around 75 calories) with 1½ teaspoons healthy spread

   1,500–1,600 CAL/DAY: Skip the healthy spread

   2,000 CAL/DAY: Have 1 cup steamed sliced zucchini topped with 1 teaspoon healthy spread

   2,500 CAL/DAY: Have 2 cups steamed sliced zucchini topped with 1 tablespoon healthy spread or 1 teaspoon olive oil, and have ¾ cup raspberries or other berries for dessert

HIGH-CALCIUM SNACK LS V

■ Celery with Creamy Herb Dip (page 195)

   1,800, 2,000, AND 2,500 CAL/DAY: Add ¼ cup more ricotta and an extra ½ teaspoon olive oil to the dip

TREAT *(anytime during the day)* LS V

■ 150 calories of light ice cream, about ¾ cup

   1,500 CAL/DAY: Skip the treat

   1,600 CAL/DAY: Have 100 calories light ice cream, about ½ cup

   1,800 CAL/DAY: Have 210 calories light ice cream, about 1 cup

   2,000 CAL/DAY: Have 280 calories light ice cream, about 1¼ cups

   2,500 CAL/DAY: Have 300 calories light ice cream, about 1½ cups

---

THURSDAY, DAY 4

BREAKFAST V

■ Scrambled egg wrap. Scramble ½ cup liquid eggs, such as Better'n Eggs, in 2 teaspoons healthy spread. Roll into 1 whole grain 100-calorie tortilla or wrap, such as Flatout Flatbread Multi-Grain.

- 1 cup fat-free milk

- 1 pear or apple

  2,500 CAL/DAY: Add ¼ cup liquid eggs and 1 teaspoon healthy spread

SNACK LS V

2,500 CAL/DAY ONLY: 6-ounce fruit-flavored, low-fat yogurt, around 170 calories

LUNCH LS

- BBQ chicken: 3 to 4 ounces cooked (or rotisserie) chicken; that's about ½ breast or 1 whole leg, or ⅔ cup pieces, coated with 2 tablespoons BBQ sauce (with no more than 250 mg sodium for 2 tablespoons). Warm it up, if desired.

- 1½ cups carrots

- 1 cup strawberries dipped in 3 ounces vanilla or strawberry yogurt

  2,000 CAL/DAY: 1 slice whole grain bread or roll, around 75 calories

  2,500 CAL/DAY: 1 slice whole grain bread or roll, around 75 calories, with 1 teaspoon healthy spread and another ½ cup strawberries with another 3 ounces yogurt

DINNER LS V

- 1 serving Broccoli, White Bean, and Leek Tart (page 152)

- 1 slice whole grain bread or roll (around 75 calories) with 1 teaspoon healthy spread

- 1 cup diced melon for dessert

  1,500–1,600 CAL/DAY: Skip the melon

  2,000 CAL/DAY: Have another 1 cup melon

  2,500 CAL/DAY: Have another 1 cup melon and another slice whole grain bread or roll, around 75 calories, with 1 teaspoon healthy spread

HIGH-CALCIUM SNACK V

- 1½ ounces reduced-fat cheese

- 70 calories whole grain crackers

  1,800, 2,000, AND 2,500 CAL/DAY: Have another 35 calories of crackers

TREAT *(anytime during the day)* LS V

■ Frozen Banana Chocolate Chip "Ice Cream" (page 200) with 1 teaspoon Hershey's Chocolate Syrup

1,500 CAL/DAY: Skip the treat

1,600 CAL/DAY: Have a little less than 1 serving

1,800 CAL/DAY: Have ⅓ of the recipe instead of ¼, as the recipe specifies, with 2 teaspoons Hershey's Chocolate Syrup

2,000 CAL/DAY: Have 2 servings with 1 teaspoon Hershey's Chocolate Syrup

2,500 CAL/DAY: Have 2 servings with 2 teaspoons Hershey's Chocolate Syrup

---

FRIDAY, DAY 5

BREAKFAST LS V

■ Irish Oatmeal with Pears and Vanilla (page 17)

■ 1 cup fat-free milk

2,500 CAL/DAY: Have 1 tablespoon unsalted almonds

SNACK

2,500 CAL/DAY ONLY: 45 calories of any whole grain cracker, such as 1 piece Wasa Multi Grain crispbread, or any other variety with the Best Life seal, spread with 1½ teaspoons light mayonnaise and topped with 1 slice (1 ounce) turkey breast and ⅓ avocado, sliced

LUNCH LS V

■ Taco Salad (page 87)

2,000 CAL/DAY: Have 1 orange

2,500 CAL/DAY: Have 1 orange and 1 cup of corn, either added to the salad or on the side

DINNER V

■ Takeout pizza: 2 slices (Check Web site nutrition information for 420 calories of vegetarian pizza, such as Pizza Hut 12-inch Hand Tossed or "The Natural" Veggie Lovers. Make this an occasional treat, as pizza is usually made with white flour, and sodium levels are often high.)

- All-vegetable salad: At least 2 cups mixed greens with 1¼ cups chopped vegetables, ½ tablespoon olive oil, and 1 tablespoon balsamic vinegar

  1,500–1,600 CAL/DAY: Have ¾ cup chopped vegetables on the salad instead of 1¼ cups and use 1 teaspoon olive oil

  2,000 CAL/DAY: Have 1 apple

  2,500 CAL/DAY: Have 1 apple and 1½ tablespoons unsalted nuts

HIGH-CALCIUM SNACK LS V

- Hot chocolate: In a mug, mix together 1 tablespoon sugar and 1½ tablespoons cocoa, such as Hershey's Natural Cocoa. Heat 1 cup fat-free milk in a microwave and gradually add hot milk to cocoa mixture, stirring until blended. Stir in ¼ teaspoon vanilla extract. (Alternately, mix all ingredients in a small pot over medium heat.)

  1,800, 2,000, AND 2,500 CAL/DAY: Have 1 banana

TREAT *(anytime during the day)* LS V

- 2 Edy's or Dreyer's fruit bars

  1,500 CAL/DAY: Skip the treat

  1,600 CAL/DAY: Have 1 fruit bar instead of 2

  1,800 CAL/DAY: Have 2 fruit bars with 1 tablespoon trail mix

  2,000 CAL/DAY: Have 2 fruit bars with 2 tablespoons trail mix

  2,500 CAL/DAY: Have 2 fruit bars with 2½ tablespoons trail mix

---

SATURDAY, DAY 6

BREAKFAST V

- 1 Zucchini Muffin (page 22) with 2 teaspoons healthy spread or butter and 1 teaspoon honey

- ½ cup blackberries mixed with ½ banana, sliced

- 1 cup fat-free milk

  2,500 CAL/DAY: Have the whole banana

SNACK LS V

2,500 CAL/DAY ONLY: 1¼ cups grapes with 1½ ounces reduced-fat cheese

LUNCH AT THE MALL

- Sandwich and side salad: Subway 6-inch Turkey Breast Sandwich with a Veggie Delight salad and a 2-ounce packet Red Wine Vinaigrette

  2,000 CAL/DAY: Have 1 small banana from home

  2,500 CAL/DAY: Have 1 small banana and 3 tablespoons unsalted nuts from home

DINNER LS V

- Baked Beans on Grits (page 158)

- Salad: 2 cups mixed greens with 1 cup chopped vegetables, 1 tablespoon olive oil, and a splash of red wine vinegar

  1,500–1,600 CAL/DAY: Use 2 teaspoons olive oil instead of 1 tablespoon

  2,000 CAL/DAY: Add ½ cup vegetables to the salad, and sprinkle with 1 tablespoon sunflower seeds

  2,500 CAL/DAY: Add ½ cup vegetables to the salad, and serve with 1 slice whole grain bread or roll (around 75 calories) dipped in ½ tablespoon olive oil

HIGH-CALCIUM SNACK LS V

- ¾ cup nonfat plain yogurt mixed with 3 tablespoons dried fruit

  1,800, 2,000, AND 2,500 CAL/DAY: Add another 2 tablespoons dried fruit

TREAT *(anytime during the day)* LS V

- 1 Lemon Oatmeal Cookie (page 206)

  1,500 CAL/DAY: Skip the treat

  1,600 CAL/DAY: Have ½ Lemon Oatmeal Cookie

  1,800 CAL/DAY: Have 1 Lemon Oatmeal Cookie with ¾ cup light vanilla soymilk

  2,000 CAL/DAY: Have 1½ Lemon Oatmeal Cookies with ½ cup light vanilla soymilk

  2,500 CAL/DAY: Have 1½ Lemon Oatmeal Cookies with ¾ cup light vanilla soymilk

SUNDAY, DAY 7

BREAKFAST LS V

- Cereal. Adults: Mix 1¼ cups Wheaties, ¼ cup Fiber One, or other 160-calorie serving of cereal that offers at least 6 g fiber: Children: Have 1 cup Kix, Cheerios, Barbara's Puffins, or other cereal children like that contains at least 3 g fiber per 100 calories.

- 1 banana, sliced

- 1 tablespoon walnuts or other unsalted nuts of your choice

- 1 cup fat-free milk (1% or fat-free for children)

  2,500 CAL/DAY: Add 1 tablespoon unsalted walnuts

SNACK LS V

  2,500 CAL/DAY ONLY: 1 medium apple sliced and spread with 1 tablespoon nut butter, such as Smart Balance Peanut Butter

LUNCH LS V

- Grilled Tofu, Lettuce, and Tomato (page 90)

- 1 orange

  2,000 CAL/DAY: Add ¼ cup lowfat vanilla yogurt mixed with 1 teaspoon chopped pecans

  2,500 CAL/DAY: Add ½ cup lowfat vanilla yogurt mixed with 4 teaspoons chopped pecans

DINNER LS

- Beef with Tomatoes and Olives Over Pasta (page 105)

- Salad: 2 cups mixed greens with 1 cup vegetables tossed with 2½ teaspoons olive oil and 1 teaspoon balsamic vinegar

  1,500–1,600 CAL/DAY: Use 1½ teaspoons olive oil instead of 2½ teaspoons

  2,000 CAL/DAY: Use 2 teaspoons olive oil instead of 2½ teaspoons. Add 1 slice whole grain bread or roll (around 75 calories)

  2,500 CAL/DAY: Use 1 tablespoon olive oil instead of 2½ teaspoons. Add 1 slice whole grain bread or roll (around 75 calories)

HIGH-CALCIUM SNACK LS V

- Chocolate milk: 1 cup 1% milk with 1 tablespoon Hershey's Chocolate Syrup with ½ cup sliced strawberries

  1,800, 2,000, AND 2,500 CAL/DAY: Have another ¾ cup sliced strawberries

TREAT *(anytime during the day)* LS V

- Apple Pie with Oatmeal Crust (page 215). Have a small piece (⅒ of the pie instead of ⅛ serving).

  1,500 CAL/DAY: Skip the treat

  1,600 CAL/DAY: Have ½ a regular serving of pie

  1,800 CAL/DAY: 1 serving Apple Pie with 1 tablespoon caramel or butterscotch sauce

  2,000 CAL/DAY: 1 serving Apple Pie with ⅓ cup vanilla light ice cream

  2,500 CAL/DAY: 1 serving Apple Pie with ½ cup vanilla light ice cream

WEEK 2

MONDAY, DAY 8

BREAKFAST LS V

- Peanut Butter and Banana "Sushi" (page 25)

- 1 cup fat-free milk

  2,500 CAL/DAY: Add ½ tablespoon peanut butter to the sushi

SNACK LS V

  2,500 CAL/DAY ONLY: 1 Kashi GoLean Crunchy! Bar, or another 150- to 180-calorie bar with at least 4 g fiber.

LUNCH

- Turkey and cheese sandwich: Spread 2 slices 100% whole wheat bread with 2 teaspoons light mayonnaise. Add 2 ounces turkey breast (with no more than 360 mg sodium per 2-ounce serving, such as Applegate Farms) and 1-ounce slice reduced-fat Cheddar, Swiss, or jack. Also add tomato slices and lettuce leaves.

- 10 baby carrots

- 1 pear

  2,000 CAL/DAY: Have another 1-ounce slice reduced-fat cheese

  2,500 CAL/DAY: Have another 1-ounce slice reduced-fat cheese, and ¼ cup trail mix

DINNER LS

- 1 medium baked potato, topped with ¼ package frozen mixed vegetables, cooked according to package directions, sprinkled with herbs of your choice, and 3 tablespoons slivered almonds

- Spinach Salad with Turkey Bacon (page 79)

  1,500–1,600 CAL/DAY: Have just 2 tablespoons slivered almonds

  2,000 CAL/DAY: Add 1½ teaspoons healthy spread to your potato

  2,500 CAL/DAY: Have a large baked potato and add 1½ teaspoons healthy spread

HIGH-CALCIUM SNACK LS V

- 7 graham cracker squares (1¾ rectangles; whole wheat, such as Mi-del if you can find them)

- 1 cup fat-free milk

  1,800, 2,000, AND 2,500 CAL/DAY: Have 2 full rectangles

TREAT *(anytime during the day)* LS V

- ½ cup light ice cream topped with 1 tablespoon Hershey's Chocolate Syrup

  1,500 CAL/DAY: Skip the treat

  1,600 CAL/DAY: Just have the ice cream

  1,800 CAL/DAY: Have ½ cup ice cream with 2 tablespoons Hershey's Chocolate Syrup

  2,000 CAL/DAY: Have ¾ cup ice cream with 2 tablespoons Hershey's Chocolate Syrup

  2,500 CAL/DAY: Have ¾ cup ice cream with 2½ tablespoons Hershey's Chocolate Syrup

TUESDAY, DAY 9

BREAKFAST LS V

- Blueberry Smoothie (page 10). If your family prefers strawberries, simply substitute them for the blueberries, or mix banana and berries.

- 1 slice whole wheat toast with 1 tablespoon healthy spread

   2,500 CAL/DAY: Add 1 tablespoon jam or jelly to the toast

SNACK LS V

   2,500 CAL/DAY ONLY: 6 ounce fruit-flavored lowfat yogurt, around 170 calories

LUNCH-ON-THE-GO LS V

- 1 part-skim mozzarella cheese stick

- 1 large apple, sliced

- ¼ cup nuts of your choice

- 70 calories of any whole grain cracker, such as 1½ pieces Wasa crispbread

   2,000 CAL/DAY: Have ⅓ cup nuts instead of ¼ cup

   2,500 CAL/DAY: Have 90 calories of any whole grain cracker, such as 2 Wasa crispbreads and ½ cup nuts

DINNER LS *(if you find lower sodium beans)* V

- Fish Taco (page 97)

- Raw Garlicky Kale (page 181)

- ½ cup canned refried beans, preferably with no more than 250 mg per ½ cup (such as Amy's Light in Sodium), with one 6-inch corn tortilla, warmed

   1,500–1,600 CAL/DAY: Skip the tortilla

   2,000 CAL/DAY: Add ¼ cup refried beans

   2,500 CAL/DAY: Add ⅓ cup refried beans and have 2 tortillas instead of 1

HIGH-CALCIUM SNACK LS V

- Cherry Milk (page 197) with 8 unsalted cashews

   1,800, 2,000, AND 2,500 CAL/DAY: Have another 5 cashews

TREAT *(anytime during the day)* LS V

- 100 to 110 calories biscotti, such as Nonni's, with café au lait: ½ cup hot fat-free milk mixed with ½ cup hot coffee (decaf or regular)

   1,500 CAL/DAY: Skip the treat

   1,600 CAL/DAY: Have just the biscotti

   1,800 CAL/DAY: Have another ½ biscotti

   2,000 CAL/DAY: Have another biscotti

   2,500 CAL/DAY: Have another biscotti and add another ½ cup each hot fat-free milk and coffee to your café au lait

---

WEDNESDAY, DAY 10

BREAKFAST LS V

- Cereal. Adults: Mix 1 cup Nature's Path Flax Plus with 3 tablespoons granola. Children: 1 cup Kix, Cheerios, Barbara's Puffins, or other cereal children like that contains at least 3 g fiber per 100 calories

- 1 cup fat-free milk

- ½ cup strawberries

- 2 tablespoons slivered almonds

   2,500 CAL/DAY: Have another 1 tablespoon almonds

SNACK LS V

   2,500 CAL/DAY ONLY: 1 small pear, sliced, spread with 1 tablespoon peanut butter

LUNCH V

- Egg salad in pita. Combine 2 hard-boiled eggs, chopped; 1 tablespoon light mayonnaise; ½ teaspoon Dijon mustard; 1 tablespoon sweet relish, and 2 tablespoons finely chopped carrots. Place in 6-inch pita with romaine leaves, coarsely broken.

- ½ cup carrot sticks dipped in 60 calories light ranch dressing (about 1½ tablespoons)

2,000 CAL/DAY: Add another ½ cup carrots and have a total of 115 calories of ranch, about 3 tablespoons

2,500 CAL/DAY: Add another ½ cup carrots and have a total 115 calories of ranch dressing, about 3 tablespoons and add 11 cashews and about 40 calories of dried fruit, such as 4 apricot halves

DINNER LS

▪ Cottage Pie (page 110)

▪ Salad: 2 cups mixed greens with 150 calories of dressing (with no more than 250 mg sodium for 2 tablespoons), or 1 tablespoon olive oil and 1 splash balsamic vinegar

▪ 1 apple, sliced, sprinkled with cinnamon

1,500–1,600 CAL/DAY: Use ½ tablespoon olive oil on the salad instead of 1 tablespoon

2,000 CAL/DAY: Add 1 tablespoon pumpkin or sunflower seeds to the salad

2,500 CAL/DAY: Add 1 tablespoon pumpkin or sunflower seeds to the salad, and 1 slice whole grain bread or roll (around 75 calories) with 1 teaspoon healthy spread

HIGH-CALCIUM SNACK LS V

▪ Apple Cheddar Melt (page 194) sprinkled with 1½ tablespoons slivered almonds

1,800, 2,000, AND 2,500 CAL/DAY: Add another tablespoon slivered almonds

TREAT *(anytime during the day)* LS V

▪ 150 calories dark chocolate for adults, any candy for children

1,500 CAL/DAY: Skip the treat

1,600 CAL/DAY: Have 100 calories of candy

1,800 CAL/DAY: Have 210 calories of candy

2,000 CAL/DAY: Have 280 calories candy

2,500 CAL/DAY: Have 300 calories candy

THURSDAY, DAY 11

BREAKFAST

▪ Turkey Bacon and Egg White Wrap (page 26)

▪ 1 cup cherry tomatoes, tossed with 1 tablespoon parsley, dash of salt, and 1½ teaspoons olive oil

▪ Café au lait: 1 cup hot fat-free milk with 6 to 8 ounces hot coffee (decaf or regular)

   2,500 CAL/DAY: Add ¼ cup shredded reduced-fat Cheddar to the wrap

SNACK LS V

   2,500 CAL/DAY: 3 tablespoons trail mix

LUNCH LS V

▪ Hummus sandwich: Stuff one 6-inch diameter pita with ⅓ cup hummus, ¼ cup chopped tomatoes, 1 ounce reduced-fat cheese

▪ 1½ cups diced melon

   2,000 CAL/DAY: Have ½ cup tomatoes instead of ¼ cup. Add another ½ ounce cheese and another ½ cup melon

   2,500 CAL/DAY: Have another tablespoon of hummus. Add ½ avocado, sliced, another ½ ounce cheese, and another ½ cup melon

DINNER LS

▪ Shrimp Curry (page 139)

▪ ¼ cup dry whole wheat couscous, such as Casbah, Fantastic World Foods, Bob's Red Mill, and Whole Foods 365 brand, cooked according to package directions mixed with 1 teaspoon olive oil. Comes to nearly 1 cup cooked

▪ Sugar Snap Peas with Peanut Dressing (page 188)

   1,500–1,600 CAL/DAY: Skip the olive oil

   2,000 CAL/DAY: Add another tablespoon dry couscous

   2,500 CAL/DAY: Add another 2 tablespoons dry couscous and another teaspoon olive oil

HIGH-CALCIUM SNACK LS V

■ ½ cup calcium-fortified orange juice and ½ cup (or a small 4-ounce container) low-fat fruit yogurt, such as Yoplait.

1,800, 2,000, AND 2,500 CAL/DAY: Have another ⅛ cup yogurt or have a 6-ounce container yogurt, total

TREAT *(anytime during the day)* LS V

■ ½ ounce (about 3) tortilla chips, such as Tostitos Natural Yellow Corn or Blue Corn dipped in 3 tablespoons guacamole

1,500 CAL/DAY: Skip the treat

1,600 CAL/DAY: ½ ounce (about 3) chips with 1 tablespoon guacamole

1,800 CAL/DAY: ¾ ounce (about 5) chips with ¼ cup guacamole

2,000 CAL/DAY: 1¼ ounces (about 8) chips with ¼ cup guacamole

2,500 CAL/DAY: 1½ ounces (about 9) chips with ¼ cup guacamole

---

FRIDAY, DAY 12

BREAKFAST LS V

■ ½ cup dry, plain oatmeal, cooked to package directions using ½ cup water and ½ cup plain, calcium-enriched soymilk or fat-free milk (add more water if you like a thinner oatmeal). Or try ¼ cup quick-cooking steel-cut oats, such as Arrowhead Mills or McCann's.

■ Top with ½ small apple, chopped, 2 teaspoons brown sugar, 2 tablespoons walnuts, and another ½ cup fat-free milk or soymilk

2,500 CAL/DAY: Have another 1 tablespoon walnuts

SNACK

2,500 CAL/DAY ONLY: 90 calories of any whole grain crackers, such as 2 Wasa Multi Grain crispbreads, topped with 1 ounce sliced turkey breast and slices from ¼ avocado

LUNCH LS V

■ Almond butter and pear roll-up. Spread 1 Flatout Flatbread Multi-Grain or other whole grain, 100-calorie wrap with 2 tablespoons almond butter or any other nut butter. Add ½ small pear, chopped. Children over 1 year of age can have 1 teaspoon of honey, as well.

- The rest of the pear

- ½ cup fat-free milk

  2,000 CAL/DAY: Have 2½ tablespoons almond butter total, and a total of ¾ cup milk

  2,500 CAL/DAY: Have 3 tablespoons almond butter total, 2 teaspoons honey, and a total of 1 cup milk

DINNER LS

- Flank Steak with Potatoes and Garlic (page 104)

- Papaya and Avocado (page 71). Substitute mango for papaya, if you like.

- 1 slice whole grain bread or roll (around 75 calories) with 2 teaspoons healthy spread

  1,500–1,600 CAL/DAY: Skip the spread on the roll

  2,000 CAL/DAY: Add 1¼ cups steamed broccoli florets spritzed with lemon juice or Wish-Bone Spritzer, any flavor

  2,500 CAL/DAY: Add 1¼ cups cooked broccoli florets spritzed with lemon juice or Wish-Bone Spritzer, any flavor, and have 1 tablespoon healthy spread instead of 2 teaspoons

HIGH-CALCIUM SNACK LS V

- Chocolate milk: 1 cup fat-free or 1% milk with 1 tablespoon Hershey's Chocolate Syrup and have ½ cup sliced strawberries

  1,800, 2,000, AND 2,500 CAL/DAY: Have another ½ cup berries

TREAT *(anytime during the day)* LS

- S'mores: 2 graham cracker squares (preferably whole wheat, such as Mi-del) topped with 1 roasted marshmallow and ½ ounce chocolate, such as Hershey Milk or Extra Dark

  1,500 CAL/DAY: Skip the treat

  1,600 CAL/DAY: 2 graham crackers and 1 marshmallow. Skip the chocolate

  1,800 CAL/DAY: 3 graham crackers, 2 marshmallows, and ½ ounce chocolate

  2,000 CAL/DAY: 3 graham crackers, 2 marshmallows, and ¾ ounce chocolate

  2,500 CAL/DAY: 4 graham crackers, 2 marshmallows, and ¾ ounce chocolate

SATURDAY, DAY 13

BREAKFAST V

- Pancakes: Using a whole grain pancake mix, such as Arrowhead Mills or Bob's Red Mill, check label—use 200 calories worth, which is about ¼ cup mix, making 3- x 4-inch pancakes. Top each serving with 2 teaspoons healthy spread, ½ cup raspberries (or other chopped fruit), and 1 tablespoon pancake or maple syrup. If your family finds 100% whole grain pancakes too "grainy," then use ½ regular pancake mix with ½ whole grain.

- 1 cup calcium-enriched vanilla soymilk or fat-free milk

  2,500 CAL/DAY: Have another ¼ cup berries and another teaspoon syrup

SNACK LS V

  2,500 CAL/DAY ONLY: 1 small pita (around 75 calories) with ¼ cup hummus

LUNCH V

- Vegetable cheeseburger: Cook a soy-based vegetable burger (with 100 to 120 calories), such as Amy's All American Veggie Burger, Gardenburger The Classic Burger, or Boca Cheeseburger, according to package directions. In the last minute or two of cooking, top with a 1-ounce slice of reduced-fat Cheddar and let melt. Place on a 170-calorie, whole wheat bun, spread with 2 teaspoons light mayonnaise, and lettuce, tomato, and 1 to 2 teaspoons each: mustard, catsup, and relish (optional).

- ½ cup red pepper sticks

- 1 orange

  2,000 CAL/DAY: Add a salad: 1 cup mixed greens, ½ cup vegetables, 1 teaspoon olive oil, and 1 splash balsamic vinegar

  2,500 CAL/DAY: Have 2 burgers, and add a salad: 1 cup mixed greens, ½ cup vegetables, tossed with 1 teaspoon olive oil, and a splash balsamic vinegar, topped with 1 tablespoon toasted nuts, such as pine nuts or walnuts

DINNER LS

- Turkey Chili (page 52)

- ¾ cup cooked brown rice (from ¼ cup raw). Make extra rice for tomorrow's Brown Rice Pudding for breakfast. For instance, if you make 4 servings for tonight's meal and 4 servings for tomorrow's breakfast, you need to cook about 2 cups of raw rice, according to package directions.

- 1½ cups romaine or mixed greens tossed with 5 sprays Wish-Bone Spritzers, any flavor

    1,500–1,600 CAL/DAY: Have ½ cup rice instead of ¾ cup

    2,000 CAL/DAY: Have another ¼ cup cooked rice

    2,500 CAL/DAY: Have 1⅓ cups cooked rice total, and top chili with 2 tablespoons reduced-fat cheese

HIGH-CALCIUM SNACK LS V

- Orange Cream Smoothie (page 197) with 1½ tablespoons unsalted nuts

    1,800, 2,000, AND 2,500 CAL/DAY: Have another ½ tablespoon unsalted nuts of your choice

TREAT *(anytime during the day)* LS V

- Chocolate Cake (page 217)

    1,500 CAL/DAY: Skip the treat

    1,600 CAL/DAY: Have ½ slice cake

    1,800 CAL/DAY: Have 1 slice cake with 2 teaspoons chocolate syrup

    2,000 CAL/DAY: Have 1 slice cake with 2 teaspoons chocolate syrup and ¼ cup light ice cream

    2,500 CAL/DAY: Have 1 slice cake with 2 teaspoons chocolate syrup and ⅓ cup light ice cream

---

SUNDAY, DAY 14

BREAKFAST LS V

- Brown Rice Pudding (page 20)

- ½ cup strawberries mixed with ½ cup raspberries, fresh or frozen, thawed, topped with 4 ounces lowfat vanilla yogurt

    2,500 CAL/DAY: Have another ½ cup berries

SNACK LS V

    2,500 CAL/DAY ONLY: ½ ounce tortilla chips (about 3 chips) dipped in ¼ cup guacamole

LUNCH v

▪ Grilled cheese sandwich: 2 slices whole wheat bread with 2 ounces reduced-fat Swiss, Cheddar, or jack. Smear 2 teaspoons healthy spread on the outside of sandwich and heat in a skillet or toaster oven and serve.

▪ 1 cup carrot sticks

▪ ½ cup diced pineapple

2,000 CAL/DAY: Add another teaspoon healthy spread and another ½ cup pineapple for a total of 1¼ cups pineapple

2,500 CAL/DAY: Add another 2 teaspoons healthy spread and another ½ cup pineapple for a total of 1¼ cups pineapple. Top pineapple with 3 tablespoons pecans or other nuts of your choice

DINNER LS

▪ Sweet-and-Sour Stuffed Chicken (page 127)

▪ Steel-Cut Oats "Polenta" (page 167)

▪ 2 cups mixed greens with 5 sprays Wish-Bone Spritzer, any flavor

1,500–1,600 CAL/DAY: Have ⅙ of the "Polenta" recipe instead of ¼

2,000 CAL/DAY: Add 1 teaspoon olive oil to the greens, along with the Spritzer

2,500 CAL/DAY: Add 1 teaspoon olive oil to the greens, along with the Spritzer, and an extra ½ serving of "Polenta"

HIGH-CALCIUM SNACK LS V

▪ Celery with Creamy Herb Dip (page 195)

1,800, 2,000, AND 2,500 CAL/DAY: Add ¼ cup more ricotta and an extra ½ teaspoon olive oil to the dip

TREAT *(anytime during the day)* LS V

▪ Grape Crumble with Frozen Grapes (page 212); have ⅕ of the recipe

1,500 CAL/DAY: Skip the treat

1,600 CAL/DAY: Have ½ serving

1,800 CAL/DAY: Have 1 serving with ¼ cup light vanilla ice cream

2,000 CAL/DAY: Have 1 serving with ½ cup light vanilla ice cream

2,500 CAL/DAY: Have 1 serving with ⅔ cup light vanilla ice cream

Basic Recipes

THIS SECTION CONTAINS BASIC RECIPES you'll find used throughout the book.

Chicken Stock

MAKES 8 CUPS

YOU CAN USE THIS as a starting point for many soups, including the recipe for Chicken Noodle Soup (page 54).

Vegetable oil cooking spray

1/2 medium onion, sliced

2 pounds chicken legs and thighs, trimmed of excess fat and cut into 2-inch pieces (or 2 pounds chicken backs, cut into 2-inch pieces, plus bones, if desired)

2 quarts water

1/8 teaspoon salt

1 bay leaf

1. Heat a large heavy-bottomed stockpot over medium-high heat. When hot, coat with the cooking spray. Add the onion and chicken pieces and sauté until the chicken is no longer pink, about 7 minutes.

2. Reduce the heat to low. Cover and cook until the chicken releases its juices, about 20 minutes.

3. Add the water, salt, and bay leaf. Turn the heat to medium-high until the broth comes to a simmer. Reduce the heat to low. Cover and simmer until the broth is rich and flavorful, about 20 minutes.

4. Strain the broth immediately and discard the solids.

5. Use the broth or cool to room temperature and refrigerate for up to 5 days, or freeze.

PREP TIME: 10 minutes   TOTAL TIME: 1 hour

PER 1-CUP SERVING, ABOUT: Calories: 12 Protein: 2 g Carbohydrate: 0 g Dietary Fiber: 0 g Sugars: 0 g Total Fat: 1 g Saturated Fat: 0 g Cholesterol: 7 mg Calcium: 0 mg Sodium: 49 mg

Vegetable Stock

MAKES 8 CUPS

YOU CAN USUALLY USE vegetable stock in recipes that call for chicken stock if you want to make a vegetarian dish.

3 cups roughly chopped vegetables, such as onion, celery, carrot, parsnip, turnip, rutabaga, mushroom, and so on

10 cups water

1/8 teaspoon peppercorns

1. Place all the ingredients in a large pot over high heat. Bring to a boil. Reduce the heat to low and let the soup simmer for 40 minutes.

2. Drain the stock and discard the solids. Use the broth or cool to room temperature and refrigerate for up to 5 days, or freeze.

PREP TIME: 5 minutes   **TOTAL TIME:** 50 minutes

PER 1-CUP SERVING, ABOUT: Calories: 5 Protein: 0 g Carbohydrate: 2 g Dietary Fiber: .5 g Sugars: 0 g Total Fat: 0 g Saturated Fat: 0 g Cholesterol: 7 mg Calcium: 8 mg Sodium: 11 mg

Quick Tomato Sauce

MAKES 3 CUPS

MAKE THIS WHEN TOMATOES are at their peak, and freeze what you don't need for a taste of summer all year-round.

3 pounds ripe tomatoes

1 tablespoon olive oil

2 cloves garlic, finely chopped

⅛ teaspoon salt

Black pepper to taste

¼ cup fresh basil, roughly chopped

1. Bring a large pot of water to a boil. Prepare a large bowl with ice water.

2. Cut a small X in the bottom of each tomato using a small knife. Plunge the tomatoes into the boiling water for 30 seconds. Remove from the boiling water with tongs and then submerge in ice water. Peel off the skins of the tomatoes; they will come off easily.

3. Cut each tomato in half and remove the core and seeds. Coarsely chop the seedless skinless tomatoes.

4. Heat a large heavy-bottomed skillet over medium heat. Add the olive oil and garlic. Cook for about 1 minute, stirring.

5. Add the tomatoes and turn the heat to medium. Cook until the sauce is thick, about 20 minutes. Add the salt, pepper, and basil. Use the sauce or store in the refrigerator for up to 5 days or freeze.

PREP TIME: 15 minutes   **TOTAL TIME:** 35 minutes

PER ½-CUP SERVING, ABOUT: Calories: 63 Protein: 2 g Carbohydrate: 9 g Dietary Fiber: 3 g Sugars: 6 g Total Fat: 3 g Saturated Fat: 0 g Cholesterol: 0 mg Calcium: 28 mg Sodium: 60 mg

Basic Vinaigrette

DRESSES 2 TO 3 CUPS SALAD

YOU CAN MAKE YOUR own "house dressing" and change it up every time.

2 teaspoons vinegar, such as balsamic,
sherry, champagne, or red wine

2 teaspoons olive oil, or any type of nut oil

Pinch of salt

Black pepper to taste

1. Whisk the ingredients together in a small bowl or shake until combined in a tightly covered glass jar.

2. Use immediately or refrigerate for up to 1 week.

PREP TIME: 1 minute   TOTAL TIME: 1 minute

PER SERVING (ENTIRE RECIPE), ABOUT: Calories: 90 Protein: 0 g Carbohydrate: 2 g Dietary Fiber: 0 g Sugars: 2 g Total Fat: 9 g Saturated Fat: 1 g Cholesterol: 0 mg Calcium: 3 mg Sodium: 212 mg

Mustard Vinaigrette

DRESSES 2 TO 3 CUPS SALAD

THIS IS DELICIOUS ON hearty greens or vegetable salads.

2 teaspoons mustard (with less than
50 mg sodium per teaspoon)

1 teaspoon red wine vinegar

¼ teaspoon honey

2 teaspoons olive oil

1. Mix the mustard, vinegar, and honey thoroughly in a medium bowl using a fork or whisk. Mix in the olive oil until completely incorporated.

2. Use immediately or refrigerate for up to 1 week.

PREP TIME: 2 minutes   TOTAL TIME: 2 minutes

PER SERVING (ENTIRE RECIPE), ABOUT: Calories: 96 Protein: 0 g Carbohydrate: 3 g Dietary Fiber: 0 g Sugars: 1 g Total Fat: 9 g Saturated Fat: 1 g Cholesterol: 0 mg Calcium: 0 mg Sodium: 101 mg

Almond Biscotti

MAKES 15 COOKIES

THESE ARE SO GOOD with a cup of tea or coffee. Craving chocolate? Use the variation below to whip up a batch of chocolate biscotti.

3 tablespoons tofu

½ cup unbleached all-purpose flour

¼ cup sugar plus 1 teaspoon for rolling

¼ cup whole wheat flour

2 tablespoons roughly chopped almonds

1 teaspoon baking powder

2 tablespoons olive oil

1. Preheat the oven to 375°F.

2. Process the tofu in a food processor until smooth, about 30 seconds. Add all the other ingredients except 1 teaspoon sugar and process for 1 more minute.

3. Remove the dough and roll into a ball. Then roll into a log with a 1-inch diameter. Pour 1 teaspoon sugar on a plate and roll log in the sugar until it is evenly coated. Place on a baking sheet and cook for 10 minutes.

4. Remove from the oven, let cool for 5 minutes, and slice into ½-inch-thick slices (it should make about 15 cookies).

5. Return the slices to the baking sheet and place in the oven. Turn the oven off and let the biscotti dry for 15 minutes in the oven or overnight in the oven before serving. (The longer you dry biscotti, the harder the cookies will be. They are delicious either way.)

VARIATION: Substitute 1 tablespoon cocoa powder for 1 tablespoon flour

PREP TIME: 5 minutes   TOTAL TIME: 35 minutes

PER COOKIE, ABOUT: Calories: 62 Protein: 1 g Carbohydrate: 9 g Dietary Fiber: .5 g Sugars: 4 g Total Fat: 3 g Saturated Fat: 0 g Cholesterol: 0 mg Calcium: 43 mg Sodium: 33 mg

Techniques

THIS LITTLE HOW-TO SECTION IS a quick tutorial on techniques we use over and over again in the Best Life recipes.

Roasting Garlic

1. Preheat the oven to 375°F.

2. Separate the head of garlic into cloves, taking care to make sure that papery skin remains on the individual cloves.

3. Lightly and evenly coat the cloves with cooking spray and place on a sheet pan.

4. Cook until the cloves are soft to the touch, about 20 minutes.

5. Remove from the oven and cool.

6. Remove the papery skin from the garlic; it will peel off easily.

7. Look for a sprout running through the clove. Cut the clove in half lengthwise and remove the sprout with a small knife. Occasionally, you will get garlic that doesn't have a sprout, or it's too small to see and remove.

8. Use the garlic or store tightly covered in the refrigerator for 5 days.

PREP TIME: 5 minutes   **TOTAL TIME:** 25 minutes

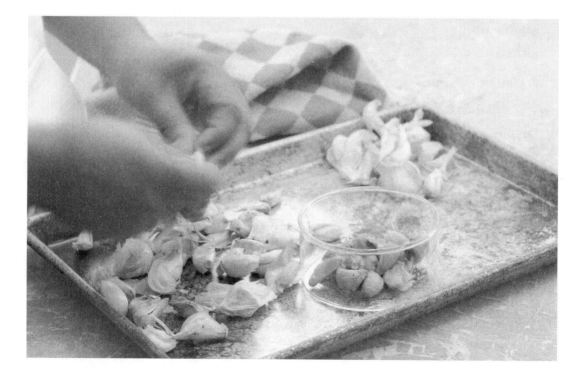

Cooking Beans

BECAUSE OF THE WIDE variety of beans, it is impossible to give exact directions. The cooking instructions that follow are simply a guide.

DRIED BEANS

1. Rinse the beans in a strainer and look them over, discarding any discolored beans or foreign material.

2. Place the beans in a large pot, cover with about 5 cups water for every 1 cup dried beans and turn the heat to high. Bring to a boil, reduce the heat to low, and simmer. If the beans become uncovered because the water has evaporated, add more water.

3. Taste the beans regularly to see if they are cooked or need additional time. They should be tender but not mushy.

4. Use the beans immediately, refrigerate covered for about 5 days, or freeze. If refrigerating or freezing, store beans with their cooking liquid.

   PREP TIME: 5 minutes   TOTAL TIME: 20 minutes for lentils and split peas to 2 hours for most other beans, such as black beans, kidney beans, and garbanzo beans; lima beans and black-eyed peas are somewhere in between.

FRESH BEANS

1. Shell the beans. Rinse the beans in a strainer and look them over, discarding any discolored beans or foreign material.

2. Put the beans in a large pot, cover with about 3 cups water for every 1 cup fresh beans and cook over high heat. Bring the water to a boil, reduce the heat to low, and simmer. If the beans become uncovered because the water has evaporated, add more water.

3. Taste the beans regularly to see if they are cooked or need additional time. They should be tender but not mushy. Fresh beans cook quickly, anywhere from 5 to 30 minutes, depending on the variety.

4. Use the beans immediately, store covered in the refrigerator for about 5 days, or freeze. If refrigerating or freezing, store beans with their cooking liquid.

   PREP TIME: 5 minutes   TOTAL TIME: 10 to 35 minutes

Toasting Nuts and Seeds

DON'T USE A HIGH temperature when toasting nuts and seeds, as they burn easily.

1. Preheat the oven to 350°F.

2. Spread the nuts or seeds on a sheet pan. Toast in the oven (or toaster oven) for 3 to 10 minutes, stirring often. They are ready just as they start to turn golden brown. Be careful not to burn; nuts and seeds can go from golden brown to burned in 1 minute.

    PREP TIME: 1 minute   **TOTAL TIME:** 11 minutes

Sectioning Citrus

THIS TECHNIQUE MAY SEEM complicated at first, but give it a try; you will quickly become a master at this useful and versatile skill.

1. Cut off a thin slice of skin at the top and the bottom of your orange, grapefruit, or lemon.

2. Place the fruit on a cutting board, sitting on one of the flat, sliced-off sections.

3. Starting at the top, with a downward motion, carefully slice off the skin using the edge of the knife, removing all the white pith but leaving as much of the fruit intact as possible. Continue until the fruit is completely peeled.

4. Remove the individual sections of fruit using a small knife leaving the pith that encases each section behind. You will get clean citrus sections without all of the pith.

    PREP TIME: 5 minutes   **TOTAL TIME:** 5 minutes

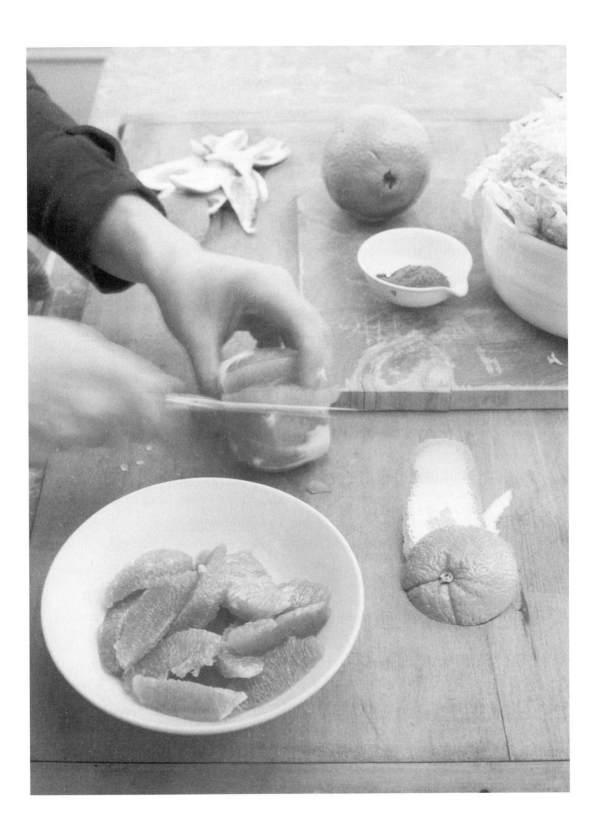

Roasting Squash or Pumpkin

COOKING TIMES VARY GREATLY, depending on the size and density of the squash or pumpkin.

1.   Preheat the oven to 375°F.

2.   Cut the squash or pumpkin in half, scoop out the seeds (they can be cleaned and roasted or used in a vegetable broth). Cut with caution since this can be cumbersome and dangerous, depending on the variety and size of the squash or pumpkin. Use a good sharp knife and keep your fingers away from the blade.

3.   Place the squash or pumpkin on a sheet pan cut side down and coat with cooking spray. Bake until soft (test with a fork), anywhere from 20 minutes to an hour.

PREP TIME: 5 minutes   TOTAL TIME: 25 minutes to 1 hour 5 minutes

Grinding Flaxseeds

FLAXSEEDS ARE THE RICHEST form of alpha-linolenic acid (ALA), the plant form of omega-3s. They're also high in fiber as well as a class of phytonutrient called lignans, which may offer cancer and heart disease protection. Their subtle, nutty taste works well in a number of recipes in this book. Although it is slightly more convenient to purchase ground flaxseeds, they can spoil quickly, are more expensive, and lose some of their nutritional value if exposed to light and air for any length of time. These simple directions let you grind the seeds as you need them.

1.   Blend the flaxseeds in a blender on high for 1 minute. Scrape the sides of the blender with a spatula and continue blending until you have a fine powder, about 2 more minutes.

2.   Store the ground flaxseeds in an airtight container in the refrigerator; they can be stored for about 1 week in the refrigerator and much longer in the freezer.

PREP TIME: 3 minutes   TOTAL TIME: 3 minutes

Slicing Beef

THE WAY YOU SLICE meat can affect how tough or tender it is. This slicing technique, which can be used for any cut of beef either raw or cooked, will make meats that are typically thought of as tough more tender.

1. If slicing cooked beef, be sure to let it rest for 5 minutes before slicing.

2. Place the meat on a cutting board, and with a sharp knife cut against the grain of the beef. The knife should be cutting perpendicular to the direction of the grain of the beef. Cut the beef to desired thickness.

Juicing a Pomegranate

DELICIOUS POMEGRANATES ARE RICH in antioxidants, especially one called ellagic acid, which has been shown in numerous studies to help fight cancer. They're a versatile fruit that can be used in salads or desserts, or paired with either meat or poultry.

1. Use your thumbs to press and soften the skin all the way around the entire fruit.

2. Insert a paring knife halfway into the side of the pomegranate to make a small hole. Hold the pomegranate over a bowl with the hole facing down, and squeeze firmly to extract the juice.

Seeding a Pomegranate

1. Cut the pomegranate into four pieces.

2. Peel away the skin. Working over a bowl of cold water, use your fingers to pry the seeds away from the membrane. Discard large pieces of membrane.

3. The seeds will fall to the bottom of the bowl and any remaining small pieces of the membrane will float to the top, making it easy to separate.

4. When you finish separating the seeds, skim membrane from the top of the bowl and discard. Strain the seeds to remove them from the water.

Clarifying Butter

EIGHT TABLESPOONS OF BUTTER will produce about 6 tablespoons of clarified butter.

1. In a medium saucepan over low heat, melt the butter slowly. Let it sit for about 5 minutes to separate. Skim off the foam that rises to the top with a spoon.

2. Gently pour the butter (the top layer) into a small bowl and discard the bottom layer of milk solids.

Blanching Vegetables and Fruit

PROPER BLANCHING CAN ENHANCE vegetables and fruits by altering texture, accentuating color, and allowing them to better absorb dressings and seasonings. Just take care not to overcook.

1. Bring a pot of water large enough to comfortably hold the veggies or fruit you wish to blanch to a boil.

2. Fill a bowl with ice and water.

3. Plunge the vegetable or fruit into boiling water for about 30 seconds.

4. Drain the vegetable or fruit and plunge into ice water to cool.

5. After the vegetables are cooled, drain before using or storing.

INDEX